hands-on sports therapy

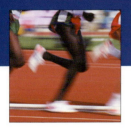 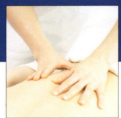 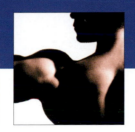

hands-on sports therapy

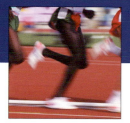 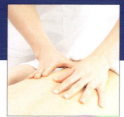 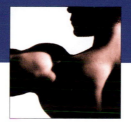

KEITH WARD

THOMSON
™

Australia • Canada • Mexico • Singapore • Spain • United Kingdom • United States

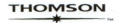

Hands-on Sports Therapy

Copyright © Thomson Learning 2004

The Thomson logo is a registered trademark used herein under licence.

For more information, contact Thomson Learning, High Holborn House, 50–51 Bedford Row, London WC1R 4LR or visit us on the World Wide Web at: http://www.thomsonlearning.co.uk

British Library Cataloguing-in-Publication Data
A catalogue record for this book is available from the British Library

ISBN 1-86152-920-1

Text design by Design Deluxe

Typeset by Graphicraft, Hong Kong

Printed in Italy by Canale

I would like to dedicate this book to my ever-caring Mom and Dad (Nina and Peter), my ever-loving and hard-working partner, Katarina, and our wonderful children, Reiss, Sara and Arielle.

contents

foreword

Injuries were part of my sporting career, as indeed they are with all sportsmen and women. Incorrect treatment at the pitch side has left me with a legacy of permanent reminders of my playing days.

When I retired from playing, sports therapy was unknown in the United Kingdom and so for the last 20 years it has become a major part of my life – I've eaten, drunk and slept it! My enthusiasm has been tried at times by the lack of informative, easy-to-read textbooks. This book I feel will address this.

The concept of Sports Therapy arrived from the United States in the early 1980s, probably via the role of the athletic trainer. However, in reality injured athletes have been cared for in treatment rooms and at pitch side since the era of the gladiators.

My early memories as a young footballer are of the trainer running onto the pitch in a long white coat and working miracles with nothing more than the 'magic sponge'! Fortunately since then there have been significant developments in the provision and delivery of sports therapy education. Pioneers in this field have worked tirelessly to achieve the recognition they justly deserve for their skills – whether as a sports massage practitioner or a highly trained individual who is able to recognize common musculo-skeletal conditions or soft tissue injuries and treat them effectively.

Keith Ward's contribution is a text which the student, tutor or experienced practitioner will find an invaluable guide, be it pitch side, or in the treatment room or teaching clinic.

Sports performers should always remember '*pain diminishes performance*'.

David J. Edge B.Ed (Hons) FHT, SMA

preface

There has been an explosion of consumer interest in health and fitness in recent years. To meet this growing demand, and as standards steadily rise, the fitness and therapy professions require ever more knowledgeable and skilful practitioners. The subject of sports therapy should appeal to all: the health, fitness and therapy students; the professionals already in practice; the sports managers, coaches and trainers; the athletes themselves; the general public.

Having taught this subject for quite a few years, I began to feel that maybe I had something good to offer budding practitioners. Following the encouragement of students and colleagues, and after considering the many and various requirements, the production of a good book on the subject seemed to be an ambition that I just might be able to achieve. When planning a structure for my ideas, I wanted to cover the more practically relevant areas of interest to the developing sports therapist. Of course, every book proposal should have a strong rationale, and our main criteria were to develop the project with a logical structure, to tackle the subject as thoroughly as possible, and to be interesting, motivating and accessible. The early feedback, during construction, from other sports therapy lecturers was strongly positive, and their comments helped to refine the final shape of this book.

Obviously, the majority of aspects around and within this subject can be explored in greater technical depth, and no book will ever take the place of a solid professional course of training. So although obviously not encyclopedic, an ambitious all-in-one book was what I wanted to produce.

The material has been developed with certain regard to students of the (level 3) sports therapy courses offered by the mainstream UK providers. The text should also provide something in the way of supplementary reading for students at undergraduate level – especially the practical aspects of assessment, treatment and rehabilitation. Qualified therapists should be able to use this book as part of their continued professional development. I feel that the health, fitness and therapy professionals, a typically highly motivated audience, will appreciate an innovative and inspirational format. Sports therapy, remedial exercise and massage therapy are practical subjects, and should on paper be treated as such for the study of the crucial aspects. Hopefully, an ideal balance between the theory and the practical applications has been struck.

We have elected to break the book up into two sections. Section one is entitled 'The theory behind the practice'. In essence, section one starts logically at the beginning and lays down the foundational knowledge and background to the subject. Although it can be seen that the crucial science and art of physical assessment involves a great deal of practical skill, the study of the actual therapeutic interventions and the many techniques available is where, probably, most people would see the practice begin. Fittingly, therefore, section two is entitled 'The practice'.

This book has a strongly pedagogical style. Some of the concepts within sports therapy are difficult to teach and often quite confusing for students. The photography, which exemplifies and accompanies the practical aspects, should bring to life the various techniques, and where relevant, are presented in a typically sequential order. Pictures (especially photographs) paint many words. Also included are many completely new reference tables, charts and illustrations, which will encourage a familiarity with essential concepts. The frequent Tip Boxes, which accompany the main body of text, point out key points of interest. At the end of each chapter there are a Chapter Summary and Knowledge Review. A selection of questions based mainly on the text should coax some thoughtful answers out of interested readers. The Glossary, towards the end of the book, should be a useful source of reference, being totally relevant to the subject of sports therapy.

The Appendices provide many special features: Student Tasks (case scenarios to solve); Major Muscle Tables (all major muscles, their origins, insertions, actions and any important notes); Measurement Conversions (easy methods for gaining familiarity with measurements and converting imperial to metric); Sample Forms (Consultation, Record Card, Physical Assessment, Fitness Test and Remedial Action Plan), which should make the task of record keeping and therapy provision more straightforward and succinct; Useful Contacts (organizations, associations, training providers, journals and equipment suppliers). The bibliography and recommended reading provides a comprehensive list that should point the reader towards texts that will fill in any referential gaps. In addition there is a companion website to the text. The details of this can be found at the end of this preface.

It is hoped that both the students and the newly qualified will consider this to be a valuable textbook, and that it will continue to be useful to them, as a point of reference, as they get deeper into their studies and into their career, and if this book becomes a commonly recommended text to assist in the study of sports therapy, then the job will clearly have been done well. It surely stands to reason, that if the professionals gain, then so will the general public. This book offers, to the aspiring therapist, an advancing territory in which to explore – a territory that they will be comfortable and progressively familiar with and one that feeds their thirst for adventure.

Although it has been a major undertaking, I have thoroughly enjoyed working on this project. A great collective effort of ideas, debate and manual labour has been produced, and I hope that this finished product lives up to both your and our expectations. As is usually the case, with any worthy endeavour, the more you put in, the more you are likely to get out.

I would like to suggest that, if you have the time and motivation, you read through the first few chapters in their sequential order. Having a clear perspective, I feel, is important, and I have attempted to set the scene in these early chapters. Subjectively, if we are focused and ambitious, we can all potentially know where we are coming from, where we currently are, where we would ideally like to be, and what we need to do to achieve our successes.

Why 'hands-on sports therapy'?

- Hands-on training is the best way to learn most things.

- Being hands-on means being proactive.

- Literally, the hands are often on in sports therapy treatment.

- Hands-on sports therapy brings the subject to life and literally illustrates the practicalities, and where the spotlight is on sports therapy, its methods, its practice.

- The reader can easily access information by simply getting their hands on this book.

- Hands-on is quite a contemporary phrase, and sports therapy is quite a contemporary subject.

However, as sports therapists, we must work as much with our brains as with our hands!

Keith D. Ward,
Cannock, Staffordshire 2004

Visit the *Hands-on Sports Therapy* accompanying website at www.thomsonlearning.co.uk/healthandfitness/ward to find further teaching and learning material including:

For Students

- Information about the book to help guide you through using the text for your studies.

- Chapter overviews to give you an indication of the coverage of the book.

- Multiple choice questions to test your understanding of each chapter.

- Assessment forms and artwork from the book for you to print out for your own use.

- Reading lists/web references to guide you towards further study.

- Answers to knowledge review exercises so that you can check your progress as you work through the text.

For Teachers

- Additional question material to use with your students in the classroom.

- Some additional cases to set as class exercises, with suggested answers to work through with your students.

author's acknowledgements

I would like to thank everyone who has personally inspired me and helped me. First and foremost I must thank my family for their continual support and for putting up with me being locked away in my office for endless hours; all of my colleagues at Walsall College of Arts and Technology (especially Val Kay, Yvonne Gogerty, Graham Coffey, Chris Harding, Derrick Eubank, Rosemary Howey); all at Thomson Learning (especially my fantastic development editor Amie Barker, Lib Wright and Irith Williams). Gerri Moore at FHT; my patient photographer Tony Middleton LBPPA, and wife Margaret. General and generous thanks must also be offered to the following: my brother Darren and his wife Rachel; all of my mates, old and new, especially Mark and Martina, Stuart and Vicky, Mike and Deana, Maria and Francoise, Sally and Martin, Lesley, Jason, Neil, Raj and Anita, Sue and Jim, Joyce, Paul and Helga, Mark and Linda, Tim, Harry, Brian, Phil and Jo, Doog, Martin, Barry, Allan and Glyn, Stan and Phyllis, Margaret, Dave and Pauline, Therlow, Maggie, Marvin and the posse; all of my teachers, past and present, especially Dr Ruth Shiner at Wolverhampton University for supporting me while I worked on this book, Professor Steven Johnson, Vicky Schwartz, Ralph Perks, Mario Paul Cassar, Paul Clusker, Paul Kitson, Tim Crossfield, Gavin Loze; all of my students, past and present; all of my clients (especially John and Jane, Suki, Ann and Bob, Lee, Tad and Marion, Kuldip, Darren, Derek, Amrik, Ted, Corrie, Lavinia, Elizabeth, Trevor, Bob, Hazel, Lol, Kevin and Lynne, Sam, Yvonne, Colin, Beverley, Sonia, Balbinder, Keith, Steve, Gary, Mark, Bernard); Gurd and Nirmla Chahal, at Duran Drive-Thru Pharmacy; Susan Mahli, osteopath; Karen Jenkins, web design; other friends and colleagues Lilas Rawling, Jo Wright, Celia Robotham, Kerry Gillott, Pat Westwood, George Clayton, Sue Parks, Louise Perry, Chris Edmunds, Jane Turner, Maggie Merrick, Beccy Newens, Pat Cyster, Lucinda Jennings, Sarah Coward, Rob Price, Harminder Midha, Jaswinder Sagoo, Gavin Blackwell, Anthony Warwick, John Richardson, John Mayer, Dean Madden, Paul Taylor, Lisa and Lorraine from West Brom.

Specific credit must go to:

- David Edge for his typically entertaining, relevant and generous foreword.
- Ailsa Higgins for contributing an excellent nutritional chapter.
- The photographer: Tony Middleton.
- Kate Randerson, Heather Cook and Maureen Evans for the invaluable advice they gave in their reviews.

The models are:

- Katarina McGuinness (fitness instructor and sports therapist)
- Derrick Eubank (fitness instructor, sports massage practitioner and lecturer)
- Steve Avery (sports therapist)
- Graham Coffey (fitness lecturer)
- Chris Harding (fitness instructor).

section one

THE THEORY BEHIND
THE PRACTICE

Foundational background and underpinning knowledge to the
   provision of sports therapy: sports therapy in context

Anatomy and physiology

Health, safety and hygiene

Legislations

The consultation process

Contra-indications

Physical and biomechanical assessment

Sports injuries

Nutrition

chapter 1

SPORTS THERAPY IN CONTEXT

Learning Objectives

After reading this chapter you should be able to:

- know what sports therapy is and what it is not
- understand at whom sports therapy is aimed
- be aware of pathways to practise sports therapy
- appreciate the history of sports therapy
- be aware of important areas of focus for the future of sports therapy

WHAT IS SPORTS THERAPY?

For simplicity's sake, the title and phrase 'sports therapy' shall be referred to in this book as a generalized term for all that it can potentially encompass. It can be considered that sports therapy is, theoretically, about understanding safe and effective principles of fitness and athletic training and injury **rehabilitation**, and, practically, about the application of a selection of manual and electrical interventions to achieve a range of therapeutic objectives.

The theories are deep and have developed in much the same way as have other scientific knowledge bases, that is by building upon early empirical endeavours, continually integrating new scientific developments and, more recently, evaluating practice and intervention through rigorous **research**. However, like many practices, sports therapy is as much an art as it is a science. Practitioners are expected to approach their work with thoughtfulness and creativity, and there is always scope for both dynamic performance and subtle technique.

The underpinning knowledge for sports therapy comes from several perspectives. Traditional natural healing has always utilized physical therapy. Massage, a fundamental aspect, has been used instinctively as a healing

TIP
Sports therapy is about putting into practice the knowledge to help improve health, fitness and sports performance. It is the assessment of **posture**, movement, fitness and injuries. It is the application of accepted principles of training and treatment.

3

TIP

Anatomical and physiological knowledge and the latest research help to shape the format that sports therapy practices take.

method by all world cultures almost since time began. Anatomical and physiological understanding is now greater than ever, and the science of sport is now well established and studied at all academic levels. All of this helps the sports therapist to develop their practice logically and specifically.

Essentially, sports therapy should be considered complementary practice, where, when technically appropriate, practitioners must work upon the advice of medical personnel. Therapy for improving sports performance or for treatment of sports injury is well documented, to a point, and may be provided by any one or more of a number of personnel. This will include physiotherapists, podiatrists, massage therapists, sports scientists, psychologists, nutritionists and, indeed, sports therapists.

Clinical sports therapy involves health-promoting treatments, exercise recommendations and particular lifestyle advice. The treatment work often incorporates many of the practical techniques utilized by physiotherapists and osteopaths; however, many sports therapists specialize in the provision of remedial soft-tissue massage and the preparation of exercise programmes. The experienced and expert practitioner will take their time to offer the best therapy and advice, and will be able to call upon a variety of skills and methods.

Sports therapy typically offers assistance with the following:

- fitness training programmes
- preparation for sports training and competition
- recovery from sport and competition
- fitness evaluation and monitoring
- postural, biomechanical and **gait** assessment
- injury prevention
- injury treatment and rehabilitation
- nutritional advice
- relaxation and well-being

A sports therapist might be someone capable of offering advice on exercise – or someone who delivers massage before and after a sporting event – or a highly trained practitioner able to recognise common orthopaedic conditions and soft tissue injuries as well as being able to complete a progressive and effective programme of treatment and rehabilitation.

MARK HUDSON (1998)

A career in sports therapy is most suitable for enthusiastic, motivated individuals. For the practitioner, it certainly demands a mature, caring approach and a willingness to continually develop professional skills.

WHY SPORTS THERAPY?

The sociological and psychological demand for sport itself is massive. The very word sport denotes so much in the way of positivity. Sport means **inter**action, health, fitness, vitality, enjoyment, fair play, ambition and success.

The quite recent upsurge in consumer demand for health and fitness facilities and facilitators is perhaps the strongest indication of the increasing awareness in society. People appear more ready to take personal responsibility for their health, and the old adage that 'prevention is better than cure' seems to be well accepted. Of course, taking more responsibility and working with and acting upon the advice of trained and knowledgeable therapists does not guarantee good health or longevity, but by being generally more responsible, individuals are more likely to instil within themselves a sense of improvement, as well as experiencing a palpable sense of well-being.

Those fortunate enough to be working in the health and fitness industry must be able to rise to the challenge of providing the increased quality of service that is now expected of them. Many people today, from all walks of life (the young, old, active, sedentary, fit, unfit, experienced and inexperienced) are now following their own individually considered exercise routines, whether at home or under the guidance of a fitness club. The public are better informed as to the benefits of being fitter and more healthy, and they know that with regular exercise and attention to lifestyle they can feel good, look good, work better, relax better and possibly live longer. For this public, the sports therapist can be an important catalyst to their improvements.

The concept of using the scientific principles of sports training as part of the provision of therapy for health and fitness improvement for the non-sporting populations, until quite recently, was not so widespread and is actually a major aspect of this growth area. Therefore, it should be made clear that sports therapy is not just for athletes! All kinds of people can benefit from the sports therapy approach: the general public; fitness enthusiasts; competitive sportsmen and women; special populations; the injured; those with medical conditions; children; elderly; **ante-** and **post-**natal women.

A conscientious and skilful sports therapist must be seen as a major asset to any health or fitness centre. A professional sports therapy service provides sporting individuals with a base of support and assistance for their pursuits – potentially it can make the difference between success and failure. Communities, and the various populations within, benefit simply because sports therapy can be a very attractive alternative to perhaps the long-term sufferance of niggling injuries and aches and pains, symptomatic medications and waiting lists. There are times when sports therapy will help and relieve when all else has failed. It also is clearly a great preventative measure.

However, sports therapy is not a cure-all. Sports therapists, unless additionally qualified, are not physiotherapists or front-line medical personnel. Sports therapists do, however, have their own particular skills and practices, which can help to bring about improvements (or at least some relief) for a variety of problems. It is ingrained into sports therapy ethical philosophy to do no harm, to work with and upon the advice of the medical profession and to take the time to provide the best and most appropriate treatments for their clients.

> If we could give every individual the right amount of nourishment and exercise – not too little and not too much – we would have found the safest way to health.
> HIPPOCRATES

General respect for sports therapy is growing for its potential to achieve many clinical objectives, particularly in the treatment of soft-tissue injuries,

TIP

A successful and skilled sports therapist is a facilitator for improvements in health and fitness, a consultant and expert on such matters, an advocate and enthusiast of the principles that he or she practices, and a respectful and patient encourager to the clients that they attend to.

TIP

Sports therapy is not just for athletes! Most people can find benefit in sports therapy, and it is often the non-exercisers who experience the most profound improvements in vitality and well-being.

postural and mobility problems, and stress-related conditions. It is common for athletes to confidently state the beneficial effects of incorporating sports therapy into their training schedule. Hands-on therapy (in its various forms) is also often used as an important palliative (relieving) treatment. Objectively, any basic improvement in fitness is normally associated with an improvement in health.

The various objectives of sports therapy:

- improved sporting performance
- improved strength, power, flexibility, co-ordination and endurance
- improved recovery from activity
- identification of individual strengths and weaknesses
- improvement of posture, body contours, body awareness and well-being
- prevention of injuries
- treatment and rehabilitation of injuries
- improved functional fitness.

Students and practitioners should find it difficult to forget the various feel-good factors that are closely associated with sports therapy. Surely it is a bonus that something that does us such good can also feel so good – from the feelings of successful participation in sports to the sense of relaxation or recovery achieved in the clinic!

PATHWAYS TO PRACTICE

TIP

Complementary therapy is therapy that works to assist and complement conventional medicine, not to replace it. This includes osteopathy, acupuncture, homeopathy, massage therapy and sports therapy. Complementary therapy often requires medical approval (when presented with medical conditions), prior to its provision.

For various reasons it is important to have some understanding of the medical hierarchy in the UK: who is responsible for the care of people's health problems and where sports therapists fit in. In simple terms, most people will visit their GP as their first port of call for most health concerns. Depending on the nature and severity of the problem, the GP will usually either prescribe medication and offer advice, or refer their patient for expert **diagnosis** (medical consultant) or treatment. Sports therapists are not medical practitioners, and it is not their responsibility to take on such a role. Sports therapists should always seek specialist medical opinion when confronted with any potentially serious health or injury problem, and this will normally involve recommending that their client visits their GP first of all so that appropriate procedures can be undertaken (obviously in emergencies, the hospital will be the immediate destination). Of course, as the respect and demand for sports therapy grow, more clients will be seeking out sports therapy for help with their problems. But it must be remembered that sports therapy is **complementary** therapy.

At the forefront of providing therapy for sports are chartered physiotherapists, who provide high-level physical assessment, diagnosis, treatment and guided rehabilitation. Physiotherapists undergo rigorous academic training to achieve chartered and state registered status, and additionally, they may undertake post-graduate study in specialist areas such as sports medicine or manipulative therapy. Because of their broad, specific and high-level educational background, physiotherapists work in close alliance with the medical profession. They may work within the NHS or in private practice, and many are attracted to work in the field of sport. GPs and consultants refer patients to physiotherapists, and private health-care insurance companies recognize their practice. Sports therapists are not entitled to practise as physiotherapists, unless they have undertaken the recognized additional training.

Professional titles in the health-care business can be somewhat confusing for the consumer. Governmental legislation and professional ethics restrict individuals from trading under the title of a profession for which they are not qualified, for example chartered physiotherapist or registered osteopath. Additionally, the professional indemnity insurance companies will not cover treatments for which the practitioner is not appropriately qualified, for example manipulative therapy or acupuncture. This leaves the independent, inappropriately qualified therapist, who pays little attention to professional ethics and trading legislations treading on dangerous ground. There is great potential for harm and legal implications when the practitioner strays from his or her professional boundaries.

Many sports therapists gain their initial professional qualifications through the Vocational Training Charitable Trust (VTCT). Formerly known as Vocational Awards International (VAI), the VTCT has a division especially for these therapists – the International Institute of Sports Therapy (IIST). Most sports therapists who train via this route become members of the Federation of Holistic Therapists (FHT), who in turn offer a specific category of membership to the International Council of Health, Fitness and Sports Therapists (HFST). Another popular organization offering entry level sports therapy and related qualifications is the International Therapy Education Council (ITEC). Membership of a professional governing body (such as the FHT, the Society of Sports Therapists or the Sports Massage Association) gives the therapist a multitude of benefits including: recognized code of practice and ethics; practitioner insurance; continuing professional development programmes; practitioner database for the general public; and professional journals.

With regard to the currently typical, full-time, further education vocational training programme in sports therapy, students are tutored and guided through a thorough one or two year course of study that is designed to prepare them for most aspects of employment. This type of training commonly includes, alongside such subject specifics as anatomy and physiology, principles of exercise, fitness testing and sports massage, delivery of key skills subjects, health and safety, science (underlying principles to therapeutic methods) and customer services. This is in line with governmental educational directives, designed to best serve both the school leaver and the mature student seeking new qualifications and a change of career (the 'return to learn' student).

A private training institute may also offer such a comprehensive package. Training at weekends, periodic concentrated study and distance learning are typical methods available to students training with private institutions. These courses are perhaps most suited to particularly motivated mature students who may find it difficult to commit to a full-time programme.

TIP

An example of statutory regulation implementation is 'The Osteopaths Act', which was introduced in the 1990s to regulate the osteopathy profession and to protect the title. It is now illegal for non-qualified persons to call themselves an osteopath or claim that they practise osteopathy.

TIP

Allied therapeutic practice is closely related to medical practice, and practitioners are probably state registered. These include physiotherapists, occupational therapists, chiropodists, podiatrists and dieticians. Sports therapists may also eventually belong to this closely regulated collection of health professionals, once official standardization of training, qualifications and titles has occurred.

TIP

Key skills are those subjects which are central to the basic requirements of any type of work or study. They include communications (written and verbal language skills), numeracy (maths, statistics, etc.) and information technology (computer study; word processing; data processing; using the internet). Key skills subjects are usually offered at progressive levels.

Prior to enrolling on a programme, prospective students of sports therapy should:

- Look at the content and syllabus of the course.
- Look at both the amount of guided learning hours and the duration of the course.
- Find out how much time is spent in a realistic working environment with genuine clients.
- Look at the cost of the course.
- Take a look at the facilities and resources.
- Find out about the tutors. Are they appropriately qualified and experienced?
- Ask to speak to current or previous students.
- Find out whether the qualification facilitates membership of a professional organization.
- Find out whether the qualification satisfies professional insurance company stipulations.
- Find out whether the qualification is recognized as an entry qualification by the higher education providers.
- Compare the various courses, qualifications, teachers, facilities and resources, and make your informed decision.

> Schools that offer training programmes of 500–1000 hours adequately prepare students… in my opinion, fewer than 500 class hours is insufficient time to cover the necessary body of knowledge.
>
> SANDY FRITZ (2000)

The Society of Sports Therapists (SoST) was established in 1990. Its inception was in order to address the increased requirements of the sports industry by developing nationally recognized educational courses for therapists, medical practitioners, coaches, trainers and the general public. The society has also been influential in the development of university level sports therapy programmes, which most certainly helps to raise the standing of the profession.

The subject of state registration and regulation is a complex one. The responsibility is placed upon the governing bodies and the training providers to offer the appropriate, externally assessed and validated qualifications. Certainly, with any standardized increase in training quality and level arises increased professional recognition. One of the main concerns held to date is the fact that there is such a disparity in the types of courses and qualifications available. This is so for most complementary practices. Hopefully, the formation of central self-regulating governing bodies demonstrates both to the general public and the potential student a suitably higher level of professional integrity. By being regulated, both the therapist's rights and the public's safety are protected. The title 'sports therapist' or 'sports massage practitioner' implies that the individual has undergone a recognized course of training to achieve this title. However, sports therapy is not yet a restricted title, and training courses can be quite varied in content and duration, to say the least. Sports therapists who are genuinely serious about their professional practice should be welcoming of statutory regulation and state registration, because with it arrives a dramatic increase in perceived confidence from the public, a greater acceptance and

TIP

Once a therapy profession is properly regulated it is subject to the maintenance of:

- a register of practitioners
- standards of education for entry to the profession
- standards of conduct and performance expected of the profession
- procedures relating to fitness to practise
- standards of continuing professional development
- a public and practitioner information service.

integration within the mainstream medical world, and a general elevation of position and standing.

In 2003, significant developments took place in the move towards state registration for sports therapists. The Health Professions Council, the official body responsible for regulating allied health professionals (e.g. **physiotherapy**; occupational therapy; **chiropody**; radiography), officially recognized SoST as the lead body to present the final petition for state registration. This complicated process, it is hoped and anticipated, could be completed by the year 2008.

The National Sports Medicine Institute of the UK (NSMI) has also taken a striking initiative with regard to the standardization of sports massage therapy. In 2000, the NSMI invited the Qualifications and Curriculum Authority (QCA) and SPRITO (The National Organization for Sport, Recreation and Allied Occupations) to present to almost 30 sports massage training schools and organizations, which resulted in an endorsed proposal for the establishment of a united professional body, and hence, the Sports Massage Association (SMA) was formed in 2001, with the basic ethos of promoting sports massage education to an acceptable professional standard. This initiative aims to give confidence to the general and sporting public, the medical profession and governmental agencies that sports massage practitioners are suitably trained to provide a quality service and to possibly help lead the sports massage profession also towards some form of state regulation. There are several other organizations and associations proactive in the furthering of the standing of sports, massage and related complementary therapies.

B.Sc. degree courses are available at a number of universities in sports therapy, as well as in bodywork, rehabilitation studies and complementary therapies, including osteopathy. Higher-level M.Sc. programmes in sports therapy are also being proposed and developed. Additionally, there are many degree courses available in sports science, exercise science and sports studies, all of which are certainly appropriate and related progression routes for sports therapists to take, depending on the individual's particular area of interest.

For those new to this exciting and rapidly developing field, a career in health and fitness or therapy can easily begin by training as a gym instructor, exercise class instructor or massage therapist. In this industry, there is great potential for continually moving up the ladder of knowledge and success. Initial skills and qualifications can (and should) be built upon. It is not unfeasible for particularly motivated fitness professionals to move into more specialized areas, such as managing exercise **referral** schemes, providing personal training, sports science, sports coaching, osteopathy, chiropractic, rehabilitation, physiotherapy, podiatry, sports nutrition, complementary medicine, centre management or further and higher education lecturing.

Individuals considering embarking upon a career in sports therapy should ideally have the attitude and characteristics that are normally associated with professional people. They should certainly enjoy physical activities, sports, and being with and helping others, and they must also be committed to preparing themselves to become caring health professionals.

TIP
Personal qualities that the sports therapists should develop: ● communication skills ● caring skills ● empathy and sensitivity ● patience and tolerance ● the ability to use initiative ● reliability, responsibility and trustworthiness ● enthusiasm, dedication and determination.

Employment/self-employment: once qualified, where do sports therapists work?

The sports therapist is faced with a choice between employment and self-employment (or a combination of the two). Typical locations for work are the sports or fitness club, gym, sports team, therapy clinic or as part of a multi-disciplinary centre.

Being employed usually dictates that the therapist receives a guaranteed regular wage. However, the positions on offer are often limited to gym instruction, group exercise instruction or massage therapy. As well as full-time posts, there will also be part-time positions, which means that the therapist could continue with studies or work at more than one location.

Self-employment is often attractive to the more confident and motivated therapist, and opportunities tend to arise once the practitioner has gained a certain amount of practical experience and developed a good reputation. The emphasis is upon the individual to plan their business. This includes assessing the viability of setting up and organizing a realistic pricing structure. The outgoings of the business should be compared against the predicted turnover. Obvious outgoings include the purchase of basic equipment, rent, advertising, clinical disposables, membership of professional organizations and insurance to practise. Marketing and promotion is an important part of developing a business. Business cards, descriptive leaflets, newspaper and magazine adverts, directory listings, practitioner databases and websites are all now commonly utilized.

One way of getting a business known is by giving talks to interested groups (consider everything from women's institutes to support groups for medical condition sufferers). Unique angles of approach should be thought through: Is there a need for a mobile service? Does the local football team require a sports therapist on training and match days? Does the local leisure centre have a resident therapist? Would it be worth renting a treatment room in an existing practice, such as in a private fitness club, complementary therapy centre or even a beautician's or hairdresser's? Often, a private physiotherapy or osteopathic practice will welcome the addition of a well-trained sports therapist to enhance their range of services. Some GPs are keen to incorporate a complementary aspect to their practice and may have a room available for rent. This will have the dual advantages of both being in a recognized location and also having the possibility of referred clients from the GP. It is not unfeasible to develop a successful business. A career in sports therapy can be incredibly rewarding in terms of both job satisfaction and financial remuneration.

A BRIEF HISTORY OF SPORTS THERAPY

Manual medicine is as old as the science of art and medicine itself.

PHILIP E. GREENMAN (1996)

The history of **massage** and physical therapy obviously includes many pioneering and influential figures. Especially important were the early works of the Yellow Emperor (*circa* 2500 BC), Hippocrates (460–377 BC) and Galen (AD 131–201), and the later innovators such as Ling (1776–1839), Mezger (1839–1909), Still (1828–1917), Palmer (1845–1913), Kellogg (1852–1943), Beard (1887–1971) and Cyriax (1904–1985). There are many more, too numerous to mention, and the profession evolves with each new generation.

The *Huang Di Nei Jing*, or the Yellow Emperor's Medicine Classic, was a compiled source of Chinese medical knowledge and philosophy. Perhaps here was the earliest documented reference to massage as a health-promoting treatment. The recorded origins of traditional Indian *Ayurvedic* medicine date back to around 1800 BC, and massage therapy, alongside diet and exercise, was and still is, seen as a fundamental aspect.

Both the words *massage* and *therapy* are of Greek origin, indeed the legendary Greek Hippocratic physicians wrote extensively of early therapeutic techniques, including massage, exercise and traction. Five centuries later, Galen, another Greek physician, and one of the most prolific writers in medical history, built upon the Hippocratic principles of health promotion. Perhaps Galen's most important contribution to medicine was provided by his observations and discoveries pertaining to the anatomy and physiology of the body.

The Swedish gymnastic educator Per Henrik Ling was an important pioneer in the systemization of modern remedial exercises and massage techniques. Ling's work helped sports and physical therapy gain early worldwide recognition. Following on from Ling, the Dutch physician Dr Johann Mezger was also a keen proponent of massage and a developer of remedial techniques. He gained great respect from the medical community for his scientific approach.

Dr Andrew Taylor Still, an American preacher and doctor, was the founder of the practice of osteopathy. In his early work as a doctor and surgeon, Still became increasingly frustrated with the inefficacy of the medical treatments of the time. He set about to devote himself to the study of health and ill-health, especially upon the fundamental anatomical and physiological principles. Eventually, Still proclaimed two basic conclusions: that the body has the ability to heal; and that the structure of the body has profound effect upon its function. Osteopathy was developed, using manipulative procedures, to optimize structural integrity and therefore improve the body's functioning.

Another American, Daniel David Palmer, is credited as the founder of chiropractic, a somewhat similar approach to health-care as osteopathy but with subtle differences in its underlying philosophies and actual practical techniques. Both modern osteopathy and chiropractic have developed into medically recognized, scientifically founded and well-utilized systems of health-care.

At around the same time, the American surgeon Dr John Harvey Kellogg, of cornflake fame, wrote extensively on the benefits of massage, exercise, hydrotherapy and diet. Kellogg could be considered somewhat eccentric: his approach to health involved strict hygiene, vegetarianism, colonic irrigation and abstinence from smoking, laziness and excessive sexual activity! He was, however, making some important observations on the causes of health problems and certainly some of his recommendations still stand strong today.

Gertrude Beard was an important early enthusiast, exponent, educator and author of massage therapy during its formative years as a mainstream complementary therapy, and her published works are still available and remain relevant.

In the 1950s, the British **orthopaedic** surgeon James H. Cyriax presented, in his textbook, as a scientifically justified intervention, the deep transverse friction technique. Frictions are now widely regarded as one of the most useful corrective soft-tissue techniques. Cyriax was most highly regarded in the field of physical examination and assessment. He developed a system of assessment aiming to accurately diagnose lesions of the musculo-skeletal system. Contemporary physical assessments still incorporate much of the Cyriax approach.

The present-day Chartered Society of Physiotherapists (CSP) began life, when set up by a small group of nurses in 1894, as the Society of Trained Masseuses. By 1920 it had become The Institute of Massage and Remedial Gymnastics, and in 1944 adopted its present name. For various reasons, the practice of contemporary physiotherapy has moved on from its formative methods of treatment – leaving an area of therapeutic practice to be taken on by other specialist practitioners.

In the modern era, because of increased awareness, acceptance and integration of therapeutic strategies, many more influential figures have entered the arena. The British naturopath, osteopath and acupuncturist Leon Chaitow has written extensively for both the general public and specialist practitioners. As an expert practitioner and educator, he has done much to add to the growth and respectability of the therapeutic professions, especially for his work in soft-tissue manipulation techniques.

Looking at sports therapy and its elevation into the field as a practice in its own right, several notable figures have emerged, including the remedial masseur Mel Cash, and the physiotherapist Joan Watt, who have both written excellent texts on aspects of the subject. Many more experts are emerging by the year in this exciting and expanding field of health-care.

THE FUTURE OF SPORTS THERAPY

Sports therapy is growing in use, in demand, in stature. The practice is fully appreciated by a complete cross-section of populations. Sports therapists help to maintain many top athletes, sports performers and dancers. Most professional football clubs use sports massage. Sports therapists operate at many leisure centres and fitness clubs. They advise beginners on the right way to exercise, and they guide more experienced exercisers into new methods and improved techniques. They teach one to one, and they teach exercise classes. Sports therapy clinics tend to differ from the GP's or dentist's surgery in that the customers will often want to be there! Fashions may fade but genres tend to prevail, and sports therapy is not a fashion, but is here to stay.

The sports therapists of today are well served with continual professional development (CPD) programmes and with access to higher education. There is a thriving equipment and supplies industry serving sports therapists and fitness professionals, and a great deal of therapeutic and exercise equipment is readily available, with new products being continually developed and marketed.

As sports therapy is becoming more widely offered, the need for improved understanding of its potential increases. The therapeutic aspects of physical, electrical and **thermal therapy** and exercise – the physiological effects, benefits, adversities, indications for use and, ultimately, the effectiveness – all clearly require continual study, practice and research to keep the best of these interventions available to the recipients.

However much research is performed and analysed with sports therapy, the need for further, high-quality trials continues. Much of the information currently available is still relatively anecdotal – with both practitioners and patients alike reporting their own successful use of the treatment. As with all respectable practices, research is taking place – perhaps not all actually determining absolute efficacy, but at least highlighting the applications that appear to be most beneficial, and in which particular settings. The important areas in which to direct future research should be in standardized format and in conjunction with, and in addition to, other related subject areas.

Areas for research in sports therapy include the following:

- Specific physiological responses to sports therapy treatment for specific conditions.
- How individuals differ in their physiological response to sports therapy treatment.
- How to determine the strongest indications for its use.
- How to get the best response from sports therapy treatment.
- The variation in effect relating to the: specific applications; duration of treatment; frequency of treatment; number of treatments.
- How to best regulate the practice of sports therapy.
- How to best integrate the practice of sports therapy into the health-care professions.

Research into sports therapy in the past has been limited, to some extent, by the lack of funding, lack of research skills and lack of academic infrastructure, which is not to say that these processes do not now exist, however. Students involved in higher-level study are expected to contribute to the research process and as more and more people are studying at university level, the knowledge base is increasing all the time.

The therapy professions are now in the process of reaping the benefits of a massive growth in worldwide practice. Physiotherapy, sports therapy, massage, bodywork, osteopathy, chiropractic, acupuncture, yoga, Pilates, Alexander technique, tai chi, aromatherapy, reflexology, shiatsu, naturopathy, herbal medicine, homeopathy, reiki and more: all have greater utilization and acceptance than ever before. The recent developments in demand for provision heralds an era of closer integration of health-care professions, where there exists a framework for more effective cross-referral and multi-disciplinary practice.

TIP

Continuing professional development normally involves the cascading of current and developing thoughts, theories and implications important to improving practice, from the experts, educators and researchers to the practitioners. CPD commonly incorporates the opportunity for practitioners to discuss and develop new skills. CPD is also about reflecting on one's own approach to practice and continually looking out for development opportunities.

TIP

High-quality research is crucial to the acceptance and continued integration of the methods of sports therapy into the business of mainstream health-care.

CHAPTER SUMMARY

Sports therapy is an aspect of complementary health-care that is growing in stature. Many of its practical methods have developed traditionally over a long period of time. It is aimed at helping individuals improve their health, fitness, and functional or athletic performance. Sports therapy is getting more popular, and can be used by all individuals, not just athletes, to help prevent and treat injuries (in addition to, or as a follow on from, medical intervention), and to help improve fitness, posture, body contours, mobility, strength, agility, relaxation, body awareness and well-being. Several organizations are now working to encourage a standardization of training and practice in sports therapy and sports massage, and statutory regulation is a definite possibility in the near future. Sports therapy may be studied in accredited private institutions, further education colleges and at several universities. Sports therapists should enjoy physical activities and helping others. Once qualified, they should aim to develop a wide range of skills, and stay updated, and above all they should always be professional. Important to the future of sports therapy is rigorous research into its methods, and the development of processes that improve the understanding of its usefulness.

WEBSITE

Visit the companion website at www.thomsonlearning.co.uk/ healthandfitness/ward where you will find the answers to these questions for you to check your progress through the book.

Knowledge Review

1 Explain what sports therapy is.

2 What are the various basic possible objectives of sports therapy?

3 What is the difference between a physiotherapist and a sports therapist?

4 What is the reasoning behind the formation of professional governing bodies?

5 What kinds of skills and personal characteristics should a training sports therapist develop?

6 List ten prominent historical and present-day pioneers of sports therapy and related methods.

7 Why is research important to the future practice of sports therapy?

8 How do you see the future of sports therapy?

chapter 2

ANATOMY AND PHYSIOLOGY FOR SPORTS THERAPY

Learning Objectives

After reading this chapter you should be able to:

- understand the basic organization and systems of the body
- understand and make practical use of anatomical and physiological terminology
- recognize the anatomical position, the body's regional anatomy, surface anatomy and potential endangerment sites
- be familiar with important musculo-skeletal structures, functions and intricacies
- be familiar with important nervous, circulatory, respiratory, digestive, urinary, integumentary and energy system aspects and concepts
- understand key differences between men and women
- develop awareness of the ageing process

WEBSITE @

Visit the companion website at www.thomsonlearning.co.uk/ healthandfitness/ward where you will be able to download some of the artwork in this chapter to use on your course.

THE IMPORTANCE OF ANATOMY AND PHYSIOLOGY

Perhaps one of the main reasons that students are attracted to the field of health and fitness is the fact that the human body is such a fascinating structure. How we move, behave, react, function and live depends upon our anatomy and physiology (A&P). Our genetic inheritances, our learned experiences and, fundamentally, our physical capabilities all affect our quality of life and mould our existence.

Vitally important to your understanding of how to help, advise and treat your clients is the subject of anatomy and physiology, which involves study of especially the skeletal, muscular, nervous, circulatory, respiratory, endocrine, digestive and excretory systems. This fundamental knowledge cannot be brushed over lightly. Once the basic concept of our systemic make-up has been absorbed, the sports therapist can begin to understand more of the body's functional relationships – the energy systems, the regulating mechanisms, the gender differences, the processes of growth and repair, the effects of exercise, the ageing process.

Sound knowledge and understanding in anatomy and physiology help us to analyse and objectify the rationale for our intervention strategies. Being a practitioner of sports therapy dictates that you integrate learned theoretical knowledge into the practice of providing treatments and exercise prescription. It is important to understand what you are trying to achieve for your client's benefit, and also to be able to translate the best plans of action to your clients in a clear and understandable (less jargonistic) manner.

This chapter does not attempt to provide a complete text of anatomy and physiology – there are many other more detailed sources for this. Presented here are some of the more practically relevant aspects, the underpinning knowledge of which should be of interest to all sports therapists. Do remember that although it is useful and convenient to distinguish the various physiological functions of the body in relation to their systems, the fact remains that all structures are related and everything is connected in some way.

> One of the major challenges to a beginning practitioner is getting the balance right between knowledge, sensing what is under your hands and the intuitions that come to you as you gain experience.
>
> SU FOX AND DARIEN PRITCHARD (2001)

THE ORGANIZATIONS OF THE BODY

The human body can be considered to be divided into a sequence of structural organizations:

- **Chemical level**: Atoms, molecules, particles and compounds. Matter is anything that has substance. (Particulate) matter is composed of chemical elements, e.g. oxygen, carbon, hydrogen and nitrogen. Chemical elements are composed of tiny atoms. Atomic chemical reactions cause the formation of molecules. A molecule is the smallest unit of an element or compound that is capable of existing independently. Atoms and molecules form the body's many and various tissue cells.

- **Cellular level**: **Cells** are the basic structural and functional units of any organism. Many kinds of cell exist, for example muscle cells, nerve cells and blood cells. Cells contain specialized structures within their **cyto**plasm called organelles. Organelles perform the specific functions of the cell. Examples of organelles include the nucleus (containing genes), the mitochondria (where ATP is generated), ribosomes (for protein synthesis) and lysosomes (containing digestive enzymes which speed up the breakdown of molecules and microbes).

- **Tissue level**: Tissues are groups of cells that work together to perform a specific function. The four basic tissues are **epi**thelial tissue (**epithelium**), **muscle** tissue, **connective tissue** and **nerve** tissue.

TIP

There are six levels of physiological organization in the body: chemical; cellular; tissue; organ; system; organismic.

- **Organ** level: Several tissues make up one organ. Organs have specific functions and usually have recognizable shapes. The major organs include the brain, heart, lungs, liver, spleen, kidneys, stomach, intestines, genitalia and skin.
- **System** level: A body system comprises several organs or tissues that work together and independently to perform specific functions, e.g. the muscular system.
- **Organismic level**: 'Structurally, the largest level is the organismic level. All the parts of the body functioning with one another comprise the total organism – one living individual' Gerard J. Tortora and Sandra R. Grabowski (1996).

> **TIP** ✔
>
> The ten main systems of the body are: skeletal system, muscular system, nervous system, circulatory system, digestive system, urinary system, respiratory system, lymphatic system, endocrine and reproductive systems, and integumentary system.

ANATOMICAL POSITIONS, REGIONAL AREAS AND DIRECTIONAL TERMS

It is important to be familiar with terms used to describe surfaces of the body, positions of structures relative to each other and the different types of movements available at joints. There is a standardized anatomical position, where the body is described and viewed, anteriorly, posteriorly and laterally, with arms by the side, but with forearms supinated (palms facing forward).

> **TIP** ✔
>
> Regional anatomy describes the body in terms of regions:
>
> - Head = cephalic/cranial/facial regions
> - Neck = cervical region
> - Shoulder = acromial region
> - Armpit = axillary region
> - Upper arm = brachial region
> - Elbow = cubital region
> - Forearm = antebrachial region
> - Wrist = carpal region
> - Palm = metacarpal region
> - Fingers = phalangeal/digital region
> - Chest = thoracic region
> - Low trunk = abdominal region
> - Low back = lumbar region
> - Groin = inguinal region
> - Hip = coxal region
> - Front of lower pelvis = pubic region
> - Buttock = gluteal region
> - Thigh = femoral region
> - Front of knee = patellar region
> - Back of knee = popliteal region
> - Shin = crural region
> - Calf = sural region
> - Ankle = tarsal region
> - Top of foot = dorsal region
> - Underside of foot = plantar region
> - Heel = calcaneal region
> - Toes = phalangeal/digital region

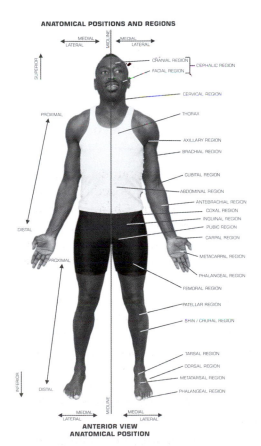

Anterior anatomical positions and regions

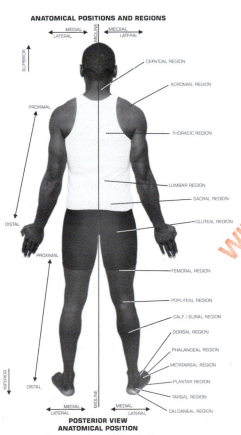

Posterior anatomical positions and regions

ANATOMICAL, POSITIONAL AND MOVEMENT TERMS

Anterior: front view
Posterior: rear view
Superior: above
Interior: below
Medial: towards the midline
Lateral: towards the outside, or side view
Proximal: near to
Distal: away from
Superficial: nearer to the surface
Deep: away from the surface
Ipsilateral: same side of the body
Contralateral: opposite side of the body
Prone: lying face down
Supine: lying face up
Internal: inward
External: outward
Flexion: bending of a joint, reducing its angle
Extension: straightening of a joint, increasing its angle
Hyperextension: increased extension
Abduction: taking away from the midline

Adduction: bringing towards or beyond the midline
Rotation: revolving movement around an axis
Circumduction: circular movement around a joint
Plantarflexion: taking sole of the foot downwards
Dorsiflexion: taking the top of the foot upwards
Pronation: turning palm of hand downwards
Supination: turning palm of hand upwards
Inversion: turning sole of foot inwards
Eversion: turning sole of foot outwards
Elevation: lifting upwards
Depression: taking downwards
Protraction: taking forwards
Retraction: drawing backwards
Radial deviation: movement of wrist from neutral towards the radius
Ulnar deviation: movement of the wrist from neutral towards the ulna
Opposition: movement of the thumb (pollex) towards the opposite fingers

Using this as a standard starting position for all other anatomical positions and directional movements, the human body's structures and movements can easily be explained and understood. Additionally, many of the body's movements are described in relation to its midline. This system enables professionals to discuss and describe the body in a common language and reduces the possibility of misunderstandings.

The concept of **planes** and sections is another important aspect to grasp. There are three planes and sections of view and movement. A frontal section divides the body into anterior and posterior sections. Movements in the frontal plane include lateral flexion, abduction and adduction. A sagittal section divides the body into left and right halves. Movements in the sagittal plane include flexion and extension. A transverse section divides the body into superior and inferior portions. Transverse plane movements are rotational. Deep anatomical illustrations are often viewed in a particular plane (or cross-section). Awareness of such planes adds to our ability to describe, understand and work with anatomy.

SURFACE ANATOMY AND ENDANGERMENT SITES

Surface anatomy is everything on the body that can be easily observed or palpated (touched). This includes the skin; superficial muscles, tendons and their fascia; bony prominences; superficial ligaments; accessible joints; superficial blood vessels; superficial lymph nodes; superficial bursae; and accessible organs.

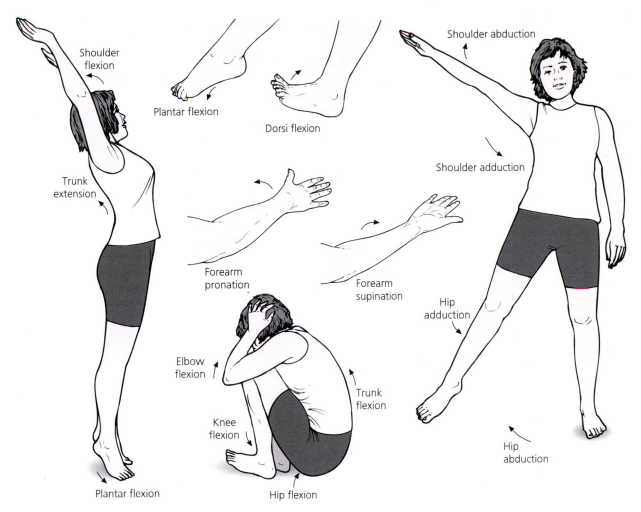

Examples of joint movements

It is all very well looking in textbooks to learn about the various structures and tissues within the body and their specific locations, but, in practice, the therapist is presented with a real person. That person presents themselves only with what is observable or palpable. Understanding surface anatomy is crucial to the successful assessment and resultant treatment of your client.

The main guides to the positions and locations of structures are the body's bony landmarks. These are the more superficial bony contours and prominences that can provide a reference point to other structures. In practical reality, the therapist should be able to confidently feel their way around the body. Once skilled in the art of assessing gross surface anatomy, the therapist can then begin to hone their skill in assessing the difference between normal and abnormal tissue appearance and structure. Examples of this in practice include understanding and assessing the difference between: a normal and a subluxed joint (partially dislocated); normal and abnormal joint contours (e.g. temperature changes, swelling); normal or abnormal (**hypertrophy** or atrophy) **muscle tone**; tightened or normal muscle **fascia**; presence or absence of muscular or fascial adhesions.

Endangerment sites are simply specific areas on the body where there is potential for harm to be caused by inappropriate pressure, movement or

TIP

Examples of movements in planes:

- Trunk rotation = transverse plane movement
- Shoulder abduction = frontal plane movement
- Hip flexion = sagittal plane movement

other technique. Being an endangerment site does not necessarily mean that no form of treatment can be applied, but it does mean that the therapist must be aware of the vulnerability of that particular area and what techniques or adapted techniques can be safely applied. Usually, an endangerment site is an area that has little in the way of skeletal or muscular protection and contains vulnerable tissues such as superficial blood vessels, nerves, lymph nodes, organs or bursae. In the early stage of a sports therapist's career, it is sensible to avoid working upon certain areas until more experience and understanding is gained. Particularly vulnerable areas include the: temporal region; facial regions; anterior neck; axillary region; abdomen; 11th and 12th pairs of (floating) ribs; kidney region; inguinal region; popliteal region. Endangerments also include some of the many and various types of contra-indications (discussed in chapter 3), such as varicose veins or phlebitis. Problems related to inappropriate or over-enthusiastic techniques of treatment are best avoided by understanding the dangers, being familiar with all the relevant anatomy, and always taking care in practice.

SKELETAL SYSTEM ESSENTIALS

As a therapist, it is important to conceptualize the systems of the body, while at the same time remembering the uniqueness of each individual aspect. The skeletal system, in particular, is very easy to conceptualize – it is the body's main structure, with well-defined components. However, deeper knowledge and understanding of its specific physical detail take longer to develop. Each **bone** is different, both in terms of structure and function. Every **joint** in the body is unique. All joints have differing physical features, supportive properties and movement capabilities.

The skeleton has six basic functions:

1 Provides a structural framework for the body as a whole.

2 Supports and protects internal vital organs (e.g. cranium protects the brain; ribs and sternum protect the lungs and heart; vertebral column protects the spinal cord; pelvis protects the bladder and genitalia).

3 Provides a surface for the attachment of soft-tissues (tendons; muscles; ligaments).

4 Acts as a biomechanical leverage system for the skeletal muscles to create joint motion.

5 Produces red blood cells, white blood cells and platelets in the red **bone marrow**.

6 Provides a store for calcium, phosphorus (in the form of phosphate), magnesium and other minerals. It helps to regulate the level of these minerals in the blood. Also stores fat in the yellow bone marrow.

Probably the most important skeletal structure is the vertebral column, the 'central pillar' of the body. The vertebral column provides so much in terms of structure, support, protection and facilitation of function. It comprises 33 vertebral bones (7 cervical, 12 thoracic, 5 lumbar, 5 sacral and 4 coccygeal).

KEY A&P FACTS: *SKELETAL SYSTEM*

Comprises: bones; cartilage; joints.

Supports and protects the body.

Bones provide sites of attachment for muscles.

Structure and shape of components facilitates body posture and movement.

Generally considered to be around 206 bones in the body.

Two types of bone: compact and cancellous.

Five classifications of bone: long; short; flat; irregular; sesamoid.

Bone contains marrow cells, which form much of the body's blood cells.

Bone stores minerals and fats.

Bone and its outer membrane – the periosteum – is living tissue and has blood, lymphatic and nerve supply.

Activity, exercise, lifestyle and accidents all have profound effects upon the development and strength of bone.

Three types of cartilage: hyaline; fibro; elastic.

Three types of joints: fibrous; cartilaginous; synovial.

Six types of synovial joints: ball and socket; hinge; gliding; pivot; condyloid; saddle.

Most vertebral bones feature a large, rounded, weight-bearing body, two laterally directed transverse processes, one posteriorly directed spinous process and two vertebral arches, which form the vertebral **foramen** (through which the spinal cord travels).

The smallest vertebrae are found in the cervical region. The first cervical vertebrae (C1 – the atlas) articulates with the **condyles** of the occipital (cranial) bone, above, and the second cervical bone (C2 – the axis) below. The occipito-atlantal joint allows 'nodding' (flexion and extension) movements. The axial-atlanto joint is a pivot joint that revolves on the odontoid peg of the axis, an upright process that allows for head-turning (rotation) movements. Obviously, the head is additionally supported by ligaments, muscles and other soft-tissues. The seventh cervical bone (C7 – vertebra prominens) has a slightly longer spinous process than the others and is a recognizable landmark. The thoracic region provides for attachment of the ribs, which, with the costal-**cartilages** and sternum, form the thorax (the thoracic **cavity** or cage). The lumbar region features the largest and strongest vertebrae. The five sacral and four coccygeal (tail) bones are fused. The sacrum articulates with the iliac bones to form the sacro-iliac joints and part of the pelvic girdle.

There are two main types of joint between each individual vertebral bone. Between the large central bodies of each vertebra are the intervertebral discs. These form the column's strong, cartilaginous (slightly movable) intervertebral joints. The discs feature two distinct layers: a tough, fibro-cartilage outer layer, the fibrosus annulus, and an inner, gel-like layer, the nucleus pulposus. The discs help the spine to bear a great deal of weight, provide it with additional shock-absorbing qualities and contribute to its curvatures. They also facilitate varying degrees of leverage to the movements of the spine.

The other type of joint, above and below the majority of each individual vertebra, is the small synovial, gliding, facet or zygopophyseal joint. These joints add to both the stability and movability of the regions of the spine. The first ten thoracic vertebrae have additional facet joints for articulation with the ribs.

There are natural curves along the length of the spine. The curves, which can be viewed in the standing position from the lateral aspect, collectively increase the overall strength and resilience of the structure. They help maintain the body's dynamic balance in the upright position and absorb shock during walking or running. The thoracic and sacral concave curves are formed during fetal development and are therefore known as primary curves. The secondary convex cervical and lumbar curves develop as the baby learns to hold its head up and, later, sit up, stand and walk. The spinal curves are of particular relevance when analysing and treating postural problems.

There are two girdles within the skeleton. The shoulder girdle comprises the clavicles and the scapulae. Together with the upper extremity bones (humerus, radius, ulna, carpals, metacarpals and phalanges), they form half of the appendicular skeleton (limbs being appendages). The clavicle communicates with the sternum at the anteriorly positioned, gliding, sterno-clavicular (SC) joint, and with the scapula, on the lateral aspect at the prominent, gliding, acromio-clavicular (AC) joint. Held within the shallow glenoid cavity of the scapula, primarily by the rotator cuff muscle group and connective tissue, is the head of the humerus. This ball and socket gleno-humeral joint has a great deal of movement available to it.

The other girdle within the body is the pelvic girdle. This comprises the two hip (innominate) bones, which are joined together by the sacrum posteriorly and the pubic symphasis anteriorly. The hip joint is an important weight-bearing joint, and therefore has a much deeper socket (the acetabulum) than that of the shoulder joint. Each hip bone is itself divided into three separate, but well-fused, bones – the ilium, ischium and pubis. On the anterior aspect, the two pubic bones form a cartilaginous joint: the pubic symphasis. The pelvic girdle, together with the lower extremity bones (femur, patella, tibia, fibula, tarsals, metatarsals and phalanges), complete the appendicular skeleton.

The structure of the lower extremity is particularly important to understand. The hinged knee joint contains both articular and fibro-cartilage. The two fibrous (medial and lateral) meniscal discs add to the stability and shape of the joint. They assist in the functional performance of knee flexion in that they help to accommodate the full weight-bearing, moving contours of the femoral condyles upon the tibial plateau. They also provide additionally important shock absorption. The menisci are slightly mobile, and the lateral meniscus more so. They are kept in position via coronary and transverse ligaments. The popliteal muscle, at the back of the knee joint, has an attachment on the lateral meniscus, which, in addition to assisting knee flexion and tibial rotation, retracts the meniscus as the knee flexes.

The ankle joint is basically a hinge joint between the tibia, fibula and talus. Further into the foot are the sub-talar (between the talus and calcaneum) and the talo-calcaneo-navicular joints, both of which are importantly involved in controlling the foot's inversion and eversion movements during gait.

An important aspect of the foot is its series of arches. Simply, there are the medial and lateral longitudinal arches, and the distal and proximal transverse arches. They help support the weight-bearing structure of the foot and allow it the biomechanical leverage required for walking, running and jumping. The arches are formed by the combined shape of all the bones involved, the ligaments supporting each joint, the intrinsic foot musculature and the plantar fascia.

It is important to discuss the synovial (freely movable) joints in a little more detail. A typical synovial joint features a joint capsule and capsular ligaments, a synovial **membrane** secreting synovial fluid and smooth articular cartilage. Synovial fluid is both an excellent lubricant for the joint and a source of nutrients to the avascular cartilage within. There are six main types of synovial joint: gliding; hinge; ball and socket; pivot; condyloid; and saddle.

A **bursa** is a synovial-like fluid-filled sac, and is commonly found situated around synovial joints. Bursae (plural) are usually sited underneath tendons adjacent to their attachment. Their purpose is to reduce friction between the moving tendon and the bony prominences that it might otherwise be exposed to. Some joints will also contain fat pads, which add to the

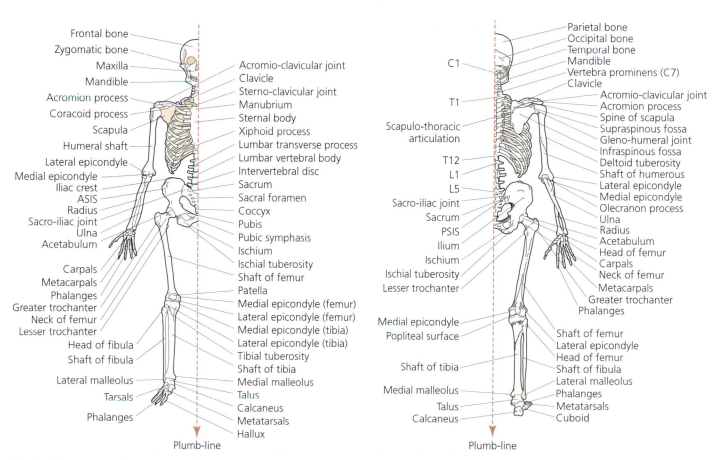

Skeletal anatomy (male): anterior view   Skeletal anatomy (male): posterior view

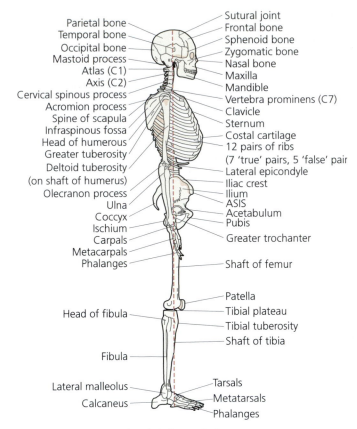

Parietal bone
Temporal bone
Occipital bone
Mastoid process
Atlas (C1)
Axis (C2)
Cervical spinous process
Acromion process
Spine of scapula
Infraspinous fossa
Head of humerous
Greater tuberosity
Deltoid tuberosity
(on shaft of humerus)
Olecranon process
Ulna
Coccyx
Ischium
Carpals
Metacarpals
Phalanges

Sutural joint
Frontal bone
Sphenoid bone
Zygomatic bone
Nasal bone
Maxilla
Mandible
Vertebra prominens (C7)
Clavicle
Sternum
Costal cartilage
12 pairs of ribs
(7 'true' pairs, 5 'false' pair
Lateral epicondyle
Iliac crest
Ilium
ASIS
Acetabulum
Pubis
Greater trochanter

Shaft of femur

Patella
Tibial plateau
Tibial tuberosity
Shaft of tibia

Head of fibula

Fibula

Lateral malleolus
Calcaneus

Tarsals
Metatarsals
Phalanges

Skeletal anatomy (male): lateral view

structure and help to fill out the joint space, therefore assisting the synovial lubrication system.

Ligaments are very much a part of the skeletal system. Wherever there is a joint there are several ligaments. Their basic role is to strap bones together

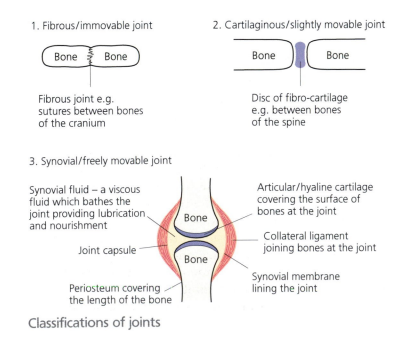

1. Fibrous/immovable joint

Bone ⟩⟨ Bone

Fibrous joint e.g.
sutures between bones
of the cranium

2. Cartilaginous/slightly movable joint

Bone   Bone

Disc of fibro-cartilage
e.g. between bones
of the spine

3. Synovial/freely movable joint

Synovial fluid – a viscous
fluid which bathes the
joint providing lubrication
and nourishment

Bone

Joint capsule

Bone

Periosteum covering
the length of the bone

Articular/hyaline cartilage
covering the surface of
bones at the joint

Collateral ligament
joining bones at the joint

Synovial membrane
lining the joint

Classifications of joints

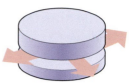

1. Gliding joint
   e.g. inter-tarsal joints

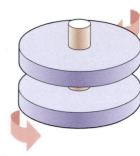

2. Pivot joint
   e.g. atlas (C1)–axis (C7) joint

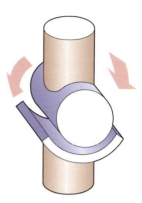

3. Hinge joint
   e.g. humeral–ulna joint

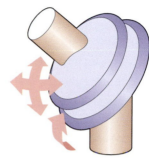

4. Condyloid/ellipsoid joint
   e.g. radio-carpal joints

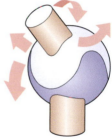

5. Saddle joint
   e.g. carpal–metacarpal
   joint of thumb

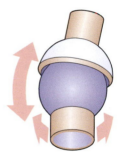

6. Ball-and-socket joint
   e.g. gleno-humeral joint

Types of synovial joints

at joints, form part of the synovial capsule, encourage optimal bone alignment and help to restrict unwanted joint movements. Ligaments are made from strong connective tissue, but lack extensibility. They also have a relatively poor blood supply, which means that if a joint is forcibly stressed beyond its normal range, the ligaments can tear and the natural repair may be slow. Prominent ligaments are: the collateral ligaments, which support the medial and lateral aspects of hinge joints; the strong anterior and posterior cruciate ligaments of the knee, which help keep the femur and tibia in close proximity and restrict unwanted forward and backward movement of the tibia; the medial deltoid, posterior talo-fibular and lateral calcaneo-fibular ligaments of the ankle; the spinal anterior and posterior ligaments, which, running from the cranium to the upper sacrum, hold all vertebral joints in close alignment; and the ilio-lumbar, sacro-iliac, sacro-spinous and sacro-tuberous ligaments, which surround the base of the spine.

**RANGES OF MOVEMENT (ROM) ASSOCIATED
WITH EACH MAJOR REGION**

Cervical: flexion; extension; rotation (left and right); lateral flexion (left and right).

Thoraco-lumbar: flexion; extension; rotation (left and right); lateral flexion (left and right).

Shoulder: flexion; extension; abduction; adduction; rotation (medial and lateral); circumduction; elevation; depression; protraction; retraction.

Elbow: flexion; extension.

Forearm: pronation; supination.

Wrist: flexion; extension; radial deviation; ulnar deviation; circumduction.

Hand: meta-carpal flexion, extension, abduction and adduction; inter-phalangeal flexion and extension; pollex flexion, extension, abduction, adduction, circumduction and opposition.

Hip: flexion; extension; abduction; adduction; rotation (medial and lateral); circumduction.

Knee: flexion; extension; tibial rotation (medial and lateral).

Ankle: plantarflexion; dorsiflexion.

Foot: inversion (rearfoot and forefoot); eversion (rearfoot and forefoot); inter-phalangeal flexion and extension.

The movements of joints

It is crucial to be familiar with the basic directional and movement terms. In addition, the sports therapist must understand which movements are normally available at each joint. A joint has a typical or normal range of motion. This range can be divided into its inner range, mid-range, outer range and full range of motion.

MUSCULAR SYSTEM ESSENTIALS

Perhaps the most interesting components of anatomy and physiology for the sports therapist are the muscles. Muscles can be classified in a variety of ways, but there are three fundamental categorizations: skeletal (voluntary or striated) muscles; smooth (involuntary) muscles; and cardiac (heart) muscle. Each category has a different structure and functional purpose.

Muscle tissue can be described as having five main functions:

1 Performance of movement (walking; running; throwing; writing).

2 Maintenance of posture (stability during sitting, standing, walking and performing other tasks).

3 Movement of substances within the body (blood; food; faeces; urine; gases; lymph).

4 Generation of heat (as muscles contract one by-product is heat, which helps maintain the normal body temperature of 37 °C).

5 Regulation of organ volume (bladder; stomach).

TIP

See the appendix for major muscle position and action tables.

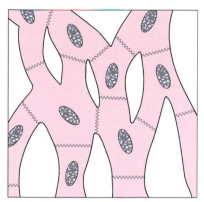
Cardiac muscle tissue

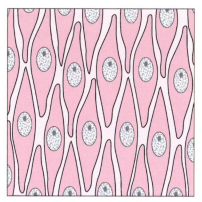
Involuntary muscle tissue

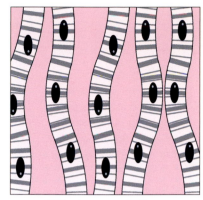
Voluntary muscle tissue

Types of muscle tissue

KEY A&P FACTS: *MUSCULAR SYSTEM*

There are over 600 skeletal muscles in the body.

Muscle tissue accounts for approximately 40% of total body weight.

There are three categories of muscle tissue: skeletal; smooth; cardiac.

Skeletal muscles maintain posture, assist in joint stability, help protect against trauma and initiate body movements.

Muscular contractions generate body heat.

Smooth muscle has different structure from skeletal muscle, having spindle-shaped cells with one centrally located nucleus. It is involuntary and is found in the walls of blood vessels, digestive tract, respiratory ducts, urinary and reproductive tubes and in the internal organs.

Cardiac muscle tissue structure is specialized to contract upon itself for production of the heartbeat. It features intercalated discs where adjacent cells meet, across which spreads the impulse to contract.

Muscle tissue has a rich blood and nerve supply, indeed muscles contain thousands of blood capillaries, which open and close according to the activity undertaken.

All muscular actions are initiated and co-ordinated by nerve impulses.

Skeletal muscle contractions assist the return, to the general circulation, of venous blood and lymphatic fluid.

TIP

Names given to the three types of muscle tissue:

1 Skeletal (because it attaches to and moves the skeleton). Voluntary (because it can be made to contract and relax, by conscious control). Striated (because striations or stripy segments can be viewed under a microscope).

2 Smooth (because of its structure and appearance when viewed microscopically). Involuntary (because its contraction and relaxation are under the influence of hormones and autonomic nerve impulses, rather than conscious control).

3 Heart/cardiac (because it is a specialized muscle tissue found only in the walls of the heart).

Muscles are often described in terms of groups (e.g. the quads or hamstrings) and individual muscles (e.g. the rectus femoris of the quad group). Individual muscles and groups of muscles are separated into compartments by the surrounding sheaths of thin fibrous, connective fascia. A similar type of fascial tissue called **retinaculum** surrounds muscles and tendons like a supportive strap to assist their positioning, and this is found around the wrist and ankle, for example.

There is a basic internal structure to skeletal muscle, which can be described as if stripping away a layer at a time. Underneath its subcutaneous, connective tissue, superficial fascia layer lie the muscle's closely approximated deeper fascial layers. The superficial fascia provides protection, reduces heat loss, stores water and fat, and provides a framework for nerves and blood vessels to enter and leave. The deeper

TIP

Muscle tissue has five basic characteristics:

1 **Excitability**: the ability to respond to stimuli (nerve impulses or hormones).
2 **Conductivity**: the ability to conduct nerve impulses along its length.
3 **Contractility**: the ability to contract (shorten and thicken) and thus produce force.
4 **Extensibility**: the ability to stretch or be stretched (within certain limits) without causing damage.
5 **Elasticity**: the ability to return to original shape following shortening or lengthening.

TIP

Basic summary of how muscles contract:

● There must be basic muscle, nerve and circulatory integrity.
● Fuel for the energy to contract is supplied by either the aerobic or anaerobic energy pathway.
● An impulse is sent along a motor nerve pathway to the neuromuscular junction.
● Stored calcium is released from the sarcoplasmic retinaculum, and diffuses into the muscle.
● Calcium binds with the protein troponin upon the actin myofilament.
● Actin filaments slide across the myosin filaments, causing the sarcomere to shorten, which generates force and movement.

fascia separates muscles into groups, allows free movement and also supports nerves, blood and lymphatic vessels. Three further layers extend from the deep fascia: the epimycium contains the muscle; the **peri**mycium surrounds the bundles of muscle fibres (the fascicles); and the endomycium separates the individual muscle fibres. Muscle tissue is made up of many muscle fibres (the muscle cells), and each muscle fibre is made up of many contractile units called **myo**fibrils. The muscle's tendon, which attaches it to bone at its origin and insertion, is a continuation of the connective tissues that surround it.

The muscle cell's membrane is called the sarcolemma, beneath which is the sarcoplasm (the muscle cell's cytoplasm). The sarcoplasm houses the cell's proteins, organelles and the threadlike myofibrils. The myofibrils, within the muscle fibres, are composed of many overlapping protein threads called myofilaments. The myofibrils are also divided along their length into a series of distinct sections called sarcomeres. The sarcomeres are the functional contractile (shortening) units of each myofibril. The overlapping myofilaments of the sarcomere are the thin actin and thick myosin. The alternating light and dark pattern formed by these myofilaments is what gives skeletal muscle fibres their characteristic striped or striated appearance when viewed microscopically.

When a muscle fibre receives a message (via a nerve impulse) to contract, the myofilaments (actin and myosin) slide across each other. In order to contract, stored calcium (in the sarcoplasmic retinaculum, which surrounds the myofibrils) must be released. This occurs when the nerve impulse action potential reaches the sarcoplasmic retinaculum. Calcium diffuses into the muscle and binds with the protein troponin, which is located on the actin myofilament. The two proteins troponin and tropomyosin (both of which rest on the actin filament) are the main regulators of muscular contractions. They do this by controlling the interaction of actin and myosin. As released calcium binds with troponin, a positional change immediately occurs in tropomyosin. This reaction results in an energized movement between the two myofilaments, which have small, bridge-like projections (cross-bridges). These projections allow the two filaments to interact with each other. As the actin filaments connect with the adjacent myosin filaments, they slide across each other, and the sarcomere shortens. The simultaneous contraction of each sarcomere results in the contraction of the myofibril. The myofibril shortens and thickens.

When a stimulus occurs that requires the muscle to contract, the muscle fibres work on an all or nothing basis; that is to say, each fibre is capable only of full contraction or no contraction when stimulated. However, during exercise, as fatigue sets in, the degree of contraction may decrease. To create a stronger contraction, more muscle fibres have to be recruited. The amount of functional force produced depends upon the number of cross-bridges created. The process described, whereby the sarcomere is seen to shorten during a concentric contraction, is commonly known as the sliding-filament theory.

In addition to nerve impulses, muscles need fuel to produce the energy to contract. ATP (**adenosine triphosphate**) is the energy currency, and fuel for muscle contraction is supplied by the aerobic and anaerobic energy pathways.

Skeletal muscle fibres are usually divided into three categories according to their structure, functional capacities and preferred energy pathway. These are commonly known as fast-twitch, slow-twitch and intermediate muscle fibres, and are primarily distinguished by their differing fibre size, speed of contraction, preferred metabolic source of energy (aerobic or anaerobic), and their capacity to perform work. The proportions of the different fibre types within muscles varies from individual to individual, and also within the various muscles of one person.

In simple terms, the classic fast-twitch fibres (also called fast-glycolytic FG or **Type IIB** fibres) have a larger diameter and are capable of generating great force quickly, favouring the anaerobic energy pathway. They have a low content of both mitochondria and myoglobin (the oxygen carrier within muscle), and therefore appear white in colour and have low resistance to fatigue.

Slow-twitch fibres (slow-oxidative SO or **Type I** fibres) rely upon aerobic metabolism. They have a smaller diameter, many mitochondria, a dense capillary network and high myoglobin content, and therefore have a red appearance. These fibres contract slowly, but have resistance to fatigue and are suited to long-duration, low-intensity work.

Intermediate fibres (fast-oxidative-glycolytic or Type IIA fibres) have a medium sized diameter, are relatively fast to contract and, although primarily anaerobic, have a greater aerobic capacity than Type IIB fibres and therefore a greater resistance to fatigue. This is because they have more mitochondria and myoglobin. They are sometimes described as being white fast fibres.

The relative proportion of muscle fibre types within an individual is, surprisingly, not necessarily a good predictor of performance capability, although there is a great tendency for elite performers to specialize in the sports and activities that their predominant fibres are best suited to. The amount of muscle fibres an individual has is determined, mainly through inheritance, during the developing years and cannot be increased through training; however, the size (cross-sectional area), strength and endurance can be. Any increase in a muscle's diameter is mainly due to an increase in both the number and size of the myofibrils within it, and also to an increase in the amount of protein myofilaments making up the myofibrils. All fibre types can be trained to improve their performance of any type of activity, but one constant that tends to remain is their speed of contraction.

The skeletal muscles can be clearly described as being **agonists** (prime movers), **antagonists** (opposing the action of their agonists), **synergists** (working together to perform particular work, and assisting the agonist) and **fixators** (stabilizing body parts). Muscles are possibly postural or **phasic**, global or local. Muscles are capable of performing contractile work in a variety of ways: isometric contractions are performed without altering the length of the muscle; isotonic contractions involve shortening of the muscle (concentric work), where the insertions of the muscle(s) move towards the origins. When a lengthening contraction occurs (eccentric work), the insertions are moving away from the origins. To illustrate this, the simple movements of the elbow joint (flexion and extension) are described: the agonist (main) elbow flexor muscle is the biceps brachii (assisted by the synergistic brachialis and brachioradialis). When the elbow flexor muscles shorten they are working both isotonically and concentrically, the angle of the joint is reducing, and the insertions are moving towards their origins. If a weight is involved (such as a dumb-bell), as the arm moves into extension the flexor muscles are called upon to control the lowering of the arm, they are working eccentrically (and still isotonically). Whether a contraction is concentric or eccentric depends on the position of the joint, the levers involved, the fulcrum of the joint and specifically where the force (or resistance) is being applied.

Levers, fulcrum, effort and resistance

- The leverage system provides us with a mechanical explanation for the ability to perform our many movements – in terms of the muscles, bones and joints, and whatever work they are being asked to do.
- The bones are the levers.
- The fulcrum (axis) is the working joint.
- Effort is provided by the muscles.
- The resistance is the load being lifted.
- In the body, there are three basic classes of lever:
    1 In a 1st class lever, the fulcrum is sits between the effort and the load (EFR). The movement is like that of a see-saw, e.g. cervical flexion and extension (at the atlanto-occipital joint).
    2 In a 2nd class lever, the resistance sits between the fulcrum and the effort (FRE). This lever performs work like a wheelbarrow, e.g. standing on tip-toes (plantarflexion).
    3 In a 3rd class lever, the effort is applied between the fulcrum and the resistance (FER), e.g. biceps brachii (and its synergists) flexing the elbow joint.

An example of muscular activity is provided by flexing your right knee (in a standing position), see p. 33. The resultant muscular activity is as follows:

- Right hamstrings contract concentrically.
- Right gastrocnemius and popliteus assist the action.
- Right quadriceps are inhibited, i.e. they relax and lengthen – so as not to resist the knee flexion.

Therefore:

- Right hamstrings are the agonists (prime movers).
- Right quadriceps are the antagonists.
- Right gastrocnemius and popliteus are the main synergists.
- Left foot and leg, right and left hip and all back and torso muscles are the fixators.

The body features a series of major pairs of reciprocally antagonistic muscles, which basically work together to provide the ability to maintain postural stability and perform co-ordinated movements. A series of reverberating neural circuits regulate the tension and work performed by

SUPERFICIAL   DEEP

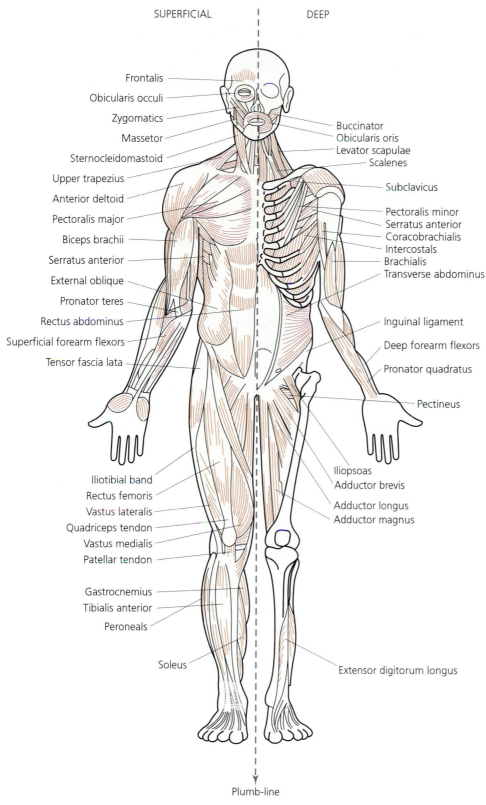

Frontalis

Obicularis occuli

Zygomatics

Massetor

Sternocleidomastoid

Upper trapezius

Anterior deltoid

Pectoralis major

Biceps brachii

Serratus anterior

External oblique

Pronator teres

Rectus abdominus

Superficial forearm flexors

Tensor fascia lata

Buccinator

Obicularis oris

Levator scapulae

Scalenes

Subclavicus

Pectoralis minor

Serratus anterior

Coracobrachialis

Intercostals

Brachialis

Transverse abdominus

Inguinal ligament

Deep forearm flexors

Pronator quadratus

Pectineus

Iliopsoas

Adductor brevis

Adductor longus

Adductor magnus

Iliotibial band

Rectus femoris

Vastus lateralis

Quadriceps tendon

Vastus medialis

Patellar tendon

Gastrocnemius

Tibialis anterior

Peroneals

Soleus

Extensor digitorum longus

Plumb-line

Major muscles (anterior view)

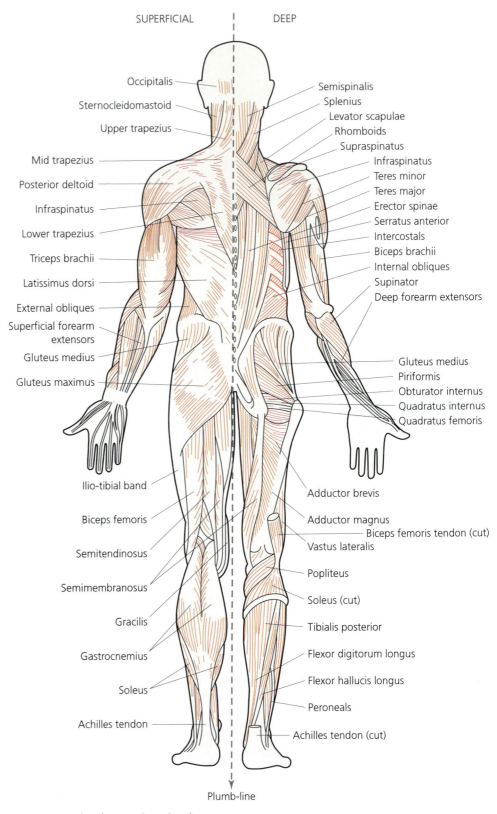

SUPERFICIAL   DEEP

Occipitalis
Sternocleidomastoid
Upper trapezius
Mid trapezius
Posterior deltoid
Infraspinatus
Lower trapezius
Triceps brachii
Latissimus dorsi
External obliques
Superficial forearm extensors
Gluteus medius
Gluteus maximus

Semispinalis
Splenius
Levator scapulae
Rhomboids
Supraspinatus
Infraspinatus
Teres minor
Teres major
Erector spinae
Serratus anterior
Intercostals
Biceps brachii
Internal obliques
Supinator
Deep forearm extensors

Gluteus medius
Piriformis
Obturator internus
Quadratus internus
Quadratus femoris

Ilio-tibial band
Biceps femoris
Semitendinosus
Semimembranosus
Gracilis
Gastrocnemius
Soleus
Achilles tendon

Adductor brevis
Adductor magnus
Biceps femoris tendon (cut)
Vastus lateralis
Popliteus
Soleus (cut)
Tibialis posterior
Flexor digitorum longus
Flexor hallucis longus
Peroneals
Achilles tendon (cut)

Plumb-line

Major muscles (posterior view)

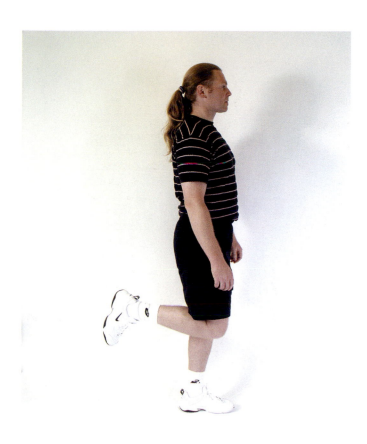

Example of the muscular activity involved in standing unilateral knee flexion

MAJOR PAIRS OF RECIPROCALLY ANTAGONISTIC MUSCLES
Biceps – triceps.
Pectoralis major – rhomboids and trapezius.
Latissimus dorsi – deltoids.
Anterior deltoids – posterior deltoids.
Infraspinatus and teres minor – subscapularis and teres major.
Forearm flexors – forearm extensors.
Rectus abdominus – erector spinae group.
Left external obliques – right external obliques.
Gluteus maximus – psoas, iliacus and rectus femoris.
Gluteus medius and minimus – gracilis, pectineus and adductors brevis, longus and magnus.
Quadriceps – hamstrings.
Gastrocnemius and soleus – tibialis anterior.

the opposing groups of muscles. During relative static posture there may be observed a state of partial equal tone in these muscle groups; however, during movement there is normally a process of contraction (in the agonist) and reciprocated relaxation (in the antagonist), automatically and neurologically controlled, that facilitates ease of movement.

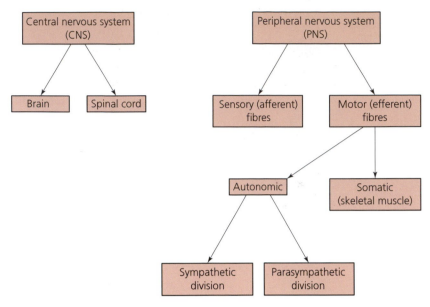

Divisions of the nervous system

NERVOUS SYSTEM ESSENTIALS

The incredibly complex nervous system, which controls most aspects of living, has two distinct anatomical divisions: the central nervous system (CNS) and the peripheral nervous system (PNS).

TIP	✔

The nervous system has several crucial functions:

- regulation of the physiological environment
- co-ordination of voluntary movements
- activation of spinal cord reflexes
- responsibility for the experiences of learning, memory, emotions and behaviour.

KEY A&P FACTS: *NERVOUS SYSTEM*

Comprises the central, peripheral and autonomic nervous systems (CNS; PNS; ANS).

Main components are: brain, spinal cord; cranial and spinal nerves; special sense organs; sympathetic and parasympathetic divisions.

The nervous system co-ordinates and regulates body activities and works in close conjunction with the endocrine system.

Typically, smooth muscle contractions (in organs and vessels) and glandular secretions are controlled by the nervous system in response to both the internal and external environment.

Has complex sensory, motor and integrative functions.

Is responsible for the experience of learning, memory, knowledge, emotions, thought, behaviour, temperature, pleasure and pain.

The functional nerve cell is the neuron, which propagates nerve impulses.

Once initiated, the impulse is generated via an action potential, which causes a wave of electrical depolarization over the surfaces of the chain of nerve cells involved in the impulse.

Each impulse is conducted neuron to neuron via a chemical neurotransmitter substance, the most common being acetylecholine.

The impulse may be to sense or integrate information or stimulate (excite) or depress (inhibit) organ, muscle or tissue activity.

The functioning unit of the nervous system is the nerve cell or neuron (sometimes called a neurone). Neurons transmit messages from one tissue to another by way of electrical impulses. Sensory (or afferent) neurons convey impulses that begin at the sensory receptors of the body's functioning tissues and end in the CNS. Motor (efferent) neurons convey impulses from the CNS to the body's various muscle tissues and glands. Neuroglial cells, specialized neural connective tissue, outnumber the neurons and work to provide them with support and protection. There are different types of neuroglial cells, some are phagocytic (engulfing invading microbes and cell debris), some are involved in the metabolism of **neurotransmitters**, some produce the neuron's insulating white matter substance myelin, and some merely line the cavities of the brain and cord.

There are two principal types of matter in the nervous system. White matter is the aggregation of myelinated processes of the neurons. Myelin, produced by the neuroglia, forms an insulating sheath around the nerve fibres which assists in the conduction of impulses. Grey matter is made up of the neuron cell bodies (including the nucleus within a cytoplasm), dendrites (tree-like branches, which receive impulses from adjacent neurons at synapses) and axons (also referred to as the nerve fibre). Axons carry the electrical impulse from the cell body to the next neuron or effector tissue. Neuroglia are also classed as grey matter.

A nerve impulse (action potential), whether sensory or motor, involves the transmission of a signal from its origin to its destination. The resting cell membrane of an individual neuron is said to be polarized or negatively electrically charged, and the energy within the cell is different from that outside the cell. In order for an impulse to be propagated, the cell's resting potential must be altered or become depolarized. The main system for regulating the potential for the rest or action of the neuron is the sodium–potassium pump, and its role in altering the concentration gradient of each inside and outside the cell. Depolarization occurs when a sufficiently strong stimulus reaches the membrane, changes its **permeability** to sodium, and causes the sodium channels to open, diffusing into the neuron and making the cell more positive. When depolarization reaches its threshold level, an action potential is generated. Repolarization and resting potential occur immediately afterwards as potassium channels open and diffuse outward. A nerve impulse is seen to be an all or nothing response. That is, if an impulse is generated then it will be transmitted along the entire length of its axon. Where an impulse must pass from one neurone to another, the signal must cross a synapse. At a synapse a neurotransmitter substance is released to open the channel. Naturally, there must exist a process for the continual manufacture, activation and removal of these chemicals.

The place where an impulse meets skeletal muscle fibres is called the neuromuscular (or myoneural) junction. The neuron and the muscle fibres it innervates are described as the motor unit. The motor end-plate is the terminal part of the axon, which is very closely approximated to the post-synaptic membrane of the responding muscle fibres (the motor point). The amount of muscle fibres stimulated by one motor neuron varies. Some muscles, such as those involved in eye or hand movements, require a great deal of control and have small motor units (few fibres per motor neuron). Large muscle groups commonly have much larger motor units. One single

Motor end plate (neuro-muscular junction)

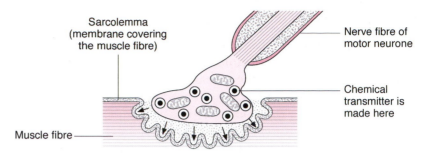

Synapse and neuromuscular junction

motor neuron could potentially stimulate up to 3000 muscle fibres. The emphasis in the major muscles is more about regulating the strength, power and endurance than fine control, and therefore recruitment is the key neurological feature. The term recruitment refers to the number of muscle fibres being activated at any one time, which is determined by the number of active motor units involved. Motor units are sometimes described as being slow or fast, which relates to the fibres they supply (Type I, IIA or IIB) the metabolic energy pathway they prefer, the size of the motor nerve and the speed of impulse conduction.

The brain and spinal cord make up the CNS. The PNS, which comprises simply all the nerve tissue outside the CNS, is further divided into the somatic and autonomic nervous systems (SNS and ANS). The brain is protected by cranial and facial bones; meninges three connective tissue membranes: dura, arachnoid and pia mater); cerebro-spinal fluid (CSF, secreted into the ventricles of the brain by the choroid plexuses, helps cushion, lubricate and nourish the brain); connective tissues, muscle and skin. The main components of the brain are:

- the brainstem (midbrain, pons varoli and medulla oblongata)
- vital CNS reflex and relay centres
- the medulla oblongata (a major regulator of heart and respiratory rate, also involved in the processes of **vasoconstriction** and **vasodilation**)
- the cerebrum, the major part of the forebrain (the two cerebral hemispheres control most mental activities such as memory, thought and reasoning, and integrate much sensory information such as sight, touch, sound, taste, smell, temperature and pain, and control most skeletal muscle contractions)
- the cerebellum (involved in the co-ordination of skilled movements, and regulation of muscle tone, posture and **balance**)
- the hypothalamus (a major regulator of the ANS and endocrine activity; secretes regulating hormones, controls anterior pituitary gland secretions, helps regulate body temperature, food and water intake, emotions, sexual behaviour, circadian rhythms, etc.)
- the thalamus (an important relay station for ascending sensory tracts of the spinal cord)
- the pituitary gland (the master endocrine gland)

- four ventricles (cavities into which CSF is secreted)
- grey matter (neurons and neuroglia)
- white matter (myelin sheath surrounding the neurons).

The spinal cord is protected by: the vertebral column; meninges, adipose and connective tissue; CSF; vertebral ligaments, muscles and skin. It consists of: inner grey matter; outer white matter; sensory (ascending) and motor (descending) tracts; anterior (ventral) horns at each spinal level, which propagate motor impulses along the spinal efferent nerves; posterior (dorsal) horns, which receive sensory impulses from incoming afferent spinal nerves; and two spinal cord enlargements (cervical and lumbar), which accommodate the extra activity of the upper and lower extremities. The cord terminates at L2, but major nerves continue, within the vertebral foramen (as the cauda equina), passing the level of L5 and anteriorly to the sacrum and coccyx.

The PNS features 12 pairs of cranial nerves (2 pairs to and from the cerebrum and 10 pairs to and from the brainstem) and 31 pairs of spinal nerves. Spinal nerves are named by the region from which they arise, e.g. C7 or L5. There are 8 cervical, 12 thoracic, 5 lumbar and 5 sacral pairs, and 1 pair of coccygeal nerves. Spinal nerves convey incoming sensory impulses from the tissues towards the spinal cord. On arrival at the cord the impulse will either travel up the cord to the brain or be subject to a reflex response (fast motor reaction). Motor impulses (efferents) travel from the appropriate cord level to their designated muscle or gland to stimulate or inhibit activity. The peripheral motor nerves originating at the spinal cord are referred to as lower motor neurons. Upper motor neurons are those originating in the CNS. All impulses occur in an instant, and there are thousands of continually reverberating neural circuits. Most tissues have many different neural connections and pathways, with most impulses occurring unconsciously and automatically.

Reflexes

A reflex is a fast automatic response of the body to a stimulus. Examples of reflex activity include the blinking of eyes when an object approaches the face or simply the swallowing of food, coughing or sneezing. The rapid movement away from a painful stimulus, such as when a hot plate is touched or a pin trodden on, is predominantly a spinal reflex, without a great deal of initial CNS involvement. However, as the various messages are processed, other reactions occur, such as verbally expressing the pain with an 'ouch!' Deep **tendon** reflexes occur naturally as a protective mechanism against over-stretching of a muscle. These are activated on stimulation of the specialized sensory receptors, the muscle spindles (proprioceptors), which are sensitive to stretch. Testing the deep tendon reflexes (such as in the knee jerk reflex) provides useful assessment information relating to nerve and muscle integrity.

Major peripheral nerves sometimes join together to form plexuses. A plexus, therefore, is where there is a collection of major nerves passing through a region in close approximation. There are four main plexuses: the cervical plexus (lying either side of the neck, supplying the muscles and

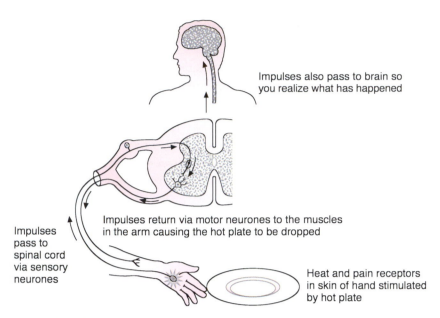

Impulses also pass to brain so you realize what has happened

Impulses return via motor neurones to the muscles in the arm causing the hot plate to be dropped

Impulses pass to spinal cord via sensory neurones

Heat and pain receptors in skin of hand stimulated by hot plate

A simple reflex arc

skin of the head, neck and upper shoulders, also the phrenic nerve from this plexus serves the diaphragm); the brachial plexus (extending from C5 to T1, passing over the first rib, behind the clavicle and continuing onto the axillary region as it serves the shoulder and upper extremity); the lumbar plexus (extends from L1 to L4, and heads outwards behind the psoas muscle and in front of the quadratus lumborum, serving the abdominal wall, genitals and areas of the lower extremities); the sacral plexus (extends from L4 to S4, mainly anterior to the sacrum, and supplies the buttocks, perineum – between the anus and urethra, and the lower extremities).

The major spinal nerves of the body are the brachial, radial and median nerves of the arm, and the sciatic, femoral, tibial and peroneal nerves of the leg. The cranial nerves are very much involved in the special senses of sight, hearing, smell and taste, as well as balance. They also supply most of the muscles of the head and face. The 10th cranial nerve (the vagus nerve) has a large role in regulating the function of the respiratory and digestive tracts, and also slows heart rate.

The SNS (somatic nervous system) is concerned primarily with controlling skeletal muscle activity. The effector tissues of the SNS are the muscles (the tissues that respond to the impulses). The SNS bases its activities upon the inputs (into the CNS) received from the skin and various other special sense receptors. A myotome is a group of muscles innervated by a single nerve root (i.e. from a spinal nerve at a particular level). Most muscles receive their innervation from more than one spinal nerve root segment. Therefore, each spinal nerve supplies more than one muscle, and each muscle is supplied by more than one spinal nerve segment. The spinal nerve roots are separate structures to the peripheral spinal nerves that they supply, i.e. they attach the nerve to the cord at a specific level by way of two pairs of anterior or ventral (motor) horns (left and right) and two pairs of posterior or dorsal (sensory) horns.

The special senses (the sense organs)

The special senses are usually referred to as being the senses of smell, taste, sight and hearing. These sensations provide us with much in the way of stimulation and enable individuals to detect changes in their immediate environment.

- Olfactory sensations – smell. The receptors for olfaction are located in the nasal epithelium, and convey impulses to the olfactory bulbs and tracts and on to the limbic (emotional) regions of the cerebral cortex of the brain.

- Gustatory sensations – taste. The receptors for gustation are found in the taste buds of the tongue. Stimulation of the gustatory receptors causes impulse transmission, along cranial nerves, to the medulla, thalamus and cerebrum.

- Visual sensations – sight. Light is absorbed by the photoreceptors (rods and cones) of the retina. Impulses are transmitted to the thalamus and cortex by the optic cranial nerves.

- Auditory sensations – hearing. Sound waves enter the external auditory canal (outer ear), strike the eardrum, then pass the through the ossicles (three ear bones in the middle ear) and eventually cause the hair cells of the inner ear to generate nerve impulses along cranial nerves to the thalamus, cerebrum and cerebellum. The ears are also important organs involved in the co-ordination of balance, working in close conjunction with incoming visual stimuli and the proprioceptive input from muscles and joints.

Sensory perception from the body, in addition to the special senses, involves a selection of afferent neural receptors which sense light touch, pressure, vibration, temperature and many different types of pain. Just as impaired motor supply to muscles can cause weakness and atrophy (muscle wasting), impaired sensory supply produces its own abnormal responses. However, sensory testing is difficult as it relies greatly upon subjective responses.

Dermatomes are specific areas of skin supplied by spinal sensory nerve roots. Each **dermatome** region on the body, relates to a specific spinal segment. The **derma**tomes can be shown on the body by way of a dermatome map. Dermatomes provide useful diagnostic information relating to problems of spinal nerve supply. They help in the assessment of the sensory signal from the periphery, and whether it is being received and processed. Aching and pain, **para**esthesia (pins and needles) or anaesthesia (numbness) are all possible symptoms of a problematic nerve supply in a particular dermatome. The nerve supply in adjacent dermatomes overlaps to some degree, however, and there are slight individual variations in dermatome regions. Also, the resulting sensory distribution of a nerve root (the dermatome) differs from that of the peripheral sensory spinal nerve (see the dermatome maps on p. 128, chapter 4).

The term **kinesthesia** is usually seen to mean conscious awareness of body position and movement rates. The awareness of one's position in space is achieved via a variety of integrated sensory pathways. Touch and pressure receptors, visual images, vestibular messages (mechanisms for recognizing balance, which are generated in the inner ear), joint receptors, muscle spindles and golgi tendon organs (GTOs) all provide the initial sensory stimuli relating to body position, and this is commonly referred to as **proprioception**. This information is integrated, analysed and acted upon, mainly in the cerebrum and cerebellum, to produce generally well-controlled, even very finely performed, intricate movements, all within an instant.

Deep within the skin, muscle, tendon and ligament tissue lie specialized sensory receptors called proprioceptors, sometimes referred to as mechanoreceptors, which may be sensitive to stretch, tension and/or pressure. Both muscle spindles and GTOs are responsive to changes in muscle length and tension.

Muscle spindles sit within the muscle, in alignment, parallel to the muscle fibres, and as the muscle stretches, so too do the spindles. The spindles typically feature tiny specialized muscle fibres (intrafusal fibres) and two separate sensory afferent fibres, which relay information relating to their stretching. When stimulated, in simple terms, they transmit impulses to the spinal cord, which results in a spinal reflex reaction, causing motor impulses back to the muscle: the muscle contracts to some degree, which reduces the stretch stimulus affecting the spindles. This is a protective mechanism, commonly called the stretch reflex. The spindles also contain a small motor efferent nerve fibre, which provides a mechanism to allow for optimal sensitivity and function of the spindles' **intra**fusal fibres at different muscle lengths. The stretch reflex is an important mechanism to help control movement and maintain posture, especially with regard to making the muscles ready to respond to changes in position and gravitational pull.

GTOs are located in the muscle's tendon, near its muscular-tendinous junction. They report back to the CNS differences in muscle tension both during active contraction, and during passive stretch. When activated, they cause a reflex inhibition stimulus to the contracting muscle, thereby acting as a protection mechanism that prevents excessive muscular force. They will also encourage a slowly stretching muscle to relax. The manual stimulation of GTOs is attempted during the application of treatment techniques such as proprioceptive neuromuscular facilitation (PNF) or muscle energy techniques (MET), which are commonly used to bring about improvements in flexibility and functional strength (see MET in chapter 9).

Testing the deep tendon reflexes helps to establish whether there is an upper or lower motor neuron deficiency. Testing these reflexes involves tapping a tendon briskly with a reflex hammer and monitoring the quality of the reflex. Normal reaction to a tap (a momentary stretch of the muscle) is to contract mildly, which produces either an observable joint movement or a palpable muscle contraction. Tendon reflexes are taken on both sides of the body and compared. Tendon reflexes are graded progressively as being absent, diminished, normal, exaggerated or clonic (very brisk). The commonly tested tendon reflexes are the: patella tendon (knee jerk) (L2/3/4); biceps (C5/6); triceps (C6/7); ankle (S1). Note: see deep tendon reflex testing in chapter 4.

The ANS, which regulates most organ activity automatically, has two separate but complementary components: the sympathetic and parasympathetic systems. The effector tissues of the ANS are the smooth muscles of blood vessels, tracts and organs, cardiac muscle and glands. Most organ tissue (viscera) has both sympathetic and parasympathetic innervation. Generally, the sympathetic system tends to stimulate or speed up specific activity, while the parasympathetic system tends to inhibit or slow activity. Therefore, the parasympathetic pathways dominate during periods of rest, enabling digestion and assimilation to occur, which encourage growth and repair. The sympathetics, which work in conjunction with the adrenal hormones, automatically prepare the body for immediate action, and dominate when the presenting situation is threatening or stressful or requires an instant physical response. In such a situation, the sympathetic nervous system is involved in increasing heart rate, blood pressure, breathing rate, blood sugar (glucose) levels and even the size of the pupils of the eyes. It will cause a reduction in digestive activity. These combined actions are often referred to as the 'fight or flight' response. The two autonomic divisions arise from separate regions of the spinal cord. Sympathetic nerves leave the cord at the thoracic and lumbar levels. Parasympathetic nerves leave at the cranial and sacral levels.

CIRCULATORY SYSTEM ESSENTIALS

The circulatory and respiratory systems provide the body with its basic mechanisms for supplying the tissues with the ingredients for activity, growth and repair (oxygen, nutrients and hormones), and for removing metabolic waste products such as carbon dioxide. It is a universal communication system involving a wide variety of tissues and structures. It is most dynamic, continually responding to the neurological and hormonal stimuli that it receives in response to both internal and external influences.

In simple terms, blood flows from the heart to the tissues, back to the heart, and then to the lungs, before being pumped out again to the tissues. The tissues require oxygenated, nutrient-laden blood. Once the blood has oxygenated the tissues and eventually returned to the heart, it has become deoxygenated. In the lungs it rids itself of carbon dioxide and

TIP

Key cardio-respiratory aspects:

- the systemic (arterial and venous) circulation
- the pulmonary circulation
- the portal circulation
- the lymphatic circulation
- the structure of the body's different vessels
- the location of main arteries and veins, and pulse points
- the structure and activity of the heart, including heart rate, cardiac cycle, cardiac output and stroke volume
- the composition and activity of blood
- blood pressure
- the mechanisms for breathing, pulmonary ventilation, external and internal respiration and capillary exchange.

KEY A&P FACTS: *CIRCULATORY SYSTEM*

Consists of: heart; blood; blood vessels.

The heart is a unique organ and has its own pacemaker system, which sets heart rate.

It receives deoxygenated blood from the tissues, pumps it to the lungs (pulmonary circulation) to get oxygenated, receives it back from the lungs and pumps it out, via the aorta, into the general (systemic) circulation.

Arteries divide into arterioles, which further divide into capillaries.

Capillaries facilitate the exchange of gases, nutrients and waste products in the tissues.

Deoxygenated blood is returned to the heart from the tissues by venules, which form into (larger) veins.

The circulatory system carries oxygen, carbon dioxide, nutrients from the digestive system, endocrine hormones, antibodies, white blood cells and heat.

Heat can be transported to the skin's surface or kept more within the body, depending upon the body's temperature requirements (a homeostatic function).

replenishes itself with oxygen. The cycle continues as the freshly oxygenated blood returns to the heart in order to be pumped out again to the tissues.

The systemic, or general, circulation is the blood supply to and from the tissues. Arteries are the vessels that carry blood away from the heart. The main artery is the aorta, the body's widest and longest artery. It exits the heart from the left ventricle, where the myocardium (heart muscle) is thickest and strongest. The body's main named arteries arise from it. The arteries that exit the aorta, along its path from above the heart to the abdomen, are generally in pairs, feeding the left and right sides of the body, and are often referred to as branches. As the systemic circulation gets more specific, to supply particular tissues, arteries divide to become arterioles and metarterioles (small and smaller arteries). The metarterioles feed blood into the capillaries, which is where the exchange of oxygen and nutrients between the blood and tissues takes place. Blood moves through capillaries via the pressure from the blood behind in the arterioles.

The main arteries are as follows:

- **Aorta**: the body's major artery. It exits the heart from the aortic valve of the left ventricle, and heads upwards (as the ascending aorta) to serve the arterial branches, which supply the head and neck. It curves downwards (at the aortic arch) to become the descending aorta. It runs deep in the torso, anterior to the vertebral column, eventually dividing into the common iliac arteries at the level of the lower lumbar vertebrae. All along its route, the aorta has branches leading off to supply specific regions of the body with freshly oxygenated arterial blood. The arch contains blood pressure-sensitive baroreceptors.
- **Left and right (L&R) pulmonary arteries**: the only arteries to carry deoxygenated blood. They run from the right ventricle of the heart to the left and right lung respectively.
- **Coronary arteries**: supply the heart.
- **Brachiocephalic artery**: the first large artery to leave the aorta. It supplies the head and arm (feeding into the right common carotid and subclavian arteries).
- **Left and right common carotid arteries**: serve the head and neck. Contain the carotid bodies (baroreceptors). An easy pulse reading can be taken here.
- **Left and right subclavian arteries**: supply the brain (via the vertebral arteries) and arms.
- **Subclavian arteries**: in the arm, divide into the axillary and brachial arteries, and in the lower arm, the radial and ulnar arteries.
- **Circle of Willis**: a cerebral arterial circle (in the brain), where ascending arterial vessels connect, equalize blood pressure, and allow for alternative pathways for blood in the brain, should damage occur.
- **Thoracic region of the aorta**: serves a collection of important arteries – the pericardial arteries (supply the pericardium); the bronchial arteries; the oesophageal arteries; the intercostal arteries (supplying chest and abdominal muscles and the overlying skin, mammary glands and vertebral canal).

- **Phrenic arteries**: serve the diaphragm.
- **Hepatic artery**: serves the liver.
- **Gastric artery**: serves the stomach.
- **Splenic artery**: serves the spleen and pancreas.
- **Renal arteries**: serve the kidneys and adrenal glands.
- **Superior mesenteric artery**: serves the pancreas and the small and large intestines.
- **Genital arteries**: supply the testes or ovaries.
- **Inferior mesenteric artery**: serves the large intestine and rectum.
- **Common (external) iliac arteries**: supply the legs, leading into the femoral popliteal, tibial, peroneal and dorsalis pedis arteries.
- **Internal iliac arteries**: supply muscles and organs within the pelvic cavity.

Venules are the tiny blood vessels that take deoxygenated blood from the capillary network of a tissue. The larger veins, which carry this blood back to the heart for pumping to the lungs, differ from arteries in that they are thin walled, having less smooth muscle tissue (the tunica media), and contain valves to stop the back-flow of blood.

The main veins are as follows:

- Usually, the deeper veins have similar names to their closely associated arteries.
- The left and right pulmonary veins are the only veins to carry oxygenated blood. They run from the left and right lungs to the left atrium of the heart.
- The main veins are the superior and inferior vena cavae, which enter the heart at the right atrium. The superior vena cava contains the venous blood returning to the heart from the head, neck and arms. The inferior vena cava drains the deoxygenated blood from the abdomen and legs.
- The coronary sinus drains venous blood from the heart, and has its own entry point into the right atrium.
- In the neck, there are the jugular and vertebral veins, which empty into the subclavian and brachiocephalic veins, before entering the superior vena cava.
- The subclavian veins, which drain the veins of the arm and the vertebral vein of the neck, have entry points for the thoracic (on the left) and right lymphatic ducts (on the right). Therefore, all lymphatic fluid eventually drains into the venous blood circulation at the subclavian veins.
- Other veins emptying into the superior vena cava are the azygos and hemiazygos veins, which lie close to the vertebral column and drain the thorax.

The main veins feeding into the inferior vena cava are: the hepatic vein (from the liver), which has itself received the hepatic portal vein (containing venous blood from the digestive tract, spleen, pancreas and gall bladder); the renal veins; the phrenic veins; the iliac veins (which have received venous blood from the saphenous, tibial, popliteal and femoral veins of the leg, and also blood from the pelvic cavity).

The return of blood to the heart, known as venous return, is not performed by the direct pumping of the heart. Blood moves through the veins, in a centripetal direction, as a result of several mechanisms:

- The pressure in arterioles, which is higher than that in the venules, pushes blood onward through the capillaries.
- The presence of valves in the veins.
- The squeezing action of skeletal muscles that surround the veins (the skeletal muscle pump).
- Venoconstriction. A narrowing of the diameter of veins, which occurs via reflex sympathetic stimulation of the vessels draining skeletal muscle. This reduces the volume capacity of veins, and helps move blood onwards.
- The alternate expansion and recoil of the chest and diaphragm during inspiration and expiration create negative pressure within the thorax and abdomen, which assists blood movement (the respiratory pump).
- The suction action of the pumping heart helps draw blood towards and into it.
- Gravity assists venous return from the head and neck when standing or sitting, and offers less resistance to blood flow from the lower body when lying down.

The deoxygenated blood enters the heart at its right atrium (the first upper chamber). It is released into the right ventricle (first lower chamber), from where it is pumped into the pulmonary artery (the only artery in the body to carry deoxygenated blood), which transports it to the lungs. Once oxygenated, the blood returns to the heart via the pulmonary vein (the only vein to carry oxygenated blood), and enters at the left atrium. This is known as the pulmonary circulation. The less expansive portal circulation is the flow of nutrient-laden blood from the digestive organs to the liver, where it is further processed.

It can be seen that the heart itself contains four chambers: the two atria and the two ventricles. Atria receive the blood, and ventricles, which have thicker muscular walls, pump the blood out, either to the lungs or to the tissues, via the aorta. The amount of blood moved from the atria into the ventricles, and from the ventricles outwards, is controlled, to some degree, by the presence

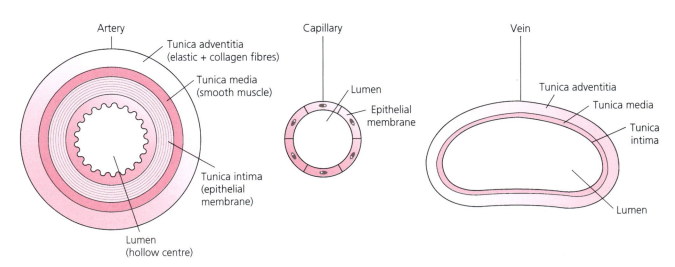

Blood vessels

of valves between the chambers and at the exit point of the two arteries. The heart is itself a highly vascular organ, and receives its blood from the coronary arteries.

The cardiac cycle is simply the repetitive alternate contraction and relaxation of the heart. Contraction is referred to as systole, and relaxation as diastole. Normal resting heart rate (the amount of heart beats in a minute) is usually stated as being between 60 and 80 **beats per minute** (bpm), but values either side of these rates can be considered acceptable if asymptomatic, indeed athletes commonly record resting rates of 60 bpm or less. Individual heart rates vary, and dominant factors include age, sex, heredity, lifestyle and state of health and fitness. Heart rate is related to oxygen consumption, in that they both increase as intensity of physical activity (exercise) increases. The maximal exercising heart rate (HR_{max}) is a scientifically estimated figure that allows safety in fitness training to be monitored (see chapter 12).

The **pulse** is a wave of distension that can be felt in the more superficial major arteries as the left ventricle of the heart momentarily contracts. The most commonly taken and accessible pulses are the radial (wrist) and carotid (anterior neck) pulses.

Stroke volume (SV) is the amount of blood pumped with each heartbeat (SV ml/beat). Cardiac output (CO) is the amount of blood pumped per minute ($HR \times SV = CO$ l/min).

The heart has both intrinsic and extrinsic influences upon its rate of contraction. The sino-atrial (SA) node, located in the upper right atrium, is the heart's pacemaker. The heart contracts as the SA node initiates a wave of electrical depolarization through its conducting tissues, which also includes the atrioventricular (AV) node, bundle of His, bundle branches and eventually the Purkinje fibres, which spread the wave of depolarization through the right and left ventricles. The normal process of alternate neurological polarization and depolarization can be observed on an electrocardiograph (ECG). ECG recordings are used to identify cardiac malfunctions and to assess heart function in response to exercise. The autonomic nervous and endocrine systems have a major (extrinsic) role in regulating heart activity through both the SA and AV nodes, especially in relation to the demands placed upon the cardio-respiratory system by exercise. The main cardio-vascular control centre in the brain is the medulla oblongata (of the brainstem), which, at rest, maintains a balance between sympathetic and parasympathetic stimulation of the heart. In simple terms, sympathetic stimulation increases heart rate, and parasympathetic stimulation slows it. There are a number of mechanisms for reporting alterations in such important parameters as blood pressure or blood oxygen concentrations to the medulla, which responds by stimulating the nerve pathways to the heart and regulating the rate accordingly.

Blood is a connective tissue. It is the plasma-based carrying substance that is pumped around the body by the heart. Plasma is a transparent fluid (90 per cent water) containing various dissolved substances (e.g. proteins, salts, nutrients, hormones, **anti**bodies and waste products). It constitutes around 55 per cent of normal blood volume. The other 45 per cent of blood volume is made up of red (erythrocyte) and white (leucocyte) blood cells and platelets (thrombocytes). Both erythrocytes and leucocytes are manufactured in the red bone marrow. There are very many erythrocytes in the blood, and these cells contain the protein haemoglobin onto which bind oxygen molecules. The vast majority of oxygen, therefore, is transported around the body in the **haemo**globin of red blood cells. Leucocytes are much fewer in number, but they are the largest blood cells. These cells are concerned with the immune responses of the body. There are three basic types of white blood cell: granulocytes; monocytes; and lymphocytes. They provide a defence against invading micro-organisms, and are phagocytic (engulfing and absorbing) at sites of injury, **inflammation** and infection.

Thrombocytes, also produced in the bone marrow, provide the blood with a mechanism for coagulation (clotting) when injury has occurred. When a blood vessel is damaged, a series of processes occur to minimize blood loss and to promote healing. This involves a reflex **vaso**constriction (narrowing of blood vessels in the affected region), platelet release and plug formation (where 'sticky' platelets adhere to damaged surfaces), coagulation (a fibrous protein mesh forms a clot), and fibrinolysis (the breakdown of the clot) and the beginning of the healing.

The term 'blood shunting' is a reference to the fact that blood flow is directed to different parts of the body according to demand. For example, during exercise, blood flow is increased to the working skeletal muscles, and following a meal, an increase in blood flow is directed towards the digestive organs.

Blood pressure is the pressure that the circulating blood exerts upon the walls of the arteries. It is higher in the main arteries, and is normally described in two phases. Systolic pressure is when the heart is contracting, forcing more blood out into the general circulation. Diastolic pressure is the relaxation phase, following the contraction. Blood pressure is externally (manually or digitally) measured in millimetres of mercury (mmHg). A normal resting blood pressure is around 120/80 mmHg (values of up to 140/85 mmHg are considered high). Blood pressure is important and dynamic, and is affected by a variety of factors, such as changes in the blood demands of the various tissues of the body, the responsibility of the circulatory, nervous and endocrine systems to meet these demands, and the underlying state of health of the blood vessels. Internal feedback systems assist in the regulation of blood pressure, and these adjust such mechanisms as heart rate, stroke volume and blood vessel diameter (vasoconstriction and vasodilation). The medulla oblongata's cardiovascular centre is greatly involved in these processes, and it receives input from various sources such as the baroreceptors of the aortic arch and the carotid bodies (which are pressure sensitive). The endocrine system has an important role in adjusting cardiac output, vascular resistance and total blood volume.

Capillaries are the smallest blood vessels. They are microscopic, consisting of only a single layer of semi-permeable cells, and branch thoroughly through whichever tissue they are serving. Capillaries are fed by metarterioles, and pre-capillary sphincters help to regulate the blood flow through a tissue – when the particular tissue is active, capillaries open for maximal flow, and when at relative rest, many capillaries are closed. The fluid outside the vessels and cells is called **tissue fluid**. It contains phagocytic cells and wastes, but no red blood cells, and is eventually

TIP ✔

The **circulating blood** carries: oxygen from the lungs to the tissues; carbon dioxide from the tissues to the lungs; digested food from the digestive tract to the cells; waste products to the kidneys for excretion; hormones from endocrine glands to target tissues and glands; heat from warmer active regions to colder less active regions. Blood also provides protection for the body against disease and infection.

deoxygenated. Oxygen and nutrients move from the blood and tissue fluid into the cells by way of **diffusion**. Carbon dioxide and other waste products diffuse in the opposite direction, and as the tissue fluid returns to the blood, around 90 per cent of it moves into venules. Any remaining fluid is drawn into the lymphatic capillaries, and enters the lymphatic circulation.

KEY A&P FACTS: *LYMPHATIC SYSTEM*

A secondary circulatory system and part of the immune system.

Comprises: lymphocytes; macrophages; lymph; lymphatic capillaries and vessels; lymph nodes; thoracic duct; right lymphatic duct; spleen; thymus gland; tonsils; adenoids; lacteals; Peyer's patches.

Lymphocytes (lymphatic B and T cells) and macrophages are phagocytes and antigen presenting.

Lymph is a straw-coloured fluid similar to blood plasma.

Lymph transports, towards the venous blood circulation: interstitial fluid; plasma proteins; metabolic waste products; bacteria; viruses; dietary lipids.

Lymphatic capillaries and vessels convey lymphatic fluid from the tissues towards lymph nodes, the lymphatic ducts and eventually the venous blood circulation.

Lymph nodes are oval structures located at specific areas where lymphatic vessels run to (also found in the digestive, respiratory, urinary and reproductive tracts).

Lymph nodes are responsible for filtration of lymph and proliferation of plasma and specialized lymphocytes, the T cells.

The two lymphatic ducts are the thoracic duct and the right lymphatic duct.

The thoracic duct is the main collecting duct. All lymphatic vessels from the left side of the head and neck, left upper limb and the whole of the lower body drain into it.

The right lymphatic duct drains lymph from the upper right side of the body.

The spleen is the largest mass of lymphoid tissue. It is a site of B-lymphocyte proliferation into plasma cells and the phagocytosis of bacteria and worn-out or abnormal erythrocytes, the red blood cells.

The thymus gland is behind the sternum and is a site of T-cell storage and maturation – having first been developed in the red bone marrow. The T lymphocytes are released into the bloodstream when required. The thymus is relatively large at birth and reaches its largest size at puberty, after which it reduces in both size and activity.

The tonsils (in the throat) and adenoids (in the nasopharynx) help protect against foreign substances that are inhaled or ingested.

Lacteals are in the walls of the small intestine; these absorb lipids.

Peyer's patches are in the small intestine and have immune functions.

Lymph travels only in one direction – from the tissues towards the heart.

Returning lymphatic fluid, like venous blood, relies upon the presence of valves within the vessels to prevent back-flow, respiratory movements and the contraction of adjacent skeletal muscles to pump the fluid onwards.

The two lymphatic ducts eventually drain into the returning venous blood circulation at the left and right subclavian veins (below the clavicles).

The major functions of the lymphatic system are to: drain away excess (interstitial) fluids; destroy bacteria and other foreign substances; help prevent and fight infection; transport dietary lipids.

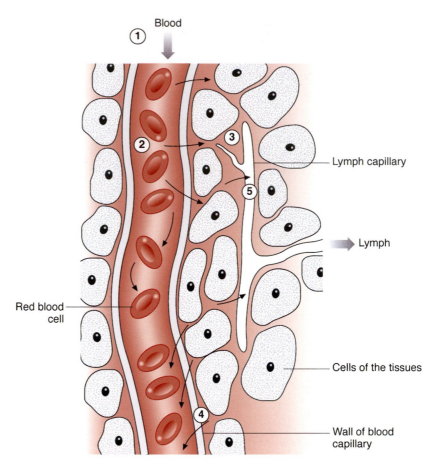

Blood

① Lymph capillary

Lymph

Red blood cell

Cells of the tissues

Wall of blood capillary

Exchange of blood, tissue fluid and lymph

TIP ✔

Lymph nodes filter lymph, and are the site of activated lymphocytes (immune responses). The main aggregations of lymph nodes are: the submandibular, cervical, axillary, supratrochlear, intestinal, iliac, inguinal and popliteal nodes.

Lymph (fluid) is formed from tissue fluid in the capillary beds. It enters, firstly, lymphatic capillaries, which gather to form lymphatic vessels. Lymphatic vessels travel towards the lymphatic ducts via the nearest lymph nodes. Lymphatic vessels have similarities to veins, in that they rely upon the presence of valves, skeletal muscle contraction, negative pressures and gravity to move their contents onwards. The term lymphatic drainage refers to the drainage of excess tissue fluid and particulate matter into the lymphatic vessels and onwards. It is encouraged by such activities as exercise, massage and electrotherapy.

The pathway of lymph is summarized as follows:

- Any excess tissue fluid and waste, not taken up into venules, is drained into lymphatic capillaries.
- Tissue fluid in the lymph capillaries becomes lymph.
- Lymph capillaries drain into lymphatic vessels.
- Larger lymphatic vessels travel towards lymph nodes.
- Lymph filters through the lymph nodes.
- From the nodes, lymphatic vessels take the lymph to either the thoracic or right lymphatic duct.
- The collected lymph then drains into either the left or right subclavian vein.

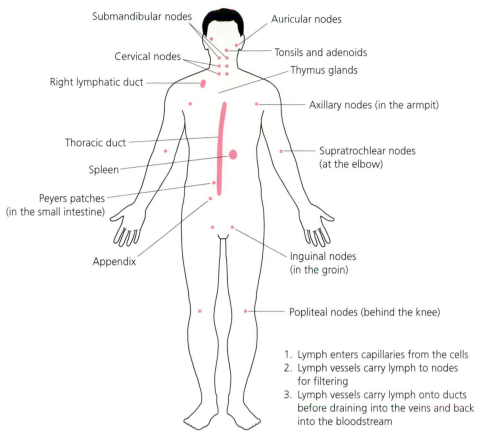

Submandibular nodes

Auricular nodes

Cervical nodes

Tonsils and adenoids

Thymus glands

Right lymphatic duct

Axillary nodes (in the armpit)

Thoracic duct

Spleen

Supratrochlear nodes
(at the elbow)

Peyers patches
(in the small intestine)

Appendix

Inguinal nodes
(in the groin)

Popliteal nodes (behind the knee)

1. Lymph enters capillaries from the cells
2. Lymph vessels carry lymph to nodes
   for filtering
3. Lymph vessels carry lymph onto ducts
   before draining into the veins and back
   into the bloodstream

Lymphatic circulatory system

RESPIRATORY SYSTEM ESSENTIALS

The respiratory system is linked very closely to the circulatory system, and
has three basic processes:

1 Pulmonary ventilation is the act of breathing in and out, i.e. inspiration
and expiration.

2 External respiration is the exchange of gases (oxygen and carbon dioxide)
within the lungs, and involves the capillary-rich alveoli. Gaseous exchange
occurs by way of diffusion across the alveolar–capillary membrane.

3 Internal respiration is the exchange of gases between the blood and
tissue cells.

During inspiration the thoracic volume increases. The major muscles of
inspiration are the diaphragm and external intercostals, which are assisted
by the scalene and sternocleidomastoid muscles of the anterior neck, and
the pectoralis minor of the anterior chest.

During normal quiet expiration the thoracic volume decreases so that air
is expelled; however this is more of a passive process, resulting from an
elastic recoil of both the thoracic cage and the lungs, rather than muscular
contraction. When breathing is more intense (laboured), such as during

KEY A&P FACTS: *RESPIRATORY SYSTEM*

The main organs of respiration and gaseous exchange are: nose and mouth; pharynx; larynx; trachea; lungs; bronchi; bronchioles; alveoli.

The pharynx is situated at the back of the mouth. It is a membranous and muscular channel for both food and inhaled and exhaled gases and contains the epiglottis, a flap of fibro-cartilage, which prevents food from travelling towards the lungs.

The larynx ('voice box') is made up of hyaline cartilage, ligaments and membranous tissue and contains the vocal cords.

The trachea ('windpipe') is composed of C-shaped rings of hyaline cartilage, connective and muscle tissue.

The bronchi are two tubes similar in structure and continuous from the trachea. They divide and enter each lung.

The bronchioles are smaller continuations of the bronchi within the lobes of each lung, but without the cartilage.

Bronchioles further divide into terminal bronchioles, respiratory bronchioles, alveolar ducts and, finally, alveoli.

The alveoli have a dense network of capillaries.

The exchange of gases during (external) respiration takes place, by way of diffusion, across two membranes – the alveolar and capillary membranes.

Breathing is the moving of air into and out of the lungs.

The actual rate of breathing depends upon the body's requirements and the intensity of activities being performed.

The pons varoli and medulla oblongata function as the brain's respiratory centre and breathing rate is affected by the concentrations of carbon dioxide in blood flowing through the brain and also by the messages relayed to the respiratory centre from the chemoreceptors of the aorta and carotid arteries.

The major muscles of respiration are the diaphragm (between the thoracic and abdominal cavities) and the intercostals (between the ribs).

The respiratory system is responsible for: inhalation; exhalation; external respiration (exchange of gases in the lungs); internal respiration (exchange of gases in the tissue cells); cellular respiration (use of oxygen within the cells – oxygen is used to release energy from glucose, which takes place in the mitochondria).

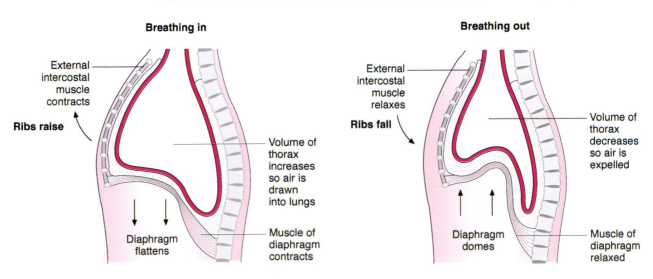

Process of inspiration and expiration

LUNG VOLUMES AND CAPACITIES

Tidal volume (TV) is the amount of air passing through the lungs during each cycle of quiet breathing, that is the volume inspired or expired per breath.

Minute ventilation (MV) is the amount of air breathed per minute.

Total lung capacity (TLC) is the volume in the lungs following maximal inspiration.

Residual lung volume (RLV) is the volume in the lungs following maximal expiration.

Inspiratory capacity (IC) is the amount of air that can be inspired with maximal effort.

Forced vital capacity (FVC) is the maximum volume expired following maximal inspiration.

Peak expiratory flow rate (PEFR) is the maximal amount (peak rate) of air expired in one forced expiration.

Forced expiratory volume in one second (FEV1) is the maximum volume expired in one second following maximal inspiration.

Forced expired ratio (FER) is the ratio of air that can be forcibly expired in one second (FEV1) to the maximal expired volume (FVC).

exercise or in the presence of respiratory problems, the muscles of (forced) expiration become involved. These are the abdominal (internal and external obliques, and rectus and transversus abdominus) and internal intercostal muscles.

The diaphragm itself is a dome-shaped muscle situated between the thorax and abdomen. It is pierced by several structures passing through it: the aorta, thoracic duct and azygos vein pass through the aortic hiatus; the oesophagus and vagus nerves pass through the oesophageal hiatus; the inferior vena cava passes through the vena caval foramen. The diaphragm has its origins at the xiphoid process, the costal cartilages of the lower six ribs, and the lumbar vertebrae. It has a centralized tendon for its insertion, which, as it contracts during inspiration, pulls downwards, flattens the dome, and increases the volume of the thorax.

The volumes and capacities of the lungs are commonly measured for the assessment and monitoring of lung function, either in the presence of respiratory **dys**function (e.g. asthma, bronchitis or emphysema) or during fitness tests. Lung volume measurements are affected by age, sex, body size and composition, lifestyle, fitness and **pathology**. Common basic tests of respiratory function include the peak-flow and micro-spirometry tests, whereby the subject breathes forcefully into a measuring device.

The respiratory tract is also responsible for the production of vocal sounds, in the larynx, and is greatly involved in a selection of other actions, including: laughing; crying; yawning (deep inspiration, related to tiredness); sneezing (spasmodic expiration, usually due to nasal irritation); coughing (strong reflex expiration often in response to a foreign body); hiccuping (intermittent diaphragmatic spasm followed by sudden closing of the glottis, often in response to digestive irritation); valsalva response (forced expiration against a closed glottis, e.g. straining to lift something, or straining at the toilet).

ENDOCRINE SYSTEM ESSENTIALS

Hormones are the body's chemical messengers released directly into the bloodstream by ductless **endocrine glands**. The endocrine system is closely linked with the nervous system in providing a physiological control and communication system. Whereas the nervous system functions by initiating direct nerve impulses, the endocrine system releases its hormones indirectly into the blood, which results in a slower response time. However, typically the response is longer-lived, and consequently, the endocrine system tends to be involved in such long-term processes as growth, development and reproduction. As much of the nervous system is concerned with responding to external stimuli, the endocrine system is more involved in the regulation of the body's internal environment, and with metabolic processes.

Three basic mechanisms stimulate or inhibit hormonal release: nervous impulses; chemical changes in the blood; other hormones. When stimulated, endocrine glands tend to release their hormones in short bursts. Increased stimulation results in frequent bursts, and reduced stimulation results in either inhibition or minimal release. Most hormonal secretions are subject to homeostatic negative feedback systems.

Feedback systems

A feedback system (or loop) is where physiological activity is internally monitored by three basic components:

1 A control centre, which reacts to information it receives (such as the medulla oblongata of the brainstem, which is the main control centre for heart and breathing rates).

2 Receptors, **specialized tissues** – the two main types being mechanoreceptors and chemoreceptors – which are able to detect changes in, for example, blood pressure or body temperature.

3 Effector tissue, which actually receives the output information from the control centre, and produces the required response (effect), for example, slowing of heart rate, increased sudoriferous (sweat) gland activity (to reduce body temperature), or vasodilation (to reduce blood pressure).

A negative feedback is where the response of the effector tissue reverses the original stimuli. A positive feedback is where the stimuli are maintained or intensified.

Hormones are formed from the nutrients of digestion. They are mainly protein-based, though some are fat-based (such as steroid hormones). Hormonal imbalance is where there is a situation of **hypo-** or **hyper-**secretion, which, if continued, results in physiological dysfunction and ill-health.

The pituitary gland (sometimes referred to as the hypophysis) is the size and shape of a pea. Located in the brain, it is normally known as the master endocrine gland, releasing a selection of hormones from its anterior and posterior lobes that either generally encourage metabolism and growth (such as growth hormone), or hormones that influence other endocrine glands to release their particular hormones. These are known as tropic

KEY A&P FACTS: *ENDOCRINE SYSTEM*

Also known as: the hormonal system.

Endocrine means secretion within. The endocrine system consists of specialized glands that secrete hormones directly into the bloodstream.

Hormones are chemical messengers, which assist in the regulation of the internal environment, metabolic processes and the energy balance of the body.

Hormones help regulate muscular contractions, glandular secretions and immune responses.

The endocrine system is greatly involved in the processes of growth, development and reproduction.

Hormonal release is controlled by the nervous system and by the detection of chemical changes in the blood.

Hormones, following their release, circulate within the bloodstream until they reach their target organ, tissue or gland.

Once they have performed their task, they travel to the liver where they are further metabolized and eventually excreted from the body.

The hypothalamus, in the brain – which has both nervous and endocrine functions – is the main integrating link between the nervous and endocrine systems.

The master endocrine gland is the pituitary gland, located within the brain.

The pituitary gland has anterior and posterior departments.

The hormones secreted by the anterior pituitary, which are regulated by releasing and inhibiting hormones produced by the hypothalamus, are: human growth hormone (stimulates body growth processes); prolactin (helps initiate milk production in the female); adrenocorticotrophic hormone (regulates hormonal release from cortex of adrenal gland); thyroid stimulating hormone (regulates thyroid gland); follicle stimulating hormone (helps regulate ovaries and testicles); luteinizing hormone (also helps regulate ovaries and testes).

The posterior pituitary gland secretes two hormones: oxytocin (stimulates uterine contraction during labour and milk ejection during breast-feeding) and anti-diuretic hormone (also known as vasopressin, which stimulates water reabsorption by the kidneys and arterial constriction).

Secretion of oxytocin is regulated by distension of the uterus and the suckling of the infant.

Anti-diuretic hormone release is regulated by the osmotic pressure and volume of the blood.

The other major endocrine glands, each with their own specific hormones, are: thyroid gland; parathyroid glands; adrenal glands; pancreas; ovaries; testes; pineal gland.

The thyroid gland is located in the throat area. It regulates metabolism, growth and development.

The parathyroid glands are found on the posterior surface of the thyroid gland. They regulate blood calcium and phosphate levels.

The adrenal (or suprarenal) glands – cortex and medulla – lie superiorly on top of the kidneys. They have a variety of actions including: regulation of sodium and water reabsorption; promotion of metabolism; anti-inflammatory response; stress ('fight or flight') response.

The pancreas lies posterior to the stomach. It primarily secretes glucagon, which increases blood glucose levels, and insulin, which decreases blood glucose levels.

The ovaries are situated in the female pelvic cavity. They regulate development and maintenance of feminine characteristics, reproductive cycles, pregnancy and lactation.

The testes are contained within the male scrotum. They help to regulate development and maintenance of masculine characteristics, and have integral reproductive functions.

The pineal gland is located within the brain. It secretes melatonin, which is involved in the regulation of circadian rhythms – the 24 hour day/night cycle.

There is also endocrine tissue to be found in the digestive tract, the placenta, kidneys and heart.

hormones (e.g. thyroid stimulating hormone, TSH, which stimulates the thyroid gland to release its hormones). The pituitary is regulated, to a large degree, by the hypothalamus, which releases its own tropic hormones that act upon both lobes of the gland, and by a variety of feedback mechanisms.

Autonomic regulation

An important concept to consider, when developing understanding of both the neural and hormonal autonomic regulatory mechanisms, is that the physiology of the body appears to function with an intelligence of its own. Because the neural and chemical messages are flowing through the body rapidly, the physiology knows: where things are (or is able to find specific tissues and locations); what should be done with them (or how to affect tissues or process substances); how to communicate appropriate information to the tissues concerned. The systems of the body normally work efficiently to maintain **homeostasis**, if the internal and external environments are conducive.

DIGESTIVE AND URINARY SYSTEM ESSENTIALS

Fluids and foods are taken into the body, are broken down, used in some way, and waste products are eliminated. All foods enter the body at the mouth. The sight and aroma of food stimulate digestive activity. Salivary glands increase the release of saliva into the oral cavity. Saliva, which is mostly water containing microscopic solutes, cleanses, lubricates and protects the mouth. The action of salivary amylase (ptyalin) starts off the digestion of carbohydrates, and lingual lipase begins the breakdown of fats. Skeletal mastication (chewing) muscles control the movements of the temporo-mandibular joint (TMJ or jaw), lips, cheeks and tongue. Teeth, which are composed mainly from hard, strong, bone-like connective tissues

---

KEY A&P FACTS: *DIGESTIVE SYSTEM*

Composed of: mouth; salivary glands; pharynx; oesophagus; stomach; small and large intestines; rectum and anus; liver; gall bladder; pancreas; peritoneum.

Various mechanical and chemical processes perform the five basic functions: ingestion (taking in food); digestion (mechanical and chemical breakdown of food); absorption (passage of food from the digestive organs into the blood); assimilation (breakdown of food on a cellular level); excretion (elimination of undigested and waste substances).

Like any other system, the digestive system requires an adequate blood supply to its functioning organs.

Digestive activity is generally stimulated by parasympathetic nerves and inhibited by sympathetic nerves.

Food components essential to health are proteins, carbohydrates, fats, vitamins, minerals, fibre and water.

(dentin, enamel and cementum), are housed in sockets embedded in the gingivae (gums). They have fine blood and lymph vessels and nerves running through their inner pulp cavity.

The main muscles of mastication, acting on the gross movements of the TMJ, are the large, strong and more superficial masseter and temporalis. The obicularis oris is the circular muscle that closes and compresses the lips. The buccinator is deeper at the side of the mouth, it contracts the cheeks, and enables the act of sucking. The medial and lateral pterygoid muscles, deep at the jaw, help to refine the chewing movements. The TMJ and the floor of the mouth are operated upon by a selection of deep suprahyoid muscles including the digastric and mylohyoid. The tongue, in addition to a selection of sensory receptors (the taste buds), has extrinsic and intrinsic muscles that control its movements.

In the mouth, food is chewed and mixed with saliva. A soft mass is produced so as to enable easy deglutition (swallowing). The soft bolus that is formed is moved into the oropharynx (back of the mouth) by the tongue. As the bolus hits the oropharynx, a series of reflexive nerve impulses (via receptors in the oropharynx, afferents to the brainstem, and efferents to the smooth muscles of the pharynx and larynx) facilitate the action of swallowing food into the oesophagus. The normally open respiratory tract must close (the epiglottis moves backwards) as food passes by, and the upper oesophageal sphincter relaxes.

The bolus is pushed through the oesophagus by way of peristalsis: a wave of smooth muscle contraction behind the bolus (and relaxation in front of it). Food enters the stomach through the lower oesophageal sphincter, which normally remains contracted to prevent gastric juice from entering the oesophagus.

The stomach is the food reservoir. Food here is mixed, by peristaltic waves, with the strongly acidic gastric juice, released from the stomach wall's gastric glands, to become chyme. Chyme is more fluid-like and deactivates the salivary digestive juices. The hydrochloric acid in gastric juice provides protection against microbes in the food. It also initiates protein breakdown and, once inside the small intestine, stimulates production of hormones which increase the release of the (digestive) enzyme-rich pancreatic juice. Movements and activities within the stomach are regulated (stimulated or inhibited) by neural and hormonal responses to the mechanical stretching of the walls of the stomach and intestine, and also, certain food particles stimulate or inhibit digestive processes. The less permeable stomach walls only absorb certain substances (some water, ions or charged particles, some medications and alcohol). Most absorption takes place in the small intestine.

The small intestine is a tube, 2–3 cm in diameter, and about 3 m long. It has three segments: the duodenum; the jejunum; and the ileum. Chyme is further churned and mixed with digestive juices in the small intestine. Intestinal juice is alkaline, which buffers against acidic gastric juice. Stored bile, from the gall bladder, and pancreatic juice both enter the duodenum, via converging ducts, at the ampulla of Vater, which is guarded by the sphincter of Oddie. Bile is a liquid, formed in the liver but stored and concentrated in the gall bladder. Although bile is partly a waste product, it is important for the emulsification and absorption of fats. Pancreatic juice contains a great deal of digestive enzymes. The digestive capability of the small intestine is greatly enhanced by having circular plicae (folds) in its walls, and villi (tiny hair-like projections) on its inner mucosal layer, both of which increase the surface area for absorption. Each villus (singular) contains an arteriole, venule and a lymphatic lacteal. Nutrients absorb through the villi to enter the bloodstream or lymphatic circulation. The digestion of carbohydrates, proteins and fats is virtually completed in the small intestine.

The large intestine, located superficially underneath abdominal muscle, is divided into the ascending, transverse and descending colons. It completes any remaining digestion (water, electrolytes and vitamins), manufactures certain B vitamins and vitamin K, and solidifies and eliminates faeces. Peristalsis continues into the large intestine forming the faecal material, which makes its way to the rectum and anus. Defecation occurs through a combination of reflex smooth muscle contraction in the rectum, and voluntary relaxation of the external anal sphincter.

The liver, situated in the upper right side of the abdomen, under the diaphragm, is the main accessory digestive organ, and is also the largest and heaviest internal organ of the body. It receives deoxygenated, but nutrient-rich venous blood, via the hepatic portal vein, which is fed by tributary veins running from the digestive tract (stomach, small intestine, large intestine, and also the pancreas).

The liver performs a selection of crucial roles:

- Filtration of the venous blood it receives from the digestive system (removing damaged and worn-out blood cells and bacteria; detoxifying some drugs, alcohol and certain hormones).
- Metabolism of carbohydrates, fats and proteins.
- Deamination (further catabolic breakdown) of amino acids (constituents of proteins) into the waste products urea and uric acid, for elimination in the urine.
- Storage of glycogen, vitamins (A, B12, D, E and K) and minerals (in particular, iron and copper), for later use in the body.
- Production of bile.
- Activation of calcitriol (vitamin D) by enzymes in the liver and kidney.

The gall bladder is a small pouch, behind the lower liver. It receives bile from the liver by way of the hepatic ducts. When stimulated, the gall bladder contracts to send concentrated bile down the common bile duct, and into the duodenum via the ampulla of Vater.

Metabolism is basically the ongoing process of chemical and physical changes taking place within the body to allow normal utilization of oxygen and nutrients for growth, repair, expenditure of energy and general functioning. Clearly, with metabolism, there is a great deal of autonomic and hormonal regulation at work. **Catabolism** is the breaking-down aspect of metabolism, where complex compounds are reduced to smaller simpler ones. This process generally produces energy (and heat for maintenance of body temperature). **Anabolism** is the building up of compounds into more complex products (for growth, repair, etc.), which generally requires energy. **Basal or resting metabolic rate** (BMR) is the rate at which the body, while at rest, breaks down nutrients to generate energy to perform its basic functions. Energy is used to produce ATP and heat. Normal core body temperature is near to 37 °C. Many mechanisms regulate body temperature, and the main thermostat of the body is the hypothalamus, which acts upon information it receives from the body's thermoreceptors. Heat production and conservation are affected by metabolic rate, which itself is greatly influenced by thyroid hormones, levels of physical activity, the ANS, food intake, age (higher in children) and sex (usually lower in females).

Directly related to the study of digestion are the concepts of hunger or appetite, and satiation (fullness or satisfaction). A selection of processes operate to assist the body in its regulation of food intake. Key factors include: nutrient levels in the blood; the hypothalamus, which has both a hunger centre and a satiety centre; mechanical signals from the digestive tract (sensory reception of stretching of the walls of organs); specific circulating hormones; photoreceptors (vision), olfactory receptors (smell) and taste receptors; psychological factors. Body weight, fat and composition, nutritional deficiency, food intolerance, eating disorders, supplementation and dietary approaches, too, are key areas to scrutinize.

The kidneys are located just above waist level on either side of the posterior torso, and are unprotected by the thoracic cage. They play a role in a variety of metabolic processes, but their main function is to regulate blood volume, composition and pressure. They are directly involved in the elimination of urine (around 2 litres per day), which is normally yellow in colour, and is about 95 per cent water with 5 per cent solutes (mainly waste products or undigested compounds, including: urea, uric acid, creatinine, hormones, enzymes and minerals).

KEY A&P FACTS: *URINARY SYSTEM*

Also known as: the renal system or (part of) the excretory system.

Consists of: two kidneys; two ureters; one urinary bladder; one urethra.

Functions of the kidneys include: purification of the blood – removal of waste substances such as urea, uric acid and other toxic substances; regulation of blood volume and concentration; assisting the regulation of blood pressure; synthesis of glucose; secretion of erythropoietin, which stimulates red blood cell (erythrocyte) production; regulation of blood pH (acid/alkaline) levels.

A proportion of blood is pumped into each kidney from the renal arteries with each heartbeat.

The functional activities of the kidneys are performed by the nephrons.

The ureters transport urine from the kidney to the bladder, mainly by peristalsis.

The bladder stores urine prior to micturation (urination).

The urethra extends from the bladder to the exterior.

In both sexes, the urethra discharges urine from the body. In males it also discharges semen.

The volume of urine is influenced by a variety of factors: blood osmotic pressure and concentration; blood pressure; medications, emotions.

The amount of water and salts that are reabsorbed or released as urine depends upon how much is needed by the blood to restore it to a normal concentration. It is regulated by various homeostatic mechanisms, predominantly involving the ANS, hypothalamus and the pituitary gland.

Anti-diuretic hormone (ADH) is released from the pituitary gland if blood is too concentrated.

Obviously, adequate ingestion of water is important to health and increased amounts are necessary if physical activity levels increase.

INTEGUMENTARY SYSTEM ESSENTIALS

Not forgetting the lungs, which expel carbon dioxide and a little water and heat, the intestines or the kidneys, the skin is the body's other main excretory organ. Perspiration, via the sudoriferous glands, assists in the removal of heat and water from the body, by way of evaporation. It also excretes small amounts of ions, urea, uric acid, amino acids, ammonia, glucose, lactic acid and vitamin C. As well as having sweating as a method for cooling the body, the skin's blood vessels constrict or dilate depending upon whether heat conservation or reduction is required. The arrector pili muscles, which are attached to hair follicles, cause goose bumps when they contract, which also helps to retain and generate a little heat.

The skin has a number of functions, which can be remembered by the mnemonic 'SHAPES':

- **Sensation**: the skin is a major sensory organ, reporting sensations of temperature, touch, pressure and pain.
- **Heat regulation**: the skin has a major role in regulating the body's temperature. Sweat evaporation and vasodilation assists in cooling the body. Vasoconstriction assists in retaining heat. Arrector pili muscle contractions help in a small way to generate and conserve heat.
- **Absorption**: the skin is able to absorb certain substances such as massage oils containing essential oils, medications such as in hormone replacement therapy, nicotine and topical analgesics.
- **Protection**: the skin protects the body against mechanical injury, invading bacteria and dehydration. The pigment melanin provides some protection against the sun's rays.
- **Excretion**: sweat helps to eliminate some waste products.
- **Secretion**: sebaceous glands secrete oily sebum, which lubricates and nourishes the skin and hair shafts.

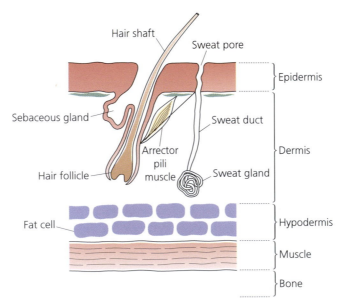

Structure of skin

KEY A&P FACTS: *INTEGUMENTARY SYSTEM*

The integumentary or 'covering' system comprises the skin, hair, nails and the various glands and nerve endings found in close association.

The skin is one of the largest organs in the body in terms of surface area and weight.

Skin consists of three basic layers: the epidermis (which can be seen and touched); the dermis; and the hypodermis (a subcutaneous layer lying under the dermis and above the skeletal muscles).

Hair, nails and skin glands are epidermal derivatives – developed from the embryonic epidermis.

The epidermis, itself a stratified epithelial tissue with no blood vessels, has four or five separate cellular layers (five where skin exposure to friction and pressure is greater, (e.g. palms and soles). The deepest of these layers is the basal layer, which is continuously in a process of regeneration and produces all other layers. The top, superficial (horny) layer is eventually shed (desquamed) and replaced.

Within the epidermis are four principal cell types: keratinocytes, which produce keratin (a protein that helps to protect and waterproof skin); melanocytes which produce melanin (a pigment contributing to skin colour, which also absorbs UV light and helps to protect the skin from the damage of sunlight); Langerhans cells are formed in the bone marrow, have immune responses and are prone to UV damage; Merkel cells are located deep in the epidermis of hairless skin and have connections to sensory nerve cells (thereby contributing to the touch sensation).

The dermis, lying under the epidermis, is predominantly connective tissue (areolar, adipose, elastic fibres and collagen).

Collagen and elastic fibres combine to offer the skin strength, extensibility and elasticity.

Hair and nails protect the body. They are made up from compressed, keratinized epidermal cells.

Commonly attached to the hair follicle, sebaceous glands secrete the skin's natural lubricant, sebum – an oily mix of fats, cholesterol, protein and salts.

Sebum helps to maintain skin suppleness and prevent hair from becoming brittle. It is mildly antiseptic, but also a source of nourishment to bacterial pimples or boils.

Tiny, involuntary arrector pili muscles are also attached to the hair follicles. These respond autonomically to cold temperatures or to short-term emotional changes. When they contract, they cause 'goose bumps' and hairs to extend.

There are over 3 million sudoriferous (sweat or perspiration) glands distributed throughout most areas of skin (except for the lips, nail beds and eardrums).

Sweat is composed mainly of water and certain waste products. It helps to regulate body temperature by way of evaporation.

The female, milk-secreting, mammary glands are specialized sudoriferous glands.

The skin is a huge sensory organ and has a variety of nerve cells, mainly in the dermis. Mechanoreceptors, free nerve endings, thermoreceptors and nociceptors convey sensory information pertaining to touch, pressure, temperature or pain.

The subcutaneous hypodermis is predominantly areolar (generalized and structural cells) and adipose (fat cells). This layer insulates the body, stores energy supplies and forms a protective structure through which blood vessels and nerves travel.

KEY DIFFERENCES BETWEEN MEN AND WOMEN

There are a selection of clear and usual, functionally relevant differences between the sexes. For the sports therapist, providing exercise recommendations or treating injuries, it is very important to recognize the main physical and physiological differences between men and women. Understanding these basic differences helps to clarify the achievable objectives. The task of recognizing, for example, the underlying causes of an **overuse injury** can become a little more straightforward, when the anatomy of the presenting individual is better understood.

- **Genetics**: the genes a child inherits are responsible for the sex of the individual (male or female) and their rate of growth and development.

- **Formative developments**: the early experiences, influences, education, conditioning and activities that a child (male or female) is exposed to have a direct effect upon their behaviour and practical abilities in later life. It used to be that males were exposed to many different experiences to females in early years, but more recently there has been more similarity (reflecting the changes occurring in society as a whole).

- **Anatomical differences**: men tend to be taller and heavier, and women tend to be shorter and lighter. Male bones tend to be heavier and thicker, female bones tend to be lighter and thinner. The surfaces of male joints tend to be relatively larger than those of females. Male muscle attachment sites tend to be more distinct than those of females. Male shoulders tend to be broader than those of females. Women have a smaller thorax than men, and have breasts. Male hips tend to be narrower. The male pelvis is deeper and has a smaller, heart-shaped, pelvic brim. The female pelvis is

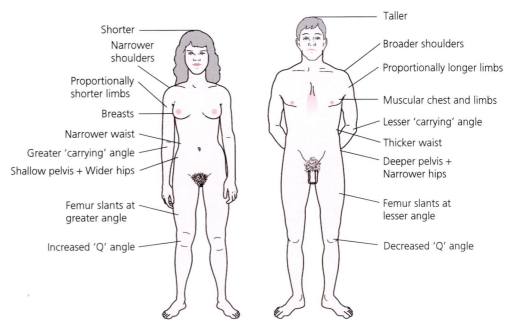

Differences between men and women

shallower and has a larger, oval-shaped pelvic brim. Male legs tend to be proportionately longer, with the neck of the femur at a lesser angle to its shaft. There is a lesser slant of the thigh to the knee on the male. Women are more likely to demonstrate genu valgus (knock-knee) posture, which means they are anatomically disadvantaged in running activities, and prone to a variety of overuse injuries. Similarly, the male arms tend to be proportionately longer, and have a lesser carrying angle (the angle of the forearm in relation to the upper arm). The increased carrying angle of the female is to accommodate the wider hips, and is, again, an anatomical disadvantage in lifting and throwing activities.

- **Body composition**: men tend to have a greater percentage of muscle tissue; women a greater percentage of body fat. Men tend to be more mesomorphic, and women more endomorphic. The average percentage of male body fat is around 13 per cent. The female average body fat percentage is around 25 per cent. Women tend to demonstrate a lower lean body mass (fat-free mass), which indicates the reduced muscle mass. Men tend to accumulate excess body fat around their waist and on the upper body, while women deposit more fat on the hips and thighs. Men tend to carry a greater percentage of blood in body fluid, and a greater percentage of water.

- **Cardio-vascular differences**: men tend to have a larger heart, with a greater stroke volume and lower resting heart rate. In blood, women tend to carry fewer erythrocytes (red blood cells) and also reduced levels of haemoglobin within the blood cells. Male blood pressure tends to be higher.

- **Respiratory differences**: male lungs tend to be around 10 per cent larger. They tend to have an increased respiratory rate and a greater vital capacity.

- **Performance differences**: men tend to be stronger, faster and more powerful than women, but women tend to be more flexible. Men also tend to have a greater aerobic capacity (by being able carry more oxygen to the tissues). Additionally, men tend to have a greater V_{O_2}**max**, which is an indication of the body's ability to take in, distribute and utilize oxygen. Women do have other aspects of their physiology to contend with in relation to physical activity (the menstrual cycle presents a selection of complications in relation to performance training, as does pregnancy, and in later life, the menopause).

ENERGY SYSTEMS

The muscles of the body require fuel to perform their work. The type of work that they perform dictates how the fuel is supplied to them. In simple terms, work is either of short and relatively intense duration (anaerobic activity) or prolonged, less intense duration (aerobic activity). The fuel that is supplied for activity arrives by either an anaerobic pathway or the aerobic pathway. Within the mitochondrion (the power-house of a cell), ATP, the fundamental fuel for energy, is generated. This continual process is called cellular (internal) respiration. Being involved in most energy exchanges

TABLE 2.1 The three energy systems

Characteristic	Anaerobic creatine phosphate system	Anaerobic lactate system	Aerobic system
Intensity of effort	Very high, up to 100% of maximal effort	High, between 60 and 90% of maximal effort	Low, up to around 70% of maximal effort
Duration	Immediate, lasts around 10 seconds	If working at higher intensity, around 30 s. At lower intensity, around 3 min	At low intensity, can provide energy for hours
Fuel and limitations	Creatine-phosphate, limited to few seconds	Carbohydrates (glycogen), limited to 3 min	Carbohydrates, fat, protein; much less limited
Waste products	No major waste product	Lactate (lactic acid)	Carbon dioxide, water
Recovery time	Very quick recovery (around 50% in 30 s; 100% in 2 min)	Several minutes to 2 h to remove and resynthesize lactic acid	Depends upon individual's ability to take in and use oxygen
Typical activities	Short bursts of explosive activity e.g. short sprint; series of heavy lifts; sudden reactions	Short bursts of intense activity, e.g. longer sprint; long series of strenuous repetitions; intense rally in tennis	Less intense, long-duration activity, e.g. walking; jogging; long-distance running; cycling; swimming; rowing

TIP

The body needs fuel to power its system:

- Fuel is needed to produce energy.
- Energy is needed to initiate, maintain and regulate movement.
- Movement is the generation and conduction of nerve impulses, the blood pumping through the arteries, the ventricles of the heart contracting strongly, the thought processes, the muscular reactions smooth and skeletal.

(muscular contractions; cellular division and diffusion; anabolic syntheses), ATP is found in all living cells, and often referred to as the body's energy currency. The basic food components of carbohydrate, fat and, to a lesser extent, protein are broken down through a series of complex metabolic processes to yield the ATP compound. ATP comprises one base molecule of adenosine (a nitrogenous sugar compound) and three phosphate groups. During the release of energy, the third phosphate group breaks away from the other components, leaving ADP (adenosine diphosphate). Stores of ATP within the muscle cells are limited and, therefore, ATP is continually being formed, conserved and resynthesized. The method by which the body generates its muscular energy depends upon the intensity and duration of activity being performed. There are three energy-providing systems – one is aerobic (in the presence of oxygen) and two are anaerobic (in the absence of oxygen). The three systems normally operate concurrently so as to offer the body great functional capacity (strength, power and endurance). They each can be described in terms of how and why they occur and how they affect the performance of activity (Table 2.1 above and Table 2.2).

The aerobic system

This system is at work, supplying the fuel for energy when the body is at rest or during relatively easy activities, or when endurance training (walking, jogging, distance running, cycling, etc.) is undertaken. During these less intensive activities, the body can normally maintain a steady supply of oxygen to the working muscles, so the aerobic pathway is a very efficient method for energy production. The main fuel for the aerobic

TABLE 2.2 Different activities and their energy sources

Activity	Duration	Energy source
One powerful movement	1–2 seconds	CP system
A short sprint	10–12 seconds	CP system (depending upon stores)
A sustained sprint	10–60 seconds	CP and lactate systems
1500 m competitive run	4–6 minutes	Probably all three systems
Marathon	2–3 hours plus	Predominantly aerobic system. Possible lactate involvement (sprint finish)
Team game (e.g. football; basketball); circuit training; exercise classes	1 hour plus	All three systems

production of ATP is provided by glycogen (the principal form of the body's stored carbohydrates) and fatty acids, both of which are normally in sufficient (or abundant) supply. The body's carbohydrates are stored, as glycogen, in the muscles and the liver. Fats are stored, as adipose tissue, subcutaneously, within and around internal organs, within muscles and inside the bone marrow. These fuels undergo the process of oxidation (combining with oxygen) inside the mitochondria, and this slowly and continually produces ATP. Typically, both carbohydrate and fat are utilized during most aerobic activities, but in different proportions. The oxidation of carbohydrate provides a faster source of energy compared to the oxidation of fat, and therefore, carbohydrates are the preferred source at higher intensities, and a greater proportion of fat is utilized during longer bouts of exercise. The predominant waste products of this system are carbon dioxide and water. These have little in the way of adverse effects upon the muscular activity (unlike the lactic acid waste product of the anaerobic lactate system), and therefore the aerobic system has a great capacity for endurance. There have, however, been some studies to demonstrate the presence of small amounts of lactic acid resulting from the aerobic metabolic pathway, but lactate removal from the muscle and the bloodstream normally equals its production rate. Like the two other energy systems, the efficiency of this system can be developed progressively, in this case through structured aerobic conditioning exercise. However, the aerobic system is not always able to generate enough ATP during more intense activities, such as a short sprint or series of heavy lifts. This is when anaerobic pathways are utilized.

The first anaerobic system: the creatine phosphate (CP) or alactic system

There is a small store of the compound **creatine phosphate** within muscle tissue. When ATP is used to fuel the energy for muscular contraction, it is reduced to ADP (adenosine plus two phosphate groups). For short bursts of energy production to continue, a phosphate can be drawn from the store of creatine phosphate to resynthesize ATP. There is, however, only enough CP to maintain energy production for around 10 seconds. Additionally, it can take 30 seconds to replenish 50 per cent of the store of CP (and ATP), and up to two minutes for it all to be replenished. Therefore, this energy pathway is best suited for high-intensity, very short duration activities such as power-lifting or the 100 m sprint. Because its main role is to provide instant energy, the CP system can be developed by employing power-based training principles. Certainly, this system is involved in the onset of exercise and the start of a race. It can be called upon to power any sudden sprint during a game or perform any other explosive action. If the intensity of the activity continues for more than a few seconds, the supply of ATP must be provided via a different pathway.

The second anaerobic energy system: the lactate or anaerobic glycolysis system

Glycogen is stored glucose. It may be accessed as a fuel both aerobically and anaerobically. Anaerobically, when exercise is quite intense and lasts longer than a few seconds, glucose is broken down within the cytoplasm of the muscle cell and converts to pyruvate, by means of glycolysis, to produce ATP. The very process of the anaerobic metabolism of glucose actually uses up some ATP, but produces more. Some of the pyruvate of this system is converted into the infamous waste product lactic acid, which breaks further down into lactate and hydrogen. The lactate causes the muscle to become more acidic, which actually inhibits some of the important processes involved in muscle contraction. As intense exercise continues, there is a build-up of lactic acid in the muscles, and this is considered to be one of the prime causes of muscle fatigue and aching. This energy system can provide energy for up to three minutes, after which activity has to reduce in intensity, and move onto the aerobic pathway. It can take anything from a few minutes to two hours to fully metabolize the lactate and therefore recover from the utilization of this pathway. To train this system (which is most suited to longer sprints and other prolonged intense activities) requires short periods of strenuous activity followed by periods of relative rest.

Certainly, how the body provides its energy to make the muscles work depends upon a variety of factors:

- The intensity and duration of the activity.
- The nutritional status of the individual both before and during the activity.
- The physiological state of the individual.
- The fitness of the individual and their ability to cope with the demands of the activity.
- Whether the individual trains to develop their ability to optimize their performance.

KEY ENERGY SYSTEM TERMS

(Maximal) Oxygen uptake: the aerobic capacity or consumption of an individual.

V_{o_2}max: a measure of aerobic fitness. Aerobic fitness tests of an individual's ability to take in, transport and a utilize oxygen during exercise. The exercise equipment is usually a treadmill or stationary cycle (ergometer). The V_{o_2}max tests are either maximal (exercising to exhaustion in a physiology lab), or submaximal (exercise at lower intensities) and predicted. In submaximal tests, which are the most commonly performed, heart rates are analysed in relation to the intensity and duration of the exercise and the results are extrapolated across a selection of validated data to predict the individual's maximal performance capability (without actually having to perform maximally). Maximal tests are more suited to more elite standard athletes.

The oxygen deficit: the delay in the uptake, or the temporary shortage of oxygen, in the tissues at the start of exercise. As fitness and oxygen uptake improves, an individual's deficit reduces (improves).

The oxygen debt: the state of elevated oxygen uptake (above resting levels) during the recovery from exercise. Light, short-duration exercise normally produces a quick recovery. Following heavy exercise it can take several minutes to repay this debt. Also referred to as the recovery oxygen uptake or elevated post-exercise oxygen consumption. Improving fitness should result in improved recovery.

Muscular fatigue: the state where the ability to maintain a certain level of intensity of exercise is greatly reduced. It has also been described as the loss of a powerful response from voluntary effort. The concept is multifactorial, the major factors being: depleted energy stores; accumulated metabolic waste products; dehydration. Other contributors include depletion of neurotransmitter chemicals, a generally poor nutritional status, the recovery from illness or a break from training, and the centrally integrated psychological factors resulting from prolonged effort, discomfort and pain. Clearly, most aspects of fitness can be improved to minimize the onset and experience of fatigue.

Anaerobic threshold: the point at which the body's demand for oxygen, during strenuous exercise, exceeds its ability to supply it.

Onset of blood lactic acid accumulation (OBLA): this is also referred to as the lactate threshold, and occurs when there is a sudden increase in lactate in the blood during strenuous exercise.

Alactic debt: this is the required supply of oxygen to facilitate all physiological processes being performed during exercise, regardless of the energy supply for the exercise. This includes the refilling of oxygen stores in both the blood and myoglobin, the maintenance of increased cardiac and respiratory activity and the various other control and regulatory mechanisms of the body (neurological and hormonal). Therefore, it is important to develop aerobic capacity for the performance of all sports.

ASPECTS OF AGEING

From birth to death occurs the ageing process. Our physical body is not immortal. Eventually, the ageing process, combined with a certain tendency to become less active, leads to a slowing down of physiological functioning, a degeneration of tissues and an increased vulnerability to disease processes. However, with the advent of widespread improvements in health-care, living environments and health awareness, life expectancy in the modern world continues to increase, as does individual functional capability into older age. Indeed, there are more older people involved in regular physical exercise (and competition) today than ever before. Exercise helps to keep us young.

Just as the very age of an individual has a strong influence upon the structure of their body and how their physiology functions, how the individual lives (works, eats, exercises, relaxes and attends to their ailments and dysfunctions) has a strong influence upon their experience of that process.

Children generally have a faster metabolic rate owing to the amount of growth and development that they need to go through. Children are not little adults. They do not have musculo-skeletal maturity, and therefore are more prone to strains and overuse injuries if sport is not taught appropriately. They also lack the benefit of great knowledge and experience, and should be monitored for postural and biomechanical (especially gait) problems. Great body and spatial awareness does not develop quickly, therefore co-ordination, balance, timing and reaction, specific skills, as well as fun and games are important components of any training programme involving children.

The earliest obvious objective signs that the ageing process is kicking in are the changes in our physical appearance. The skin becomes thinner, less elastic and supple (lines and wrinkles develop) and less protective. The hair tends to dry, become brittle, thin out, turn grey and become lacklustre. Postural changes occur as we lose height, gain (or lose) weight, lose muscle mass and strength, lose bone mass, experience wear and tear (arthritis, degenerative disc disease, etc.) and develop compensatory movement patterns to off-set pain and discomfort.

A whole variety of neurological changes occur as we age, and we actually lose nerve cells. Reductions occur in our mental functioning as sensory, integrative and motor messages become less efficient. There is generally a deterioration in the senses of vision, audition, olfaction and gustation. Reactions slow, co-ordination becomes more impaired, and memory becomes less clear.

Circulatory and respiratory systems slowly develop a general reduced efficiency. Stroke volume, and therefore cardiac output, falls. The myocardial wall hypertrophies. The maximal exercising heart rate falls. Blood pressure has a tendency to rise. Blood vessels tend to become less elastic, more brittle and congested. Lung capacities reduce. Oxygen supply to the cells reduces. Venous and lymphatic return become less efficient. There is increased susceptibility to infection and disease due to impaired immune responses. Weakening of superficial skin capillaries means that we bruise more easily.

In the digestive system, enzyme production reduces and the effective absorption of nutrients is compromised. The liver and kidneys become less efficient. Basal metabolic rate decreases. Incontinence of the urinary system can also develop.

Subjectively, how we tend to feel changes as we get older. Life is a very experiential process. Each stage of life brings with it new revelations and realizations. The elderly, by having lived to an older age, will have gone through every range of human emotion and certainly will have experienced most circumstances (love, success, failure, happiness, sadness, hardship, comfort). These experiences, and the processes involved in our coming to terms with the multitude of life situations, are really what life is all about. Older people still have a great deal to offer, and must only be respected and never disregarded: we will all be old one day. Old-age wisdom can be attained only by those who have lived a lifetime.

It is just as important to maintain a good level of fitness into older age as it is in younger years, and it is often the older generation who get the most benefit from therapeutic intervention. However, awareness of the practical effects of ageing must be taken into account when planning exercise and treatment for older people.

CHAPTER SUMMARY

This chapter has looked at the anatomy and physiology of the body, and how sound knowledge and understanding of this helps us to plan and provide our therapeutic strategies, and analyse and objectify the outcomes. The human body can be described on chemical, cellular, tissue, organ, system and organismic levels. It is very important for the sports therapist to understand well the main structures, functions, processes and relationships that go into making our body work efficiently.

TIP

A philosophical thought: our anatomical structure, to a certain extent, is a great governor to our physiological functioning. Disregarding all the individual genetic factors, the illnesses, accidents and other misfortunes that we experience, perhaps we could add our learned behaviour as one of the greatest influencers of our health. Behaviour, although obviously psychologically and sociologically complex, is how we live. Although there are always other constraints, behaviour determines where we live, the quality of our diet, how we work, rest and react to situations, and how we choose to be.

Knowledge Review

1 What is meant by the following terms: (a) medial, (b) proximal, (c) flexion, (d) contra-lateral, (e) sagittal plane, (f) endangerment site?

2 List ten facts about the skeletal system.

3 What are the typical features of a synovial joint?

4 Provide one example of each of the following joints: (a) fibrous, (b) cartilaginous, (c) ball and socket, (d) hinge, (e) gliding, (f) saddle.

5 What are the key differences between striated, smooth and cardiac muscle tissues?

6 Describe the structural breakdown of skeletal muscle tissue from the superficial fascia inwards.

7 Describe, in one paragraph, how muscles contract.

8 List the main components of the nervous system.

9 Describe the systemic, pulmonary and portal circulatory systems.

WEBSITE

Visit the companion website at www.thomsonlearning.co.uk/ healthandfitness/ward where you will find the answers to these questions for you to check your progress through the book.

10 What are the main components and functions of the lymphatic system?

11 What is lymphatic drainage?

12 List the main organs of respiration.

13 What is (a) breathing, (b) external respiration, (c) internal respiration and (d) cellular respiration?

14 Which skeletal muscles, major and accessory, are involved in respiration?

15 List the main and accessory organs of the digestive system.

16 List the main endocrine glands.

17 List five functions of the endocrine system.

18 List ten anatomical or physiological differences between men and women.

19 Describe the aerobic energy system.

20 List some of the common effects of ageing on the body.

chapter 3

PREPARATION FOR THERAPEUTIC PRACTICE

Learning Objectives

After reading this chapter you should be able to:

- develop knowledge of health, hygiene and safety, legislation and ethical issues
- understand the importance of communicating and responding appropriately to all colleagues, clients and workplace events
- understand the consultation and record-keeping process
- develop awareness of sensitivity issues
- have knowledge of all important contra-indications and contra-actions to sports therapy

Sports therapy is a caring profession and, for successful practice, one where safety and quality must go hand in hand. The provision of therapeutic services for the general public requires a great deal of health, hygiene, safety and ethical knowledge, as well as ensuring that all legal essentials are satisfied. All of this is simply to protect both the client and the therapist, and it must be considered a very important part of the professional development of the sports therapist. As such, it should prepare them for safe, effective and successful practice. It is unfortunately beyond the scope of this book to cover all aspects of law, ethics and health and safety. The aim of this chapter is simply to heighten the therapist's awareness of the importance of working with absolute professionalism.

The process of preparing for the provision of therapy treatments or exercise involves a whole selection of criteria:

- Being properly qualified and insured to practise sports therapy.
- Understanding your responsibilities to both colleagues and clients in the workplace.
- Keeping strictly in line with essential legal requirements and the ethical standards set by governing bodies.
- Keeping high standards of health, hygiene and safety in the workplace.

- Being aware of all the potential hazards posed by treatment, exercise, equipment and products.
- Effectively communicating with colleagues, clients and other concerned health practitioners.
- Recording and storing appropriate personal client details, and in keeping with legal requirements.
- Generating a respectful and responsive attitude.
- Understanding who the client is.
- Having awareness of absolute, possible and localized contra-indications to treatments.
- Having awareness of possible contra-actions (adverse reactions) that may occur.
- Staying abreast with the latest developments in the field of sports therapy practice.

The active practice of working safely, responsibly and effectively, and in line with all legal, ethical and professional standards is as important in the training environment as it is in the working environment. By working correctly to such standards, the student develops their professional skills properly, gaining good working practice and experience, which demonstrates to their assessors that they have the competence to work in such a manner.

LEGISLATION ISSUES

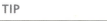

TIP

Health and safety legislations are continually updated. It is therefore important to stay aware of the latest changes.

All legislation, whether local, national or international, must be abided by. Laws, regulations and establishment rules are implemented in workplaces to protect all those concerned. During their study of this area, the sports therapist should be suitably furnished with the important legal aspects and requirements that directly affect their practice and are laid down in law. **Legislations** guide the health, hygiene and safety essentials of the sports therapy business and, therefore, the way in which the services are provided.

ETHICAL ISSUES

Professional representative therapy bodies exist to promote good practice for the benefit of the general public and their practitioner members. The promotion of sound ethical practices and the limitation of some types of practices are all in the professional therapist's long-term interests, and are for the protection of the public. It is strongly recommended that sports therapists join a reputable and well-established body, either as a student, associate or full member. For acceptance, it is usual to have to provide specific evidence of training and qualifications, including an up-to-date **first aid** certificate.

IMPORTANT LEGAL ACTS AND REGULATIONS OF RELEVANCE TO THE PRACTICE OF SPORTS THERAPY	
Health and Safety at Work etc. Act 1974	ECHR (The Human Rights Act 1998)
Management of Health and Safety at Work Regulations 1999	RIDDOR (Reporting Injuries, Diseases and Dangerous Occurrences Regulations) 1995
Health and Safety (First-Aid) Regulations 1981	PUWER (Provision and Use of Work Equipment Regulations) 1998
Employers Liability Act 1969	
Consumer Protection Act 1987	Environmental Protection Act 1990
Trades Descriptions Act 1972	Cosmetic Products (Safety) Regulations
Sales and Supply of Goods Act 1994	COSHH (Control of Substances Hazardous to Health) Regulations 1999
Local Government Miscellaneous Provisions Act	Manual Handling Operations Regulations 1992
Data Protection Act 1998	Personal Protective Equipment at Work Regulations 1992
Performing Rights Act 1988	
The Children Act 1989	Electricity at Work Regulations
Social Services Act 1970	Gas Safety Regulations
Protection of Children Act 1999	Workplace, Health and Safety, and Welfare Regulations
Youth Justice and Criminal Evidence Act 1999	Provision and use of Work Equipment Regulations
Crime and Disorder Act 1998	Fire Precautions (Workplace) Regulations
Sex Offenders Act 1997	Local Authority Licensing Regulations
Care Standards Act 2000	

A representative therapy organization will usually be able to provide:

- industry codes of practice and ethics
- specialized and competitive rates of professional practitioner insurance
- strong and active promotion of the profession
- support base
- professional conferences and events
- continuing professional development programmes
- subsidized products
- practitioner register and database
- information website for the general public
- professional journal or newsletter
- latest news and developments in the therapy field.

A **code of ethics** is guided by legal regulations, and aimed at maintaining high, safe and correct standards of practice. It is drawn up to regulate the members of a professional organization. Breaking the code of ethics may result in an official warning, possible suspension, expulsion or prosecution, depending upon the breach in question.

A typical code of ethics will state clearly the rules and obligations of the members:

- Perform all consultations and treatments in a professional manner.
- Maintain consistently high standards of hygiene.

TIP

It is important to continually reflect upon your own practice and identify weaknesses and development needs.

- Health and safety and security strategies are regularly monitored and action planned.
- Do not treat in the presence of contra-indications until medical approval has been obtained.
- Where medical advice is considered important, therapists should advise the client of this and record the advice given.
- Treatment times and costs are appropriate and consistent.
- Only perform those services for which you are qualified.
- Respect all clients and all other health-care professionals.
- Make no false claims regarding the effects and benefits of treatments.
- Maintain absolute client confidentiality, and any information gained during consultation or treatment must not be divulged to any other person or organization without the client's consent (except when required by law).
- Store all client records in a manner in keeping with the Data Protection Act.
- The premises and equipment must be suitable for the services provided.
- Professional indemnity and public liability insurance must be appropriate to the services on offer, and up to date.

HEALTH AND SAFETY ISSUES

Safe working practice helps prevent accidents and provides strategic protection for staff and clients. The sports therapy workplace may be either a purely clinical or a purely exercise environment, but it is more likely that it will incorporate aspects of both. Whatever the nature of the workplace, it must be suitable for the services and activities that are to be provided. This includes appropriate: ventilation; lighting; heating; noise levels; privacy; space; and cleanliness. The people working at the establishment must all be trained and regularly updated with regard to all of the health and safety strategies implemented by the management.

A hazard is simply a danger or risk, and there are three basic categories of hazard:

- physical hazards, e.g. lifting heavy or awkward items; burns; cuts; slipping or tripping over; electric shock
- chemical hazards, e.g. cleaning products; application (treatment) products
- biological hazards, e.g. coughs and colds; fungal infections; contaminated waste.

Hazards are always best avoided. As a therapist it is very important to work in a manner that minimizes the potential for hazards, and you should also be familiar with appropriate actions to take in the event of hazards occurring. Obviously, minimizing risk is crucial to safe practice, and regular categoric risk assessments should be undertaken and acted upon in the establishment.

In establishments, team meetings that work to develop and implement in-house strategies will help to improve the efficiency of maintaining good standards of health and safety. Noticeboards and posters help to remind workers and clients of their various responsibilities. If an atmosphere is generated where everyone helps one another, then an effective process develops.

Simple things to encourage health and safety in the workplace include:

- safe manual handling
- asking for help when required
- using all equipment correctly, in accordance with training and manufacturer's instructions
- performing all treatments in the correct manner (knowledge of contra-indications; choice of equipment and settings; sufficient space to work effectively; appropriate intensity and duration; client understanding and feedback)
- cleaning and putting equipment away properly when finished with
- reporting faulty equipment
- provision and wearing of protective clothing when necessary
- operating an effective clean laundry system
- efficient stock control
- dispensing of products hygienically
- disposing of waste products hygienically
- swift cleaning up of breakages and spillages
- efficient and regular handwashing
- awareness and avoidance of the possibility of cross-infection
- keeping all personal belongings in a secure place (locker)
- keeping all client records in a secure place (locked cabinet)
- regular fire drills
- first aid training for all
- responsibility and co-operation.

> **TIP**
>
> The main health and safety issues relating to each therapeutic method, whether massage, thermal therapy, taping and strapping or remedial exercise, are discussed in each of the appropriate chapters of this book.

The clinic differs from the gym, with each having its particular risks and safety issues. In the gym, exercise equipment needs monitoring for its suitability and function, and all the exercising stations and areas must be kept clean and clutter-free. Exercisers need to be training correctly and observed and monitored for signs of distress.

In the clinic, therapists need to work with safety in mind. Correct techniques, appropriate equipment settings, and certainly each treatment must be tailored specifically to the individual concerned. Clients need to be informed of the treatment methods that they are going to receive. Hazards, such as trailing electric cables, clutter in aisles or electrical equipment being left switched on, need immediate action to minimize the potential for accidents. Massage oil and cleaning product bottles need to be sealed immediately after use to reduce the possibility of spillages.

In the spa area, often a feature of a therapy or fitness centre, strict hygiene rules need to be enforced. These include regular documented checking,

TIP

As part of an effective health and safety strategy, it is important to ensure clients do not use any therapeutic equipment unsupervised, unless it has been considered appropriate and fully explained to them.

testing, cleaning and maintenance of whirlpools, hydrotherapy pools, steam rooms, saunas, baths, showers and toilets – often part of the sports therapist's job.

Emergencies must be promptly dealt with. Sports therapists should be qualified to provide basic first aid, and therefore they should know the importance of prioritizing and gaining appropriate assistance if necessary. Any accidents of significance that do occur (e.g. cuts; burns; falls) must be recorded in the accident book, along with details of any first aid treatment provided, and by whom.

Fire and evacuation procedures

It is vital to implement strict fire precautions in the workplace, and sports therapists must be aware of their responsibilities. These include:

- Making sure that all fire and evacuation procedures prescribed both by the establishment and the local authority are understood by all, and are implemented.
- All corridors, stairs and fire exits in the working area are always kept free from obstructions.
- Action is taken to ensure that with actual or potential hazards, warnings are given to others on the premises.
- The locations, uses and limitations of different types of fire containment is understood (includes fire blankets, fire-hoses and different types of extinguisher, for electrical and non-electrical fires).
- Evacuation procedures (fire drills) are understood and practised regularly.
- Appropriate assistance must be provided for clients and visitors in the event of evacuation.
- The importance of notifying the establishment authorities and fire-fighting services in the event of a fire is fully understood.

HYGIENE ISSUES

TIP

Hygiene is the practice of maintaining health and preventing disease through cleanliness.

Hygienic practice in the workplace is crucial. Every fitness or therapy room must have hygiene procedures rigorously implemented, and all necessary cleaning and sterilizing products must be available. All centres must have adequate hot and cold running water. All towels, whether for cleaning and drying purposes, or for use in client treatments, must be cleaned to a high standard. Towels must be changed after each treatment session. All equipment and work surfaces must be regularly cleaned or wiped down with hot water and detergent (this includes couches, trolleys, sinks and stools). Electrical equipment must also be cleaned, but care taken so as not to damage the working parts. Waste bin liners should be tied up and disposed of properly, regularly during the day.

There are various types of cleaning products available, but whatever is used, it must be strong enough and used for long enough to be effective.

Disinfectants kill most pathogens to a level where they can do no harm. Antiseptics do not kill pathogens, but they do stop them from multiplying.

Disinfectants include:

- Surgical spirit (ethanol and water), which sanitizes (and acts as an antiseptic), rather than disinfects, and can be used to wipe down tools and equipment, and on the skin (e.g. wiping the feet prior to massage).
- Savlon will disinfect, but it is neutralized by soap.
- Coal-tar derivatives, such as Dettol and Lysol, can be used to soak tools or for swabbing floors.
- Chlorine-based bleach or Milton fluid is effective against viruses and bacterial spores.

> **TIP**
>
> Germs are spread by: unclean hands; contaminated equipment; shared used of towels, pillows, cups, etc.; close contact with infected skin; contaminated waste products; contaminated blood or tissue fluids; breath; lack of care.

To prevent cross-infection or contamination, the cleaning (sanitizing) of hands (and nails) must be very thorough, especially before and after each client. This is to prevent pathogens from multiplying or being transferred. Cuts, abrasions and any other minor skin disorders must be covered with waterproof dressings. Disposable latex gloves are used for complete covering, and are useful when dealing with any contaminated waste.

The storage of products and equipment where stated should be in line with manufacturer's instructions. Oils, creams and gels must be dispensed hygienically. This can mean use of a special dispenser tube, which inhibits contamination and can be sealed after use, or simply removal of sufficient product, by way of pouring or using a spatula, to put into a single-use container or vessel.

There must be immediate and appropriate clean up of spillages and breakages. Care must be taken to handle breakages and any contaminated waste correctly, and both should be disposed of in accordance with health and safety regulations.

In the treatment room, a clean couch cover should be put on the couch each working day (and this should be changed during the day if the need arises). Pillowcases and towels must also all be in good supply for regular changing. Paper couch roll should be laid out on the couch for each new client. There should also be plenty of paper towels or tissues and cotton wool for small cleaning jobs or available for the client's use.

Therapists themselves must obviously demonstrate extremely high levels of hygiene, both in terms of their personal image and in their working practice. By being very clearly well presented and clean (long hair tied back; nails kept neat and short; jewelry and make-up kept to an understated minimum), a positive image is generated. A neat appearance suggests efficiency and professionalism, and generates confidence. Sports therapists may choose to wear a clinical tunic (typically white or blue) or plain sportswear, e.g. polo shirt with tracksuit trousers or shorts, and clean white training shoes. It is important to feel comfortable in your 'uniform' because sports therapy is a practical job involving a lot of manual activity. Therapists should also refrain from smoking, eating certain types of foods or wearing strong perfumes prior to providing treatments, because of the obviously unpleasant odorous experience for the client. Demonstrating hygienic

TIP

TIP

The success of the workplace, where all concerned work together efficiently, professionally and productively, results in security of employment.

procedures in the view of the client definitely helps to promote confidence and foster reassurance.

It only improves the overall image of the therapist and their workplace if they work with great professional conduct and develop an attitude of always being punctual and prepared, ready for work.

COST-EFFECTIVENESS

Cost-effectiveness in the workplace is crucial to the overall success and longevity of the business. Efficient working practices also help to enhance the client's experience and their overall satisfaction. Minimizing waste is very important, because products and disposables are not cheap. Therapists and all other employees should work with awareness of the importance of looking after equipment, especially as most items of clinical or exercise equipment tend to be very expensive to replace. Another aspect to cost-effectiveness is for therapists to work to commercially acceptable treatment times. Depending upon the types of service on offer, and the pricing structures in place, some treatments might take 20 minutes, but others an hour and a half. It is important to try to keep to allocated time schedules. Customers get to know what to expect from a treatment, and the next appointment should not be kept waiting. It is usual to allow a few minutes between each appointment so that a clean-up and set-up can take place. If the therapist is not efficient in keeping to time schedules it can work very much against them. Time must also be allowed for breaks and record keeping.

COMMUNICATION ISSUES

TIP

Telephone communications require that the therapist is particularly careful to be clear and informative, and to have good tone of voice and manner.

Clear and effective communication is crucial to successful practice. Therapists need to be able to communicate, by verbal and written means, to their superiors (i.e. practice managers; team managers; employers), colleagues (i.e. fellow therapists; receptionists; coaches; maintenance workers), other practitioners and medical personnel (i.e. physiotherapists; osteopaths; chiropractors; podiatrists; GPs), external statutory authorities (i.e. local council; sports associations; support groups), the general public, and not least their clients.

Face-to-face communication is something always to develop. Although it is founded on individual background and personality, it is most effective when the therapist is alert and responsive, and able to assess the immediate appropriate approach. Recognizing body language, attentive listening and sensitive, appropriate questioning encourages good communication. Being generally pleasant, offering a smile and being able to engage in a modicum of appropriate small-talk makes everything much easier.

In the workplace, when communicating with superiors and colleagues, being clear and to the point, but always polite, helps to generate productive working relationships, efficient responses, and keeps the atmosphere calm and reliable.

When attending to clients, the therapist should try to develop their skill in adapting their vocabulary, the pace and tone of speaking so as to meet the needs of different clients. For example, some clients will be hard of hearing, some not completely fluent in English and some slow to understand.

It is important to position yourself and the client appropriately so as to encourage effective communication, and typically for the consultation this involves being seated either next to each other at the side of the treatment couch or opposite each other. Sometimes difficulties arise with communication. It is the therapist's responsibility to try to recognize and overcome any barriers that are apparent: this is all about careful use of language and tone, and remaining courteous, clear and professional at all times. By always remaining respectful, clear, polite and responsive, professional integrity will be maintained, and clients should feel comfortable and gain confidence with such an approach. Every attempt should be made to sort out any minor problems, misunderstandings or dissatisfaction with the service, before they become a bigger problem. Try to remember that your customers will be paying good money for a good professional service, and that running a successful business is very much about developing a good reputation.

Occasionally, a situation may arise where the therapist has to respond to conflicting advice given to their client by another practitioner. In such an instance, tact is the key, and certainly to dismiss the advice out of hand would not usually be considered appropriate. Probably, if suitably qualified and experienced, offering your own professional advice with explanation of your reasoning would be the best response.

Body language is non-verbal communication. Body language can sometimes tell us a lot about how an individual is feeling: for example, nervousness might by demonstrated by the individual avoiding eye contact, looking down and staying quiet. Bolder body language such as when the individual is visibly angry or impatient might involve the person having a tense frowning facial expression, standing up, pacing up and down, tapping fingers on a table, huffing and sighing, or trying to gain the therapist's attention with eye contact.

It is important, though, not to prejudge people purely on the basis of their (apparent) body language, as it is easy to mistake certain behaviour for something that it is not. Therapists should try to read each new situation in light of the body language portrayed, and also the initial words of verbal communication.

Communicating with other professionals is a different matter. Should the need arise, any personal information regarding clients must always be released with their written consent. There can be instances where sports therapists have clients referred to them by other practitioners, and there will be times when the therapist will want to refer their client to another therapist or medical practitioner. In such cases of a client being referred for sports therapy, it is often required that the therapist produces a status (progress) report, detailing such information as their assessment findings, treatment methods employed, evaluation of the therapeutic

---

TIP

Always try to maintain good customer relations: be responsive to clients' feelings; give the client opportunity to convey their feelings; try to assess if the client is nervous or anxious; deal with complaints constructively; be positive; be polite; demonstrate good manners; show confidence; be supportive; be flexible; explain any limitations or problems honestly; try to meet the clients' needs; never display a complaining attitude.

TIP

The therapist must have awareness of all of their various responsibilities to their supervisors, colleagues, clients and the workplace in which they all work.

effectiveness, and any particular recommendations regarding future treatments.

When a client is presenting with possible contra-indications or with problems that the sports therapist is not qualified to treat, they should refer them to an appropriate professional. Doctors, however, cannot be expected to take full responsibility for their patient's suitability to receive therapeutic treatment (after all it is the patient's choice), but they should be able to offer relevant advice about whether their condition could be exacerbated by such an approach. Unfortunately at present, many GPs are still in the dark about the potential benefits and adversities of sports therapy, and many will prefer to recommend more medically recognized approaches, such as physiotherapy. By developing very professional practices, and by communicating formally and effectively, general awareness will continue to grow.

Where a contra-indication is evident, and medical advice is deemed necessary, the sports therapist may choose to provide the client with a 'consent' form to take to their GP; however, it is not recommended to use the words 'consent' or 'permission' to a doctor because it can affect their professional insurance, and also it is against the advice of the BMA. A simple form explaining the proposed treatments, listing safety measures, with a tear-off slip would be more appropriate. For example: 'I have no objection to my patient .... having sports therapy treatment'.

An acceptable alternative approach to gaining the GP's approval would be to ask the client to discuss the situation with their GP. When the client reports back to the sports therapist, they can provide an account of their GP's opinion, which should then be recorded on their consultation form. The client's signature should be obtained to clarify this statement.

SENSITIVE ISSUES

There are a variety of sensitivity issues for the sports therapist to be aware of. In contemporary politically correct Britain it is crucial to always work with non-discriminatory practice, and to actively encourage equality for all. This nation has a diverse range of communities, and it is important to generate respect for all our cultural differences. No one must be discriminated against or judged, for their ethnicity, religious or spiritual beliefs, gender, age, sexual orientation, occupation, disability, body type or any other individual characteristic. Certainly, a therapist, someone who professionally helps and cares for people, should be the last person that any one could accuse of being discriminatory.

There are times when a child (a minor), an elderly person, someone with special needs, or a member of the opposite sex will present for sports therapy treatment. In such cases special care and planning (protection strategies) will be required. A minor is any person under the legal age of consent, normally said to be under 16 years. Treatment for minors, which in itself is a delicate issue, must be provided in the presence of a parent or guardian, or if they are not in attendance they should provide written

TIP

Whenever it is felt necessary to recommend referral to the GP, it should be done without causing any undue alarm or concern.

permission and have a chaperone present. Treatment of the opposite sex poses some risk in terms of the possibility of allegations of inappropriate treatment, and therefore it is recommended that such clients are treated with either a companion or appropriate adult present, or at least in the near vicinity. Similar precautions should be adopted when dealing with clients who are considered to be infirm, or have special needs. It is important to identify such needs before any treatment or examination takes place.

The sports therapist is sometimes ideally positioned to be able to suspect signs of physical or mental abuse. Abuse can be sexual, neglectful, self-harming, bullying or discrimination. The therapist may notice bruising or marking on the client's body, or the client may reveal certain information about something that has happened to them (whether true or false). This can be a particularly awkward and sensitive situation to deal with. The therapist should avoid making judgements, but it is professional to document any explanations given by the client and report any abnormal statements, events or observations to the senior person in the establishment. They may also choose to request advice, if in any doubt about how to proceed. Care must be taken with any advice given to the client in regard of their situation, but the therapist may like to recommend recognized organizations that an adult client may wish to contact.

Inappropriate behaviour from a client can sometimes occur in the sports therapy centre. This can include: actions or statements from a minor that really are not appropriate; very withdrawn or introverted behaviour; sexual innuendo; verbal harassment; inappropriate contact or statements. Any kind of offensive behaviour from clients is completely unacceptable and must be strongly discouraged, clearly but politely. The therapist should not normally experience much of this type of behaviour if their practice is run professionally. Wherever it is felt that there is even the slightest possibility of an undesirable situation occurring, the therapist should perform their work with colleagues or other responsible adults present.

Another issue of sensitivity is being able to preserve the client's dignity during treatment. Clients require privacy for physical assessment procedures and therapy treatments. The therapist must try to minimize the potential for embarrassment, especially when removing clothing. It is a professional responsibility to help make them feel at ease at all times. Remember that few people enjoy the scrutiny of a consultation, or a physical assessment for that matter, and therefore it is important to keep such procedures to as short a period of time as possible.

Clients must also have all proposed treatments and procedures explained to them before they are begun, and the client should also understand and agree to what is being proposed (informed consent).

SECURITY ISSUES

Effective security in the workplace is essential. Security relates not just to the protection against theft and damage, but also against personal harm.

Security strategies must be instigated so as to protect the staff and clients, the premises and its equipment and stock, client's records, the day's takings and the personal belongings of both staff and clients. Systems need to be in place both during and after working hours, and also strategies must be implemented so that staff know how and who to report to in the event of problems or breaches of security. It is important that complete, accurate and up-to-date records of security incidents are kept.

Examples of appropriate security measures might include:

- locks and bolts on all doors and windows
- burglar alarms fitted
- minimum number of key holders to the premises
- leaving a light on during the night and having security lights in operation
- not leaving money in the till overnight (and leaving the drawer open)
- implementing specific opening-up and locking-up strategies (particularly so that there is never one person on their own)
- installing lockable cupboards (lockers) for the use of staff and clients
- keeping all equipment, products, disposables and client records in locked cupboards or rooms
- effective stock control helps protect against pilfering by staff
- periodic random audits of money and stock.

TIP ✔

Keeping the client's valuables safe, either with them, in their sight (watches and jewelry can be placed in a small bowl on a table adjacent to the treatment couch), or locked in a cupboard, is the responsibility of the therapist.

THE CONSULTATION PROCESS: WHO IS THE CLIENT?

The client could be the person making enquiries, buying items or using the services of the sports therapist and their workplace. Once the client has made the decision to visit the sports therapist for the first time for treatment a consultation must take place before any services are provided.

> Written documentation is an important part of what establishes a holistic therapist as a professional practitioner. It confirms their educated assessment, choice of treatment and ongoing evaluation of the client's progress towards health and well-being.
> HELEN MCGUINNESS (2000)

The consultation need not take more than 15 to 30 minutes, depending upon the complexity of the individual case. The first session should allow time for a consultation period. It is an opportunity to discuss and document appropriate aspects of the client's life, in particular: the history of their health, including particular conditions and injuries, medical and therapy treatments (past and present), medications (past and present), their lifestyle (including diet, sleep, exercise, sports – past and present), their occupations (past and present) and their initial objectives (e.g. injury treatment; improve fitness; improve posture or body contours; relaxation). The client must be put at ease during the consultation, and it is normal to perform this in a relatively private atmosphere. Typically, the consultation is performed by the treatment couch, cordoned off with a curtain or portable screen. The therapist should attempt to generate a professional but friendly and informal atmosphere.

It is common for clients to present to the sports therapy clinic with a wide variety of conditions, and expect them to be treated effectively, especially when 'remedial therapy' is on offer. These can include emotional or stress-related conditions, musculo-skeletal and sports injury problems, lymphoedema, long-term illness, even terminal illness. In many of these cases the therapist must gain medical approval before providing any form of treatment, and in the case of complicated and serious medical conditions they should not attempt to provide treatment unless they have taken additional specialized training and qualification in the area. Even if the therapist is properly trained and experienced, they should still have a full understanding as to the nature of the presenting condition, and they should be confident in their ability to provide safe and helpful therapy.

There can be instances where the client is reluctant to provide the therapist with the necessary information required to provide the treatment that they are requesting. In such circumstances, the therapist should explain: that the information is required so as to make a full assessment; that the information is confidential; that it is essential for health, safety and legal reasons; that if the information is not provided, then the treatment or exercise cannot take place.

In the process of providing sports therapy, and monitoring a client's progress, there will be a number of forms (or one large dossier) onto which all relevant information is documented.

Typically, for record keeping, the following forms will be used:

- consultation form (date; name; address; telephone numbers; date of birth; GP's name and practice; occupation; exercise history; medical history; current medications; presenting problems; complementary therapy treatment history; lifestyle; initial objectives; statement of consent)
- record card (details of each sports therapy treatment and advice provided)
- physical assessment form (date; height; weight; BMI; body circumferences; postural assessment; range of movement assessment; gait analysis; analysis of whole; reviewed objectives; recommendations)
- fitness test form (date; resting heart rate; blood pressure; **body fat percentage**; lung function; aerobic tests; flexibility tests; muscular strength and endurance tests; power tests; analysis of all tests; reviewed objectives; recommendations)
- remedial action plan (date; objectives; methods to achieve objectives; specific exercise recommendations; other specific recommendations; review for progression).

Sample forms covering the above criteria can be found in the appendix to this book. Records should be complete, accurate and legible so that they are effective and usable, and confidentiality is absolutely essential in all matters of personal and medical information that has been offered by the client.

TIP

Informed and written consent is a legal requirement. This means explaining fully to the client all details relating to the proposed treatments and exercise, and what benefits they are likely to experience, making sure they fully understand what it entails. The therapist must then gain the client's signature so as to state that they agree to the proposed treatments.

TIP

Some therapists like to make use of 'SOAP' notes on their consultation form. This stands for: Subjective (the client explains experiences); Objective (what the therapist observes); Analysis (the results – what worked, what didn't); Plan (for the session, for the next session, for homework).

TIP

There may be instances, in the absence of contra-indications, when the therapist still chooses not to provide therapy treatment, for example when the treatment is unlikely to benefit the client, or when the client is demonstrating inappropriate behaviour.

TIP

Keeping accurate, legible, up-to-date records is an insurance against any possible complaints.

CONTRA-INDICATIONS AND CONTRA-ACTIONS

Contra-indications

A contra-indication is a condition that, potentially, could become adversely affected by any particular treatment or action. Contra-indications can be 'absolute' (e.g. client has history of heart problems), where treatment must not be given under any circumstances, 'possible' (e.g. client taking blood pressure medication), where medical advice must be sought beforehand, or 'local' (e.g. a wound or bruise), where the treatment may be adapted, so as to avoid the problem area.

Medical and injury conditions can be loosely graded into two categories:

1. long-term conditions (e.g. heart problems; circulatory disorders; diabetes; epilepsy; nervous system dysfunction; debilitating musculo-skeletal disorders)

2. short-term or temporary conditions (e.g. cuts; burns; influenza; feeling unwell; pregnancy; current medical treatment such as antibiotic medication; recent surgery; fractures; sprains; strains).

Different contra-indications and safety issues apply to different treatments and exercises. Sports therapists must familiarize themselves with the special precautions relating to each different aspect of their service.

Once contra-indications have been identified, the therapist has to make the decision as to what action to take, of which there are three basic options: (i) no treatment at all, (ii) treatment once medical advice has been obtained and (iii) adapted treatment.

Contra-actions

Contra-actions (adverse reactions) can sometimes occur, even though all main health issues and previous treatment experiences have been fully investigated. Contra-actions are often unavoidable, because it is so difficult to predict when somebody is going to react to a treatment in an unusual way. The therapist will know that the sensitive, the frail, the pregnant, the elderly or children, and many of the people having their first treatment, should be offered a relatively lower intensity of treatment, whether it is massage, thermal therapy or remedial exercise. Examples of contra-actions include: fainting; increased discomfort and pain; tiredness; headache; emotional response; tissue damage; increased swelling; skin reaction.

So long as the therapist works with great awareness and responsibility during their treatment of clients, any adverse reactions that do occur will usually be minor. If and when they do occur, they need to be discussed with the client, and the therapist must act reassuringly. Correct action must be taken in the event, and the client should be advised of how this might be prevented in the future.

GENERAL, ABSOLUTE, POSSIBLE AND LOCAL CONTRA-INDICATIONS AND REASONS TO PROCEED WITH GREAT CAUTION	
Acute injuries (first aid required)	Tumours or unrecognizable lumps
Severe sports injuries	Melanoma (skin cancer)
Severe pain	Haemophilia
Skin disorders (including: cuts; burns; sunburn; bruising; rashes; warts; folliculitis; dermatitis; fungal infections)	Diabetes
	Epilepsy
Contagious illness	Dysfunctional nervous system
Coronary heart disease	Severe osteoarthritis/rheumatoid arthritis/osteoporosis/gout/ bursitis/ankylosing spondylitis/spondylosis/spondylolysis/ spondylolisthesis
Circulatory disorders (including: varicose veins; thrombosis; phlebitis; atherosclerosis; arteriosclerosis; severe oedema)	
Hypertension	Metal pins and plates
Strong medications	Pacemaker
Recent surgery	Pregnancy
Inoculations (wait 24 hours)	First two or three days of menstruation
Acute hypothermia/hyperthermia	Heavy meal
Myositis ossificans	Alcohol/recreational drugs
Hernias	Any other condition requiring medical supervision

AFTER-CARE

After-care, which is discussed further in later chapters, should always be offered, even if it is just a recommendation to take it easy for a while after treatment, drink some water, and avoid alcohol. If the client has experienced any adverse reactions to their treatment then extra-vigilance and particular after-care might be required. Other advice might relate to: relaxation techniques; time management; posture; diet; training modifications; specific exercises; rehabilitation exercises; heat or cold applications; **taping**, strapping or support; self-massage; follow-up treatments.

EVALUATING THE EFFECTIVENESS OF THERAPEUTIC TREATMENTS

The evaluation of the effectiveness of the therapy treatment, which is very important, involves the monitoring of immediate and short-term (positive or negative) responses. Whether subjectively experienced or objectively observed, positive responses might include improved well-being and relaxation, easier range of movement, reduced fatigue, pain relief or improved performance. Follow-up sessions allow for a more equitable evaluation, because the client will have had time to consider their initial response and how they felt during the days that followed their treatment.

They may also have been implementing the after-care recommendations. Additionally, the therapist will be able to repeat physical assessments and tests and compare the client's previous results.

Client feedback during treatment is particularly important, and the therapist must encourage this, and respond to it accordingly. Evaluation must also incorporate assessment of whether the (realistic, achievable) initial objectives have been achieved.

There can be a wide variety of reasons as to why a client might not wish to continue with their treatment programme. These can include: failing to establish a comfortable relationship with the therapist; being dissatisfied with any aspect of the service; preferring to visit another practitioner; financial reasons; time constraints; failure to gain effective benefit from the treatments, or frustrated at the rate of improvement; experiencing adverse reactions to the treatment. If the therapist keeps these issues in mind it can help to minimize the incidence of clients not continuing with their treatments. It should be remembered, though, that many people will choose to only visit their sports therapist on an occasional basis anyway, and for various reasons, which is fine.

CHAPTER SUMMARY

This chapter has looked at the all-important health and safety, legislative, ethical, communication and sensitivity issues that underpin all aspects of sports therapy practice. If such professional standards are not maintained, problems will soon arise. All such regulations, rules and recommendations are made simply to protect the standing of the industry, the individual therapy businesses and all of their clients.

WEBSITE

Visit the companion website at www.thomsonlearning.co.uk/ healthandfitness/ward where you will find the answers to these questions for you to check your progress through the book.

Knowledge Review

1 Why are health, hygiene, safety, legal and ethical rules, regulations and recommendations so important?

2 List ten legal acts of relevance to the practice of sports therapy.

3 What benefits can a professional representative body offer its members?

4 What are the three basic categories of hazard?

5 In what ways can health and safety be encouraged in the workplace?

6 Why is working with cost-effectiveness important?

7 Describe the ideal professional image and attitude that the sports therapist should have.

8 How should the sports therapist respond to a client they suspect is a victim of abuse?

9 Why is security important in the workplace?

10 List ten contra-indications to sports therapy treatment.

11 Provide three examples of contra-actions.

12 In what ways can the effectiveness of therapeutic treatment be evaluated?

chapter 4

PHYSICAL ASSESSMENT TECHNIQUES

Learning Objectives

After reading this chapter you should be able to:

- understand the purpose, objectives and implications of physical assessment for sports therapy
- be aware of the equipment required to perform physical assessment
- be able to perform a basic physical assessment
- clearly record physical assessment findings

BACKGROUND, METHODS, OBJECTIVES AND EQUIPMENT

TIP

Biomechanics: the study of the posture, movement and physical functioning of the body. The influences upon an individual's biomechanical efficiency are multifactorial, but basically are physical, physiological and psychological.

Being able to assess the musculo-skeletal (biomechanical) system is crucial to providing sports therapy. The physical assessment for sports therapy follows on from the initial consultation, and takes place providing there are no particular concerns or contra-indications to the client's participation.

Performing a detailed physical (medical) assessment in order to form a full diagnosis can be a very complex process involving a wide selection of personnel, techniques, equipment and data gathering. Medical examination must be left to those with appropriate medical qualifications. Examinations and assessments of patients by medical personnel adhere to generally accepted and validated methods. The approach must, every time, be professionally (ethically) correct. The exact same applies to sports therapists when they are performing assessments.

Individuals with health concerns can normally be expected to visit their GP as their first port of call. The GP will listen to the patient, discuss and assess the problem, and make a decision for action. The patient, at this point, will probably be offered: advice and possibly some immediate treatment; prescription for medication; referral to a specialist (consultant or

COMMON BIOMEDICAL INVESTIGATIONS

Blood tests, e.g. cholesterol levels; urea levels; glucose levels; haematocrit levels (ratio of red blood cells to blood volume); haemoglobin levels; erythrocyte sedimentation rate (ESR, an indicator of rheumatoid arthritis); rheumatoid factor (antibody implicated in rheumatism).

Scans, e.g. plain/contrast X-ray; magnetic resonance imaging (MRI); computed tomography (CT); ultrasound.

Functional tests, e.g. electrocardiogram (ECG); electromyogram (EMG); electroencephalogram (EEG).

Biopsy (microscopic examination of extracted tissue).

Endoscopy (internal visual examination).

Arthroscopy (internal visual examination of a joint).

Spirometry (lung function tests).

Urinalysis.

Allergy tests.

practitioner). The GP is an expert in his business and is skilled in physical assessment.

Sometimes individuals will bypass their GP, and may choose to visit a physiotherapist or other allied professional in the first instance. Certain front-line health professionals are qualified to perform physical examination and assessment. The diagnosis reached may be straightforward, such as with a mild muscle strain, or it may be more complicated where further investigations are required.

Physical tests performed manually in the clinic, even though widely used and accepted, still often only provide the therapist with pointers and suspicions as to the full nature and severity of a problem. The sports therapist should not consider that they have the sole responsibility to make an absolute decision on the nature of the presenting problem, in fact, this is not their role at all. Suitably qualified medical personnel are responsible for forming a diagnosis, based upon all appropriate information. The patient acts upon the advice of the medical profession, and whether to begin or continue with conservative methods (therapy, exercise, diet, etc.), or possibly opt for medications or surgery, is a decision that they must make.

Whether working for a sports club or team, or fitness gym, there is always potential for injury or other emergency to occur. The sports therapist will often be the on-site (or on-field) person to deal with the administration of first aid or to help manage the situation. Should an injury occur during a game, the sports therapist will be expected to assess the nature and severity and take appropriate action (continue participation; stop participation; first aid; hospitalization).

The physical assessment alters somewhat in response to the individual's situation, which could be acute (on or off-field), post-acute (few days after incident) or chronic. It can be very comprehensive even though only using minimal equipment. It can be very exacting, identifying problems with

TIP

Diagnosis: to determine the definite nature of the presenting problem. A considered opinion based upon a series of assessment methods.

TIP

Differential diagnosis: during the initial stages of making a diagnosis, sometimes the clues may lead the practitioner to have to consider more than one possible diagnosis. For example, non-specific shoulder pain could result from a problematic cervical spine, rotator cuff tendonitis, from the gleno-humeral capsule or from any one of a number of other disorders. Further questions, assessments, monitoring, tests or scans usually moves the diagnosis on from being probable or provisional, to being conclusive.

TIP

Prognosis: the probable duration, progress and outcome of the presenting problem.

PHYSICAL ASSESSMENT TECHNIQUES

TIP	

Sign: an objective, physical finding that can be felt, heard or seen by the therapist during assessment (e.g. bleeding; swelling; malalignment).

TIP	✔

Symptom: a subjective finding provided by the subject relating to their perception of the problem (e.g. numbness; shooting pain; cold).

specific body parts. It can take between 5 and 30 minutes to run through the appropriate tests for a particular problem. A more comprehensive whole body physical assessment may take an hour or more if involving posture, **range of movement** (RoM), manual muscle testing and gait analysis. The physical assessment may also be linked with a fitness test to complete the picture, if the subject is able. (On and off-field injury assessments are discussed further in chapter 5.)

The physical assessment is combined with knowledge of the history of the client and all general observations made during the initial consultation. This then provides the therapist with the necessary information in order to offer the best advice, treatment and exercise. If the assessment reveals serious injury or leads the therapist to suspect certain problems, then they should tactfully inform the client and take appropriate action. Where the nature or severity of the injury or problem is beyond the sports therapist's boundaries of practice, the client must be recommended for medical investigation. As discussed in chapter 3, the sports therapist must be able to liaise well with other professionals, and act in their client's best interests. They must be alert to the intricacies of each presenting case.

> An expert is not the one who thinks they know everything and can treat everyone but the one who knows when to refer.
>
> JAMES BRIGGS (2001)

During the consultation and physical assessment, the sports therapist should be alert to the information provided by the client, and the signs and symptoms that could indicate the need for medical assessment or intervention.

SIGNS AND SYMPTOMS POSSIBLY INDICATING THE NEED FOR MEDICAL ADVICE

Malaise (feeling generally unwell).

Pallor (paleness) or cyanosis (bluish skin discoloration).

Nausea or vomiting.

Dizziness, vertigo, syncope (fainting) or seizure.

Visual or auditory disturbances.

Dyspnoea (difficult breathing).

Severe pain, radiating pain, constant pain or night pain.

Persistent or progressively worsening headache.

Widespread pain and tenderness.

Acutely distorted posture.

Bony malalignment or abnormal development.

Severe bruising or swelling.

Severe hypomobility (restricted movement).

Anaesthesia (numbness) or paraesthesia (pins and needles).

Unexplained extreme fatigue or weakness.

Flaccid (poor tone) or spastic (high tone) paralysis.

Unexplained recent muscle atrophy.

Extreme or rapid weight gain or loss.

Palpitations, abnormally fast, slow or erratic heart rate.

Angina (chest tightness and pain).

Hypertension (high blood pressure).

Psychosis (serious delusions, paranoia or schizophrenia), neurosis (apparent depression, anxiety, confusion or hypochondria).

Skin conditions (rashes, warts, lesions, itching and irritations).

Unusual lumps or thickening.

Enlarged lymph nodes.

Enlarged organs or glands (e.g. liver, spleen or thyroid).

Unexplained peripheral oedema.

Intermittent claudication (pain in legs when walking).

Persistent abdominal tenderness or pain.

Dysmenorrhoea (painful menstruation) or amenorrhoea (absence of menstruation).

Persistent dyspepsia (indigestion), constipation or diarrhoea.

Dysuria (painful urination), haematuria (blood in urine) or persistent incontinence.

Abnormal responses to any physical assessments.

Of course, if no assessment is performed at all, then the therapist cannot proceed safe in the knowledge that both they and the client are aware of the current presenting situation, nor can goals and objectives be properly set. In the main, physical assessment for sports therapy is based upon accepted orthopaedic principles of examination and is largely musculo-skeletal in focus. Once completed, the therapist should review, discuss and agree with the client, achievable objectives in light of the assessment findings.

During clinical physical assessment for sports therapy, the following methods and techniques are commonly employed:

- Discussion of medical history, current problems and objectives.
- Explanation of the proposed procedures to follow.
- Observation of body language, body type, postural alignments, body contours, muscle tone, RoM, gait, functional activities (activities of daily living: ADLs), and comparison of other, adjacent and contra-lateral body parts.
- Palpation of tissues (skin; fascia; muscles; tendons; ligaments; bones; joints; bursae; organs; glands).
- Measurement of height, weight, posture, RoM, strength, body circumferences, body fat, leg lengths, lung function.
- Performance of special tests. These include: neurological tests (sensations; reflexes; reactions); ligament stress tests; circulatory tests (heart rate; pulses; blood pressure); regional integrity tests (for specific muscles and joints).
- Inspection of footwear and sporting equipment.

Essential equipment for physical assessment includes:

- consultation form
- physical assessment form
- height measure scale
- calibrated weight scales
- tape measure
- goniometer/flexometer
- **dynamometer**
- **sphygmomanometer**/blood pressure monitor
- stethoscope
- plumb-line
- reflex hammer
- couch
- exercise mat.

Useful additional equipment includes:

- large (full height) mirror
- wall grid
- camera
- camcorder
- anthropometer
- computer with biomechanical software

THE VARIOUS OBJECTIVES OF PHYSICAL ASSESSMENT

To assess acute and post-acute injuries and chronic problems.

To assess postural problems.

To assess gait efficiency and identify problems.

To identify musculo-skeletal imbalances.

To measure major joint RoM, and compare against accepted norms and identify hyper- or hypomobility.

To assess muscle integrity, nerve supply and functional strength and flexibility.

To help identify problematic tissues.

To develop client awareness and understanding of how the body is put together, how muscles and joints work, and what is ideal for them.

To help the therapist formulate achievable objectives for the client.

To recommend specific action (sports therapy treatment; exercise; orthotic device).

To present specific relevant information to other health-care practitioners.

To provide a starting point to treatment.

To help improve sporting performance and reduce the potential for injury.

To help improve functional performance (movement; gait; breathing; circulation; appearance).

To monitor the client's progress and improvements when continuing on a programme of treatment and exercise.

TIP	

Observation: visual analysis and comparison of overall and specific appearance. Symmetry of the body, skin condition, muscle tone, structural components, general function and gait may all be normally observed. Some of the first things to observe include the client's sex, age bracket, body type, body language and behaviour, and any obvious distinguishing features. But it is very important not to judge or presume.

- isokinetic dynamometer
- treadmill.

The physical assessment is of use only if it is performed accurately and reliably. Accepted techniques can only be used to ensure validity. The practitioner must take great care to perform tests in the correct manner and record both the result of each test and also the particular technique utilized. Because a certain amount of physical assessment is performed with each visit of the client to the clinic, the tests must be performed in the same way each time, especially where there may be more than one therapist performing the assessments. If strictness is applied to the techniques of assessment, then monitoring of the client's progress can be reliably maintained.

Recording information relating to the client's history and presenting condition is crucial. In clear and simple terms, for whichever assessments, tests or measurements are being performed, the particular method, result and resultant analyses (the therapist's educated assessment) should all be documented. Once all appropriate assessments have taken place, the plan of action can be formulated.

BODY TYPES

Somatyping is the very basic categorization of people into the three body types (soma means body): ectomorph; mesomorph; or endomorph. This particular method of assessment was developed in the 1940s. Some authors have also described, perhaps controversially, relationships of **somatype** to personality type. For example, ectomorphs have been described as having a tendency to introversion or quiet thoughtfulness, mesomorphs as being more active, energetic people, and endomorphs as being more sociable and extrovert.

- A classic ectomorphic person is tall and slim, with long limbs. They tend to have difficulty gaining weight (muscle bulk or excessive body fat). These body types tend to fare better in sports such as distance running, cycling and high jump.
- The mesomorph is well proportioned and muscular. They tend to be able to gain muscle bulk more easily. They usually have broader shoulders and narrow waist, and are suited, or more adaptable, to most sports, especially football, hockey and sprinting.
- The typical endomorph is more rounded, stocky and shorter in stature, with a susceptibility to being overweight. Weight gain tends to be easy, weight loss difficult. Their sporting dominance is seen in rugby, wrestling, shot-put and discus.

Most people show aspects of each of the somatypes. The type of body an individual has is determined by various factors: sex; genetics; physiological functioning and metabolism; lifestyle; diet; activity levels. Their somatype does have an effect upon their functional abilities, posture and movement, and best choice of physical activities. Somatyping is by no means the only way to categorize the sporting performance potential of an individual, but it can provide rough pointers, and may also assist in the formulation of realistic goal setting.

HEIGHT, WEIGHT, BMI AND WHR

Height measurements are preferably performed with a sliding wall scale, without footwear. Weight scales must be accurately calibrated, and minimal clothing should be worn. Recording in metric (height in metres, weight in kilograms) is the most relevant method, although it may also be worth recording in imperial as well because some clients will be more familiar with that (height in feet and inches, weight in stones and pounds). Measurement conversions can be found in the appendix. Ideally, the therapist will develop his or her awareness of rough conversions, so as to be able to inform the client easily.

Body mass index (BMI) is a rather limited, but commonly used estimate of an individual's fatness. It was developed in America from two population surveys between 1960 and 1990. The simple formula takes the individual's weight (in kg) and divides this by their height (in m) squared:

BMI = Weight (kg)/Height^2 (m^2).

The resulting figure is then compared against a small scale of generalized norms:

- A BMI of around 20 is considered acceptable or average.
- A BMI of around 25 is considered overweight.
- A BMI of 30 or above is considered obese.

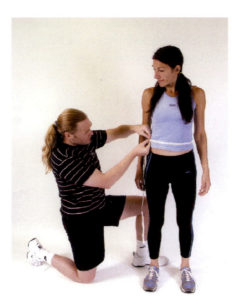 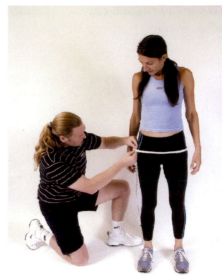

Waist measurement   Hip measurement

For example, an individual weighs 63 kg and is 1.73 m tall:

$$BMI = 63/1.73 \text{ m}^2$$
$$= 63/2.99$$
$$= 21$$
$$= \text{average and acceptable.}$$

Although a better indicator of obesity than weight alone, as it also takes into account the individual's height, the BMI formula does not make allowances for very muscular individuals (whose greater proportionate weight can be due to the fact that muscle tissue is heavier than fat), nor for the elderly with low muscle mass (where their BMI could be underestimated, and may appear to be inappropriately normal). Some authors have produced separate BMI tables for men, women and children.

The **waist to hip ratio** (WHR) helps to identify patterns of fat distribution in the upper and lower body. Waist circumference, measured just above the iliac crests across the umbilicus, in centimetres, is divided by hip circumference, measured at the widest point just above the level of the greater **trochanters**:

WHR = Waist (cm)/Hip (cm).

A WHR score of >0.8 for females and >0.9 for males is considered as a risk factor for coronary heart disease. Some authors have again produced charts which allow for sex (male and female) and age (young, middle-aged and elderly) to be taken into account, and for the level of risk to be gauged (low, moderate, high and very high risk). Additionally, a high waist measurement in relation to the hip measurement is also a cause for concern. The WHR score is prone to invalidity by the therapist's poor skill in technique, by inappropriate equipment or by client factors.

For example, a male's waist measurement is 100 cm, and hip measurement is 108 cm:

WHR = 100 cm/108 cm

    = 0.93

    = moderate risk.

A high BMI or WHR score is generally considered as a risk factor for coronary heart disease (CHD), hypertension, respiratory problems, musculo-skeletal disorders, metabolic disease (such as adult-onset diabetes) and other health-related problems, and is usually a reason to pursue other assessments and lifestyle evaluation.

Other methods used in the assessment of body fat and obesity include the measurement of specific skinfold sites and the resultant calculation of kilograms and percentages of body fat and lean body mass (LBM). There are also bioelectrical impedance methods and hydrostatic weighing techniques. Chapter 13 discusses these methods further.

BODY CIRCUMFERENCE MEASUREMENTS

Also known as girth measurements, body circumference measurements are useful in that they assess the size of body areas (trunk and limbs), determine patterns of fat distribution, allow for comparison against both contra-lateral limbs and generally accepted norms (as in WHR), and also enable tracking of changes to body shape in response to training (i.e. reductions in body fat and/or increases in muscle tone).

As with all tests and treatments, girth measurements should be taken with the absolute minimum of fuss and embarrassment to the client. It is usual to take the measurements from the side of the client, and for the therapist to position himself so that eyes are level with the tape. The tape measure itself should be both flexible and durable, and not stretch with repeated use. Specialized anthropometric tape measures are best. The tension of the tape, during measurement, should be tight enough to fit securely without indenting or compressing the skin and superficial tissues.

Anthropometers are sliding callipers that usefully allow for accurate measurements of bone and joint widths, and body breadths. They are useful for comparing limbs, especially at joints, and for monitoring changes to

---

BODY CIRCUMFERENCE MEASUREMENT SITES

Chest: at the level of the 4th intercostal space. Measured at the end of an expiration.

Waist: at the narrowest part of the torso, just above the iliac crests.

Hips: at the widest circumference, just above the greater trochanters.

Upper arms: at the mid-point between the acromion process and olecranon process, with arms hanging in a neutral, relaxed position.

Upper legs: at the mid-point between the lateral inguinal crease and the proximal patella, supine, with knee flexed to 90°.

Lower legs: at the widest circumference of the calf, sitting, with legs hanging freely.

body contours and posture. Examples of measurements taken using an anthropometer include: shoulder or biacromial width (the distance between the acromion processes); chest width; pelvic width; hip or bitrochanteric width (distance between the greater trochanters); distal femoral width; ankle width; distal humeral width; wrist width.

PALPATION

Palpation is therapeutic assessment of tissues by way of touch or feel, performed in the main by the hand, tip of thumb and fingertips. Palpation is a skill to develop, and is as much part of treatment as it is assessment. Indeed, during any treatment palpation continues to help the therapist monitor the effects of applied techniques and further develop their understanding of the presented condition. Palpation of tissues during initial assessment adds crucial diagnostic information to what the client has told the therapist. It should be performed systematically, so as to include all appropriate tissues, and it is obviously combined with close observation or inspection of the tissues. Palpation normally begins at a distance to a problem area, and gradually and carefully works its way in, both in terms of proximity and depth. The therapist should be careful to try to identify the problematic tissues and the severity of the problem without causing undue discomfort to the client or aggravation of the problem. An iatrogenic problem is one where a condition is worsened as a result of examination or treatment.

Before beginning palpation, the client should be informed and the affected tissues relaxed and supported. Gain feedback during assessment, and observe for facial expressions and other body language. Compare affected tissues with surrounding tissues and also contra-laterally. It is often a good idea to assess the non-affected side first, so as to have an idea of what is normal for the client.

The more superficial tissues lend themselves perfectly to palpation. These include: skin; subcutaneous fat; superficial fascia; muscles, tendons and ligaments, and their attachment sites; bones and bony prominences; joint lines; bursae; lymph nodes; some organs and glands; some superficial blood vessels and nerves. The therapist should try to develop their understanding of relative normality in tissues, so as to differentiate normal with what may be abnormal.

The signs and symptoms of problems in tissues revealed by palpation can be generalized, such as oedema or widespread tenderness. More usually, palpation is used to assess locally. An overworked or injured problematic muscle can commonly be palpably taut, dense and unyielding, probably tender to the touch (point tenderness), and perhaps with a 'twitch' response, which demonstrates the hypersensitivity of the tissue. There may be active or latent trigger points within the muscle tissue or surrounding fascia, which may refer their characteristic pattern of aching when pressed.

If there is a moderate partial tearing of the muscle (2nd degree strain), there will probably be a palpable indent in the tissue, possibly with a small lumpiness behind the indent. Muscle strains also often show ecchymosis (bruising and discoloration), which tracks below the injury site. A weak spot in a muscle is often its musculo-tendinous junction, a common site for tearing. Muscles may be palpated systematically along their length. Some muscles will not be accessible, while others will only be palpable in certain aspects and with specific positioning. The therapist should take their time feeling their way through the various fibres of a painful soft-tissue (muscle, tendon or ligament in particular), so as to identify the specific location of a micro-trauma. This localizing will obviously allow the correct and most direct treatment strategy to be formulated. Obviously, deep friction massage or ultrasound, for example, can be of any use only if directly applied to the affected tissues. Manual resisted muscle testing helps to complete the assessment of muscle tissue and differentiate between, for example, a muscle or a ligament injury.

Compartment syndrome is where the muscle bulk has become too great for the compartment in which it is housed. Circulation and nerve conduction can become impeded as the condition worsens. Commonly seen in the lower leg and forearm, it will show itself with tightness, swelling, pain on stretch, pins and needles, numbness and possibly absent peripheral pulses.

Tendonitis (inflammation of a tendon) often shows itself with distinct tenderness. **Tendinosis** is not always characterized by having gone through an inflammatory phase, and may be more likely to be a result of **collagen** (its predominant connective tissue) degeneration, with **adhesions** and poor quality blood vessels. It will demonstrate localized tenderness and thickening, possibly combined with swelling and crepitus. Paratendonitis (also teno**synovitis** or tenovaginitis) is a general term for the other common tendon overuse injuries, which generally affect the sheath surrounding the tendon itself. It is often associated with point tenderness, thickening and crepitus, and is therefore difficult to differentiate from tendinosis. Treatment strategies are often quite similar.

Look for how the layers of tissues move upon each other during palpation. Adhesions, a sticking together of normally separate tissues, often resulting from micro-trauma or from a general lack of suppleness, are commonly discovered within adjacent muscle fibres or their surrounding connective tissue fascia. **Scar tissue**, predominantly collagen fibres from injury repair, whether to muscle, tendon, ligament or skin, can also be felt as a lumpy knot in the affected tissue. The presence of adhesions or scar tissue is sometimes referred to as a fibrosis in the tissues.

Often areas of temperature changes are palpated, especially in comparison to adjacent or contra-lateral tissues. Increased warmth in an affected area is indicative of inflammation (as is point tenderness, redness, swelling and impaired functioning). Reduced temperature is more likely to be associated with a chronic problem or an impaired blood flow through a region. Over-activity of the sympathetic nervous system, for various reasons, can contribute to temperature changes as well as other abnormalities such as increased sudoriferous (sweat) gland activity.

Joints are obviously often in need of assessment. A dislocation is easily observed, but a subluxation (partial dislocation), with minimal deformity, may require more careful investigation. Try to develop a working knowledge of the normal contours of joint lines and **articulations**. Be aware that arthritic changes to joints include osteophyte (bony projection) formation, hard swelling, pain, crepitus, inflammation and reduced mobility. **Sprains** routinely show with swelling, which restricts movement, and ecchymosis, often inferior to the injured ligaments. Swelling often shows itself with less clearly defined contours over the superficial structures. Stress tests help to confirm assessment of ligaments.

Most fractures result from one traumatic incident and are assessed at the scene. They will usually show immediate pain and swelling, crepitus, deformity and possibly exposed bone ends. The pain from a fracture will normally increase with percussion (tapping on the suspected bone), vibration (using a tuning fork) and compression (from one end of the bone towards the other). The pain may decrease with distraction. A stress fracture, usually resulting from repetitive stress to the bone, often has a deep ache and will be distinctly tender in the affected region. **Periostitis** (inflammation of the outer membrane of bone), as in shin splints, usually has a more diffuse tenderness.

Bursae (fluid-filled sacs) are located around the body's joints, usually at sites where friction of moving parts needs to be minimized. They become irritated (inflamed) by repeated or excessive stress of movement or compression. Common sites for **bursitis** include the subacromial, olecranon, trochanteric, infra-patellar, ilio-tibial and calcaneal bursae, especially when related to biomechanical misalignment during repetitive activities. Classic bursitis presents itself with a smooth but distinct swelling, localized tenderness and pain.

Oedema is a swelling resulting from an abnormal accumulation of fluids within tissues. It can be local or general, acute or chronic. It can be lymph or synovial based. When there is bleeding within a joint capsule, it is referred to as a haemarthrosis. Oedema may result from problematic lymphatic drainage, trauma to tissues (such as a sprain) or, quite commonly, secondary to underlying pathology such as coronary heart disease or vascular disease, where the swelling often occurs at the ankles. 'Pitting' oedema is a boggy swelling, where finger pressure leaves an indent in the swollen tissue which remains for a few seconds after the pressure has been applied. Chronic oedema may be accompanied by thin, fragile skin and impaired sensation.

Various unusual lumps and other tissue abnormalities can often be discovered within the superficial tissues, and these need to be identified, possibly by medical personnel.

It is important to remember that there is often more than one tissue injured during any incident, and that palpation is a technique to be performed carefully. Palpation exercises such as feeling for a hair between layers of paper, or examining a specific body region with eyes closed can be very useful learning techniques.

POSTURE

Our posture is the skeletal alignment of our body. It is dynamic in that the muscles provide maintenance and movement of position to suit requirements. The force of gravity causes stress to the structures of posture:

Gravity places stress on the structures responsible for maintaining the body upright in a posture. For a weight-bearing joint to be stable, or in equilibrium, the gravity line of the mass must fall exactly through the axis of rotation, or there must be a force to counteract the force of gravity.

CAROLINE KISNER AND LYNN ALLEN COLBY (1996)

Good posture encourages good health. Improvements in body awareness are important to develop in clients. With good body awareness, care is taken in how we move, sit, lift, walk, run, work, play sport, drive and sleep. With the practice of good posture comes improved muscle tone and response, and muscle balance is generated. Ideal body alignment should always be encouraged. Good posture = balance. Poor posture = imbalance.

There are a basic series of requirements of the individual in order for them to be able to demonstrate ideal posture and perform efficient movements. These include optimal integrity of the muscles, bones, joints and skin, and a selection of sensory and motor mechanisms. The nervous system is obviously totally involved in our functional abilities. Crucial senses are visual, auditory, tactile and proprioceptive, each greatly influencing our movements. Perception is our ability to be aware of something (via our senses). Body awareness is the awareness of our self, positioning and movement, and spatial awareness is the awareness of our self in relation to the environment, distances and size. Cognition is the acquired knowledge and understanding that we have within us, which includes experience, memory, learning, adaptability, intuition and judgement. Emotions affect our mood, interest and motivation.

Therefore, when all things are considered, there are very many factors influencing our functioning. When all is in good order, then we may enjoy the ability to be able to balance, have focus, co-ordination and agility, good reactions and timing, endurance, strength and speed, suppleness and skill.

Most postural problems involve the postural muscles and the weight-bearing spine, pelvis and lower limbs and the associated joints.

Muscle imbalance occurs with skeletal malalignment: either can be the cause of the other. Muscle imbalance means that:

- some muscle groups tighten and shorten
- some muscle groups lengthen and weaken
- stress to the underlying tissues (ligaments; joints; nerves; blood vessels; bursae)
- musculo-skeletal stress results in deformities, stiffness and pain; maximum efficiency is lost
- ADLs become more difficult.

Structural postural abnormalities (as opposed to functional abnormalities) such as those resulting from congenital deformity, serious injury, disease processes or musculo-skeletal patterns that have become well set over many years will rarely be corrected by sports therapy. Improvements, however, and reduced suffering and worsening are often achieved via an increase in body awareness, guided remedial exercise and a course of massage therapy. Functional postural problems are mostly the result of muscle imbalance, and may sometimes lend themselves to complete correction.

TIP

Good posture is important because it:

- maintains muscle balance
- improves body shape and appearance
- prevents muscle tension and spasm
- prevents undue stresses on joints
- prevents skeletal deformities and the associated pain
- provides for good breathing technique
- improves efficiency of the circulatory system
- improves working and sporting performance
- reduces the risk of musculo-skeletal injuries
- promotes healthy ageing.

COMMON CAUSES OF POSTURAL PROBLEMS

Congenital deformities (which are not always known).

Injury.

Physical defects (e.g. poor eyesight or hearing can cause habitual postural tilting).

Sedentary lifestyle (can lead to muscle atrophy and low resistance to gravity).

Inappropriate or excessive exercise (can lead to muscle imbalance, e.g. excessive resistance work to the chest muscles can lead to rounding of the shoulders).

Lack of flexibility training (can lead to chronic shortening of certain muscles).

Occupation (repetitive work can lead to muscle imbalance).

Poor ergonomics (ergonomics is the assessment of the efficiency of the individual to their working or resting positions, and the resultant optimization of work stations, equipment and furniture).

Disease and degenerative processes (e.g. arthritis, osteoporosis, asthma, neurological disorders).

Lengthy periods of illness or recovery from surgery (can lead to muscle atrophy and weakness).

Emotional disturbance (e.g. depression, low self-esteem, stress, worry or anxiety).

Inappropriate clothing (e.g. high heels; tight shoes).

Certain sports (e.g. gymnasts can be prone to lordotic postures and hypermobility).

Pregnancy (postural changes occur during the middle stage of pregnancy, particularly stresses to the lumbo-sacral region).

Being overweight (additional stresses are placed upon the weight-bearing bones and joints and restricted RoM can occur).

Being tall (this can cause the individual to develop a forward head and kyphosis of the thoracic region).

Chronic fatigue and weakness.

Poor nutrition (eating disorders or a nutrient depleted diet can lead to a variety of musculo-skeletal problems).

Poor body awareness and postural habits generally when sitting, standing, walking, carrying, lifting, pulling, etc.

Failure to consult a therapist when problems begin to manifest (and to take appropriate action).

TIP

The main postural muscles are:

- erector spinae group
- sternocleidomastoid
- deep abdominals
- iliopsoas
- gluteus maximus
- quadriceps
- hamstrings
- gastrocnemius and soleus
- tibialis anterior.

Postural muscles are responsible for the support of the body in gravity. They have a greater proportion of Type I fibres and are slower to contract but less prone to fatigue than phasic muscles. They tend to shorten and increase their tension when under strain and are more prone to cramp and trigger point development.

A plumb-line (a suspended, weighted-string), full-height mirror or wall grid are all very helpful when assessing posture. It is normal to assess standing posture from the front (anterior view), from behind (posterior view) and from both sides (left and right lateral views). Postural assessment enables the therapist to see which particular body regions are away from the norm. It is important to remember that the client's overall structure is formed from a series of related segments. The client should wear minimal clothing and have bare feet for postural assessment. During anterior and posterior **plumb-line assessment**, the client is asked to stand, upright but relaxed, close to the line with the feet equal distances from the line. In the lateral view, the client stands close with the line just anterior to the lateral

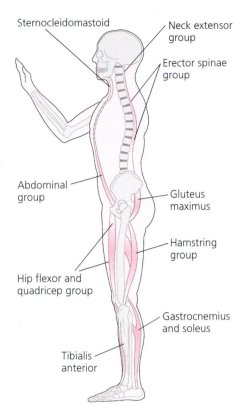

- Sternocleidomastoid
- Neck extensor group
- Erector spinae group
- Abdominal group
- Gluteus maximus
- Hip flexor and quadricep group
- Hamstring group
- Gastrocnemius and soleus
- Tibialis anterior

Main postural muscles

TIP ✔

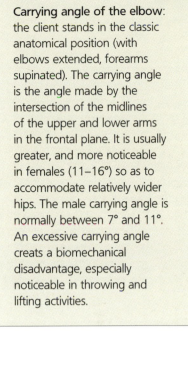

Carrying angle of the elbow: the client stands in the classic anatomical position (with elbows extended, forearms supinated). The carrying angle is the angle made by the intersection of the midlines of the upper and lower arms in the frontal plane. It is usually greater, and more noticeable in females (11–16°) so as to accommodate relatively wider hips. The male carrying angle is normally between 7° and 11°. An excessive carrying angle creats a biomechanical disadvantage, especially noticeable in throwing and lifting activities.

malleolus. All points are assessed in reference from the base point of support because this is the only fixed part of the standing posture. The therapist should be prepared to assume different positions to assess the client's posture, so as to get as good a perspective as is possible.

Deviations from what can be considered ideal arise for a multitude of reasons. There are many relatively common postural deviations, conditions or types that can be both described and viewed.

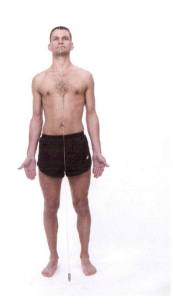

Anterior postural assessment

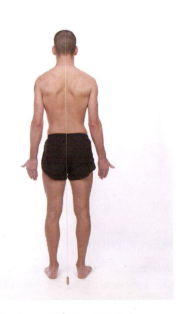

Posterior postural assessment

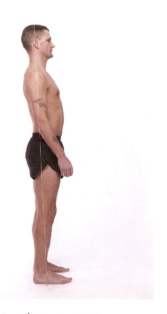

Lateral postural assessment

IDEAL POSTURAL ALIGNMENTS

Head and neck

The lateral plumb-line should travel through the ear down to the acromion process.

The posterior plumb-line travels midway through the occiput and cervical spinous processes.

The anterior plumb-line travels midway through the head and face.

Shoulder

The lateral plumb-line should pass through the acromion process and head of the humerus.

The posterior plumb-line should fall midway between the scapulae.

The anterior plumb-line travels midway down through the neck to the manubrium of the sternum.

Thoracic region

The lateral plumb-line should travel midway through the upper trunk.

The posterior plumb-line should travel through the thoracic spinous processes.

The anterior plumb-line should travel through the sternum and xiphoid process.

Lumbar region

The lateral plumb-line should travel midway through the trunk.

The posterior plumb-line should travel through the lumbar spinous processes.

The anterior plumb-line should travel midway through the middle of the torso.

Pelvis and hip

The lateral plumb-line should travel just anterior to the sacro-iliac joint and through the greater trochanter.

The posterior plumb-line travels through the middle of the sacrum and gluteal cleft (as the iliac crests, gluteal folds and greater trochanters are seen to be level).

The anterior plumb-line should travel midway through the pelvis (public symphasis).

Knee

The lateral plumb-line travels slightly anterior to the middle of the knee.

The posterior plumb-line should be midway between the knees.

The anterior plumb-line should be midway between the knees.

Ankle and foot

The lateral plumb-line travels just anterior to the lateral malleolus.

The posterior plumb-line should be midway between the medial malleoli.

The anterior plumb-line should be midway between the medial malleoli.

TIP

Remember that postural problems can result from congenital deformities, disease processes, musculo-skeletal injuries or simply bad postural and working habits.

Remember that sometimes just the slightest but certain and specific malalignment, whether it occurs in an accident or over a period of time, can result in a great deal of discomfort and poor function. It is easy to stress a problematic unprepared under-conditioned body. Once problems have begun, further problems often ensue: movements become painful, restricted and compensatory, and the vicious circle continues.

Where there are found to be deviations from the norm, they should be double-checked and then recorded. Range of motion testing and gait analysis help to complete the basic biomechanical picture.

COMMON POSTURAL DEVIATIONS, CONDITIONS AND TYPES

Forward head, where the head is situated more anteriorly to the plumb-line in the sagittal plane. This posture is often in conjunction with rounded shoulders and an exaggerated cervical lordosis.

Excessive cervical lordosis, in the sagittal plane.

Flattened or reduced lordotic cervical curve, in the sagittal plane.

Head tilt, where the head sits more to one side, in the frontal plane.

Head rotated, where the head is rotated to either side, in the transverse plane.

Clavicle asymmetry, where the relative position or shape of the clavicles varies. Causes include: subluxation (usually presenting with a prominent sterno-clavicular/acromio-clavicular, SC/AC, joint); old fracture of the clavicle; osteoarthritis (with prominent AC joint).

Rounded (forward) shoulders, where the acromion process is seen to lie anterior to the plumb-line, in the lateral view. There may be kyphosis, and the scapulae may possibly be abducted or protracted.

Dropped or elevated shoulder, where one shoulder is lower or higher than the other. This can result from a dominant handedness (dominant shoulder may be lower), scoliosis, pelvic tilt or short-leg.

Medial rotation of shoulder. This posture can sometimes be detected by the relative position of the distal humerus, as the medial epicondyle may be situated more posteriorly than medially.

Lateral rotation of shoulder. This posture can sometimes be detected by the relative position of the distal humerus, where the olecranon process of the ulna is seen to face more posteriorly.

Cubitus valgus. The carrying angle of the elbow is significantly greater than normal.

Cubitus varus. The carrying angle of the elbow is significantly less than normal.

Cubitus recurvatus. There is hyperextension of the elbow joint.

Adducted scapulae. The shoulder blades are closer to the thoracic vertebrae.

Abducted scapulae. The scapulae are further away from the midline. This posture is often seen with rounded shoulders and kyphosis.

Winging scapula(e). The medial border of the scapula is more prominent (it is especially noticeable when in the press-up position). The commonest cause of this posture is weakness of the serratus anterior.

Kyphosis. In the lateral view, there is seen to be an exaggeration of the normally kyphotic thoracic spine. An increased posterior convexity, accompanied by other deviations such as excessive cervical lordosis or as part of a general swayback posture.

Funnel chest (pectus excavatum), where the sternum is depressed and the ribs and costal cartilages curve inwards.

Barrel chest, where there is an increase in the overall diameter of the rib cage.

Pigeon chest (pectus carinatum), where the sternum protrudes forwards.

Scoliosis. In the posterior view, the spinous processes are not seen to be in alignment (there is a rotational deviation). Often showing an S-shaped curve, it is usually part of a sequence of related biomechanical abnormalities such as with a true or apparent leg-length discrepancy. Shoulders and/or pelvis are normally seen to be unequal. A scoliosis also is often described as being structural (with bone abnormalities) or functional (with soft-tissue shortening).

Lordosis. An increase in the normal lumbar curve is seen in the lateral view. Increased lumbo-sacral angle, an anterior pelvic tilt, hyper-extension of the lumbar spine, a sagging abdomen and hyper-flexion of the hips are all possibly observed.

Swayback. The pelvis is seen to be positioned more anteriorly than normal in the lateral view. This usually results in hyper-extension of the hip, exaggerated lumbar lordosis, and an increased kyphosis, with forward head. Often a result of weakened postural muscles and bad (lazy) postural habits.

Flat back. A reduced curvature in the lumbar region, possibly with posterior pelvic tilt and decreased lumbo-sacral angle. The upper kyphotic curve of the back can also sometimes be seen to be flattened.

Anterior pelvic tilt. The anterior superior iliac spines (ASISs) are observed to be more anterior to the symphasis pubis, in the lateral view. This posture is associated with an increased lumbar lordosis.

Posterior pelvic tilt. The symphasis pubis is seen to be more anterior to the ASISs, in the lateral view. This posture is associated with a flat back.

Lateral pelvic tilt. In the anterior and posterior views, the pelvis is seen to be higher on one side than the other. It may result from a leg-length discrepancy or structural changes of the pelvis.

Pelvic rotation. The pelvis is deviated in the transverse plane. It may be unilateral or bilateral. The plumb-line does not pass level with the gluteal cleft. It may be a lateral or medial rotation. The patellae may be seen to be facing more inward with medial rotation, or more outward with lateral rotation.

Coxa valga. An excessive angulation of the femoral head to its shaft (greater than 135°). Can result in genu vara of the knee. Difficult to assess, but can explain the reason for some postural abnormalities.

Coxa vara. A reduced angulation of the femoral head to its shaft (less than 120°). Leads into genu valgus of the knee. Difficult to assess manually.

Hip (femoral) anteversion. The forward angle of the femoral trochanters relative to the condyles is excessive (greater than 16°). Usually leads to increased Q (quadricep) angle, genu valgus and 'squinting patellae'. Difficult to assess.

Hip (femoral) retroversion. The forward angle of the femoral trochanters relative to the condyles is reduced (less than 13°). May result in a toe-out gait. Difficult to assess.

Genu varus (bow legs). As the knees are further apart, the lateral angle of the femur to the tibia is reduced. Can sometimes be unilateral. Commonly results from hip pathology (such as arthritis) or malalignment.

Genu valgus (knock-knees). The knees angle more inwards from the hips (i.e. increased lateral angle of the tibia relative to the femur). Females have a natural tendency towards increased genu valgus due to having relatively wider hips.

Genu recurvatum. The knees are seen to be hyper-extended in the lateral view, and the gravitational stresses are anterior to the joint's axis.

Patella alta. Where the patella is naturally situated higher (more superiorly) on its femoral groove than normal. It is usually more prone to instability.

Patella baja. Where the patella is lower (more inferior) in relation to the femur than normal. Less common.

Internal tibial torsion. The tibia is twisted or torsioned along its length (longitudinal axis) so that the foot or feet face directly forwards or inwards. Gives appearance of pigeon toes, and toeing in. Normally the feet angle outwardly with an external torsion of around 25° (during gait this is referred to as the foot angle). Having the subject sit with lower legs hanging freely typically assesses the amount of tibial torsion. Allowances must be made for the pull of such muscles as the peroneals and dorsiflexors, and also the structure and position of the tarsal bones, which also have an influence upon foot angle.

External tibial torsion. The tibia is twisted or torsioned along its length so that the foot or feet face excessively outwards (more than 25°), causing an exaggerated toeing out stance.

Tibial valgus. An outward curving of the tibia from its proximal to distal end, observed in the frontal plane.

Tibial varus. An inward curving of the tibia along its length, observed in the frontal plane.

Pes planus (flat foot). The medial longitudinal arch is reduced, is not providing much in the way of stability, and is hypermobile. Usually results in over-pronation during gait and poor shock absorption.

Pes cavus. High arching of the foot. Usually means a more tight or rigid foot, with poor shock absorption, hypomobility, claw toes and callus formation (hardened areas of skin).

Hindfoot/rearfoot valgus (valgus heels). In posterior view, the calcaneal (heel) bone is seen to be situated in an everted position (facing outwards slightly), meaning that the heel rolls out laterally during gait. The Achilles tendon will curve outwards at its distal section. There may also be pes planus with excessive pronation.

Hindfoot/rearfoot varus (varus heels). The calcaneum is observed to be situated in an inverted position (facing inwards slightly). The heel, therefore, rolls inwards medially during gait. There may also be pes cavus and general rigidity.

Forefoot valgus. Where the metatarsal (forefoot) region has an eversion misalignment (laterally raised), often part of an over-supinating syndrome.

Forefoot varus. Where the metatarsal region has an inversion misalignment (medially raised), often part of an over-pronating syndrome.

Hallux valgus. Prominent medial (valgus) deviation of the first metatarsophalangeal (mtp) joint. Quite common, and sometimes the second phalanx is forced up over its adjacent toes. A bunion (chronic bursitis) can form due to repeated friction on footwear.

Hallux rigidus. Stiffness and pain at the first mtp joint, usually of arthritic causation. Compensatory gait patterns normally follow, mainly because of a painful propulsion.

Splay foot. Where there is a widening across the forefoot. Sometimes associated with hallux valgus and pes cavus.

Claw toes. Hyperextended mtp joints, with hyperflexed interphalangeal (itp) joints. Often related to pes cavus.

Hammertoes. Like claw toes, in that there is hyperextension of the mtp joints, and flexion deformity of the proximal itp joints. The distal phalanx, however, is usually in a neutral position.

Plantar flexed first ray. The 'first ray' of the foot is the line made by the first metatarsal and phalanges leading to the hallux. When plantar flexed, it is angled downwards in relation to the other metatarsals. It may be a structural congenital deformity, and may occur with hindfoot varus or pes cavus. Supination of the foot, during gait, usually follows to compensate.

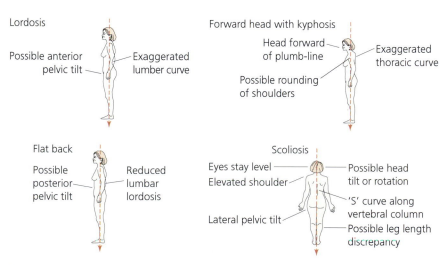

Postural problems

RANGES OF MOVEMENT

Joint movements are important to understand. Beyond awareness of which movements are normally available at each major joint (flexion, extension, rotation, etc.), the therapist needs to have knowledge of what is the normal RoM.

RoM norms provide a general guide to assessment. Do allow a few degrees either side of the stated norms, especially if the discrepancy is observed bilaterally (on both sides of the body). Marked restricted movement should encourage the therapist to further investigate the affected tissues, and to consider the possible causes (e.g. pain; arthritic changes; subluxation; muscle spasm; hypertonicity; swelling). The therapist should try to refine their skills in assessing the tensions, restrictions and qualities presented at joints at the end-range of passive movements. The soft-tissue *ease-bind* and joint *end-feel* twin concepts can assist with the therapist's assessment strategy.

The ease-bind assessment concept relates to the amount of easy, painless stretch (ease) available in the soft-tissues, and the point during passive movement (transition point) at which tissue tension or resistance (bind) sets in. Observation combined with palpation and client feedback provides the relevant information. Having an awareness of this concept helps the therapist to gauge the affected region's functional quality of movement.

RANGE OF MOVEMENT NORMS

Cervical
Flexion, 45°, hyperextension 45°, rotation 75°, lateral flexion 50°

Shoulder
Flexion 170°, hyperextension 50°, abduction 175°, adduction 180°, medial rotation 75°, lateral rotation 90°, horizontal abduction 30°, horizontal adduction 120°

Elbow
Flexion 145°, extension 145°–0°

Forearm (radio-ulnar)
Pronation 90°, supination 85°

Wrist
Flexion 85°, hyperextension 75°, adduction (radial deviation) 25°, abduction (ulnar deviation) 30°

Hip
Flexion 125°, hyperextension 20°, abduction 45°, adduction 25°, medial rotation 45°, lateral rotation 45°

Knee
Flexion 130°, extension 130°–0°

Ankle
Dorsiflexion 20°, plantarflexion 45°

Foot
Inversion 30°, eversion 25°

The end-feel of a joint is how the therapist perceives the point at which the full available passive range of movement is ended at a particular joint, and can be a useful assessment method. Common end-feels include: hard (bone onto bone); springy (mechanical blockage inside the joint); yielding (soft-tissue approximation); elastic (muscular tension restricting further movement). In normal health, a joint will have a typical end-feel, the type of which is dictated by its anatomical structure. When there are malalignments, muscle imbalances, arthritic degeneration or injuries the quality of end-feel may alter.

Hypermobility should also be assessed, as this can often be problematic. Where excessive joint motion is noted, such as in knee or elbow hyperextension, the number of degrees beyond normal should be recorded. Be aware that older clients will normally demonstrate more restrictive ranges of movement.

Ranges of movement are commonly measured with a **goniometer**. Therapists with a keen eye will, with experience, be able to assess some of the ranges simply by observation. Some body movements, such as the thoracic and lumbar movements, are perhaps best measured with a tape measure.

A goniometer (or arthrometer) is a standard piece of orthopaedic equipment, similar to a basic protractor. It is used to assess joint ranges of movement. There are several different types. The commonest is the inexpensive two-armed clear plastic goniometer, which comes in different sizes suited to measuring different joints. It consists of two arms: one is normally stationary, and the other is moved as the joint moves. The body of the goniometer is the protractor, which has the complete 360° scale marked upon it. The axis (centre) of the goniometer is also the intersection of the two arms, and is placed over the main axis of the joint's movement.

TIP
A goniometer is useful for measuring joint ranges of movement, as well as particular structural angles of the body, for example the carrying angle of the elbow and the Q angle of the knee.

Basic principles of goniometry

- Most sagittal plane measurements have the goniometer aligned to the lateral side of the joint. Frontal plane movements are measured anteriorly or posteriorly. Transverse plane measurements are usually taken superiorly or inferiorly.
- The therapist should explain the procedure to the client and decide whether an active or passive measurement is to be recorded.
- Estimate expected RoM prior to measurement (this helps the therapist position both the client and goniometer, and helps minimize the possibility of causing undue discomfort or recording a faulty measurement).
- The movement being measured is performed (passively or actively) carefully once or twice.
- The therapist should view the goniometer at eye level.
- Align the goniometer correctly.
- Any limitations to the starting positions should be recorded.
- Try to stabilize the body from unwanted movements.

- Record whether the measurement was an active or passive movement, and any particular information relating to the quality of movement and end-feel (e.g. painful; bony; springy; yielding; crepitus).
- Using the correct techniques each time ensures that results are reliable and valid.

Sometimes it is easier and more appropriate to record a range of movement in centimetres. The thoracic and lumbar regions are normally assessed as a combined unit which is what, structurally and functionally, they are. Using a tape measurement taken from specific bony landmarks before and after movement is a straightforward method. Some movements, such as trunk (thoraco-lumbar) rotation, are sometimes best recorded from observation.

Range of movement assessment techniques

Cervical

Flexion
Normal RoM: 45°.
Position: sitting.
Axis: centre of ear.
Stationary arm: 90° to the floor.
Moving arm: parallel to inferior border of nose.
Alternatives: measure distance from occiput to C7 with tape measure (record the difference between start and end position). Functionally, observe to see if chin can touch sternum.
Notes: stabilize trunk and shoulders. Flexion of the cervical region can occur through the whole region, or with more emphasis upon the upper region. Observe for segmental restrictions.

Hyperextension
Normal RoM: 45°.
Position: sitting.
Axis: centre of ear.
Stationary arm: 90° to the floor.
Moving arm: parallel to inferior border of nose.
Alternatives: measure distance from chin to sternum (record the difference between start and end position).
Notes: stabilize trunk and shoulders. Observe for segmental restrictions.

Rotation
Normal RoM: 75°.
Position: sitting.
Axis: over centre of top of head.
Stationary arm: point towards acromion process.
Moving arm: point towards nose.
Alternatives: measure distance from chin to acromion process (record the difference between start and end position).
Notes: stabilize trunk and shoulders. Compare left with right. Observe for segmental restrictions.

Lateral flexion

Normal RoM: 50°.
Position: sitting.
Axis: C7.
Stationary arm: along the thoracic spinous processes.
Moving arm: towards the occipital protuberance.
Alternatives: measure distance from mastoid process to acromion process (record the difference between start and end position).
Notes: stabilize trunk and shoulders. Observe for segmental restrictions.

Thoracic and lumbar

Flexion

Normal RoM: around 10 cm.
Position: standing.
Notes: measure distance from C7 to S1 (record the difference between start and end position).
Alternatives: measure 'lumbar excursion' from L1 to S1 (record the difference between start and end position) normally around 5 cm.
Be aware and allow for the additional influence the hip and thigh muscles have on this movement. Observe for segmental restrictions or **scoliosis**.

Hyperextension

Normal RoM: around 5 cm.
Position: standing.
Notes: measure distance from C7 to S1 (record the taut difference between start and end position, shortening the tape to take the measurement).
Alternatives: can be performed in the prone, supported position.
Be aware and allow for the additional influence the abdominal and anterior hip muscles have on this movement. Observe for segmental restrictions.

Lateral flexion

Position: standing, hands resting on side of thigh.
Notes: measure distance from tip of middle finger to lateral malleolus (record the difference between start and end position). Compare left with right. Observe for segmental restrictions and smoothness of movement, by looking at the contours of the spinous processes and erector spinae muscles. Avoid trunk rotation and thigh movement.

Rotation

Position of client: standing, therapist stabilizing the pelvis.
Notes: the client is asked to turn trunk and shoulders around to the left and to the right. The therapist observes and records the quality of movement, and compares the two. Most of the rotation occurs at the thoracic region.
Alternatives: the client can be seated, which stabilizes the pelvis. In sitting, a goniometer can be aligned over the centre of the top of the head, with both stationary and moving arms in line with the acromion process. Around 45° is the norm.

Shoulder

Flexion

Normal RoM: 170°.

Position: supine, hips and knees flexed, elbow extended, palm and forearm pronated.

Axis: through head of humerus.

Stationary arm: in line with midline of lateral trunk.

Moving arm: along lateral midline of upper arm.

Notes: compare left with right.

Hyperextension

Normal RoM: 50°.

Position: supine, elbow flexed, lying at the side of the couch, with arm able to freely move off the side.

Axis: through head of humerus.

Stationary arm: in line with midline of lateral trunk.

Moving arm: along lateral midline of upper arm.

Notes: compare left with right.

Alternatives: prone or sitting, elbow flexed.

Abduction

Normal RoM: 175°.

Position: supine, hips and knees flexed, arm in anatomical position.

Axis: through head of humerus.

Stationary arm: parallel to sternum, over lateral side of chest.

Moving arm: anterior aspect of upper arm, parallel to midline of humerus.

Notes: avoid shoulder elevation. Compare left with right. Be aware that the first 90° is mostly gleno-humeral movement, and the second phase is mainly scapulo-thoracic movement.

Alternatives: prone, sitting.

Adduction

Normal RoM: 180°–0°.

Position: as for abduction.

Axis: as for abduction.

Stationary arm: as for abduction.

Moving arm: as for abduction.

Notes: record any restriction or pain in adduction. Compare left with right.

Medial rotation

Normal RoM: 75°.

Position: supine, hips and knees flexed, shoulder abducted to 90°, elbow flexed to 90°, forearm in neutral.

Axis: olecranon process.

Stationary arm: parallel to top of couch.

Moving arm: along ulna border.

Notes: stabilize shoulder. Compare left with right.

Alternatives: prone, with elbow flexed over table. Excessive medial rotation of the shoulder can also be observed by assessing the client in standing, with arms hanging relaxed. The relative position of the medial **epicondyle** is noted. If directed more posteriorly, it is in greater rotation.

Lateral rotation

Normal RoM: 90°.
Position: as for medial rotation.
Axis: as for medial rotation.
Stationary arm: as for medial rotation.
Moving arm: as for medial rotation.
Notes: as for medial rotation. Excessive lateral rotation of the shoulder can also be observed by assessing the client in standing, with arms hanging relaxed. The relative position of the olecranon process is noted. If directed more medially, it is in greater rotation.

Horizontal abduction

Normal RoM: 30°.
Position: as for horizontal adduction.
Axis: as for horizontal adduction.
Stationary arm: as for horizontal adduction.
Moving arm: as for horizontal adduction.
Notes: as for horizontal adduction.

Horizontal adduction

Normal RoM: 120°.
Position: sitting, shoulder abducted to 90° and internally rotated, elbow flexed to 90°.
Axis: above acromion process.
Stationary arm: along midline of shoulder towards the neck.
Moving arm: along midline of upper arm.
Notes: avoid trunk rotation. Compare left with right.
Alternatives: supine.

Elbow

Flexion

Normal RoM: 145°.
Position: supine, arm in anatomical position.
Axis: lateral epicondyle.
Stationary arm: along lateral midline of upper arm.
Moving arm: along lateral midline of forearm.
Notes: compare left with right.
Alternatives: standing, sitting.

Extension

Normal RoM: 145°–0°.
Position: as for flexion.
Axis: as for flexion.
Stationary arm: as for flexion.
Moving arm: as for flexion.

Notes: record any restrictions in extension, or the degree of hyperextension. Compare left with right.
Alternatives: standing, sitting.

Carrying angle

Normal angle: Male 7–11°, Female 11–16°.
Position: standing.
Axis: middle of cubital (elbow) crease.
Arm 1: along midline of upper arm.
Arm 2: along midline of lower arm.
Notes: compare left with right. The female carrying angle is normally naturally wider.
Alternatives: supine.

Forearm (radio-ulnar)

Pronation

Normal RoM: 90°.
Position: sitting, elbow flexed to 90°, upper arm held close to trunk, forearm resting on couch, thumb extended.
Axis: just lateral to the ulnar styloid process.
Stationary arm: in line with thumb.
Moving arm: in line with thumb.
Notes: avoid shoulder or trunk movement. Compare left with right.

Supination

Normal RoM: 85°.
Position: as for pronation.
Axis: as for pronation.
Stationary arm: as for pronation.
Moving arm: as for pronation.
Notes: as for pronation.

Wrist

Flexion

Normal RoM: 85°.
Position: sitting, elbow flexed, forearm resting on couch in pronation, hand off couch.
Axis: lateral wrist.
Stationary arm: lateral midline of ulna.
Moving arm: lateral midline of 5th metacarpal.
Notes: avoid elbow extension. Compare left with right.

Hyperextension

Normal RoM: 75°.
Position: sitting, elbow flexed, forearm resting on couch in pronation.
Axis: as for flexion.
Stationary arm: as for flexion.
Moving arm: as for flexion.
Notes: avoid elbow flexion. Compare left with right.

Adduction (radial deviation)

Normal RoM: 25°.

Position: sitting, elbow flexed, forearm resting on couch in pronation.

Axis: over centre of wrist.

Stationary arm: along dorsal midline of forearm.

Moving arm: along dorsal midline of 3rd metatarsal.

Notes: avoid elbow movement. Compare left with right.

Abduction (ulnar deviation)

Normal RoM: 30°.

Position: as for adduction.

Axis: as for adduction.

Stationary arm: as for adduction.

Moving arm: as for adduction.

Notes: as for adduction.

Hip

Flexion

Normal RoM: 125°.

Position: supine.

Axis: greater trochanter.

Stationary arm: parallel to midline of trunk.

Moving arm: lateral midline of femur.

Notes: allow knee to flex. Keep contra-lateral limb extended to control posterior pelvic tilt, but differentiate for any flexion deformity (restricted normal extension).

Hyperextension

Normal RoM: 20°.

Position: prone, knee extended.

Axis: as for flexion.

Stationary arm: as for flexion.

Moving arm: as for flexion.

Notes: compare left with right.

Alternatives: side-lying, lower (non-tested) leg flexed for support.

Abduction

Normal RoM: 45°.

Position: supine.

Axis: anterior superior iliac spine (ASIS).

Stationary arm: pointed towards contra-lateral ASIS.

Moving arm: along midline of thigh.

Notes: avoid pelvic tilt. Compare left with right.

Alternatives: abduction can also be assessed with hip flexion to 90°.

Adduction

Normal RoM: 25°.

Position: supine, non-tested leg either flexed and crossed over tested leg, or passively abducted to allow full RoM.

Axis: as for abduction.
Stationary arm: as for abduction.
Moving arm: as for abduction.
Notes: as for abduction.
Alternatives: adduction can also be assessed with hip flexion to 90°.

Medial rotation
Normal RoM: 45°.
Position: prone.
Axis: through centre of femoral shaft.
Stationary arm: parallel to couch.
Moving arm: along tibial crest.
Notes: avoid hip adduction. Compare left with right.
Alternatives: supine, knees flexed, hanging off couch, or with hips flexed to 90°. Rotation can also be assessed with legs extended.

Lateral rotation
Normal RoM: 45°.
Position: as for medial rotation.
Axis: as for medial rotation.
Stationary arm: as for medial rotation.
Moving arm: as for medial rotation.
Notes: avoid hip abduction. Compare left with right.
Alternatives: as for medial rotation.

Knee

Flexion
Normal RoM: 130°.
Position: prone.
Axis: lateral epicondyle of femur.
Stationary arm: along lateral midline of thigh.
Moving arm: along lateral midline of lower leg.
Notes: record any restrictions from normal extension.
Alternatives: supine, hip flexed to 90°.

Extension
Normal RoM: 130–0°.
Position: prone.
Axis: as for flexion.
Stationary arm: as for flexion.
Moving arm: as for flexion.
Notes: record any restrictions to normal extension.
Alternatives: any excessive hyperextension (genu recurvatum) can be assessed by having the lower leg extended off the end of the couch.

Q (quadriceps) angle
Normal Q angle: Male 10–15°, Female 12–19°.
Position: supine.
Axis: centre of patella.

Arm 1: on a line running from centre of patella to ASIS.
Arm 2: on a line running from tibial **tuberosity** to centre of patella and beyond.
Notes: the Q angle is the angle of quadriceps pull on the patella, and is also influenced by both hip and lower leg alignments. The female Q angle is normally naturally wider. An excessive Q angle is implicated in maltracking of the patella. Compare left with right.

Ankle

Dorsiflexion
Normal RoM: 20°.
Position: supine, knee flexed on cushion to 25°.
Axis: lateral malleolus.
Stationary arm: along the lateral lower leg.
Moving arm: along lateral aspect of 5th metatarsal.
Notes: avoid inversion or eversion. An equinus deformity is a restricted dorsiflexion. Compare left with right.

Plantarflexion
Normal RoM: 45°.
Position: supine, knee extended.
Axis: as for dorsiflexion.
Stationary arm: as for dorsiflexion.
Moving arm: as for dorsiflexion.
Notes: compare left with right.

Foot

Inversion
Normal RoM: 30°.
Position: supine, knee extended, ankle relaxed.
Axis: over dorsal surface of foot, midway between the malleoli.
Stationary arm: along crest of tibia.
Moving arm: along dorsal surface of 2nd metatarsal.
Notes: avoid lower leg movement. Allow some plantarflexion. Compare left with right. Most inversion occurs through the subtalar and midtarsal joints; however, when the foot is in plantarflexion, the ankle joint also contributes. Therefore, to isolate assessment of the subtalar and midtarsal joints, it may be appropriate to do so in dorsiflexion.

Eversion
Normal RoM: 25°.
Position: as for inversion.
Axis: as for inversion.
Stationary arm: as for inversion.
Moving arm: as for inversion.
Notes: avoid lower leg movement. Allow some dorsiflexion. Compare left with right. Most inversion occurs through the subtalar and midtarsal joints; however, when the foot is in plantarflexion, the ankle joint also contributes.

Examples of RoM assessment techniques

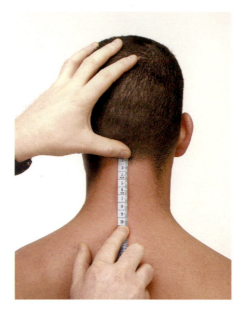

Measuring cervical flexion:
start position

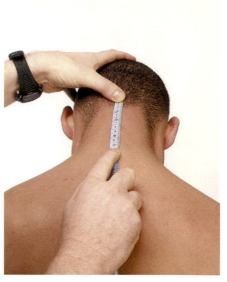

Measuring cervical flexion:
end position

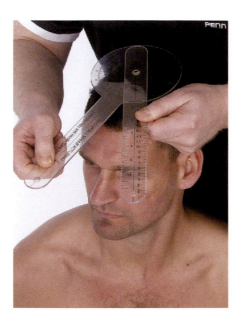

Measuring cervical rotation:
end position

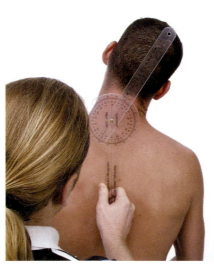

Measuring cervical lateral flexion:
end position

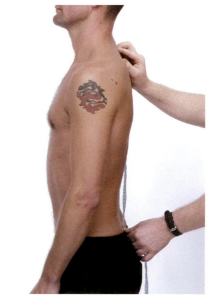

Measuring trunk flexion:
start position

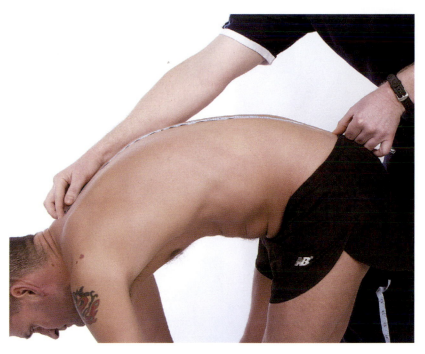

Measuring trunk flexion: end position

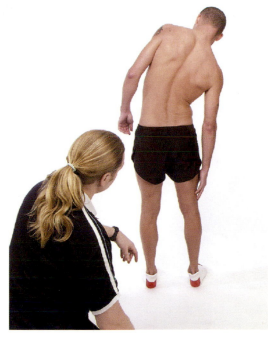

Assessing trunk lateral flexion

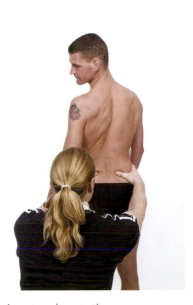

Assessing trunk rotation

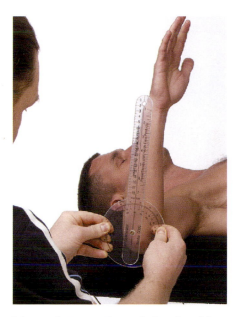

Measuring rotation of the shoulder: start position

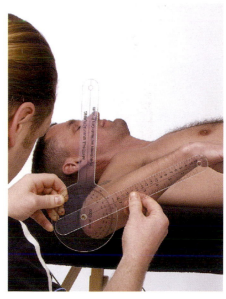

Measuring medial rotation of the shoulder: end position

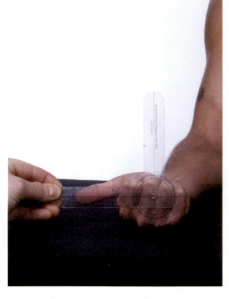

Measuring forearm supination:
end position

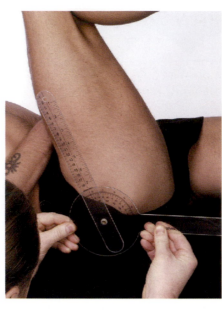

Measuring hip flexion:
end position

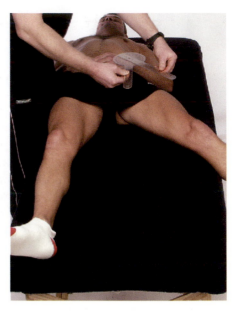

Measuring hip abduction:
end position

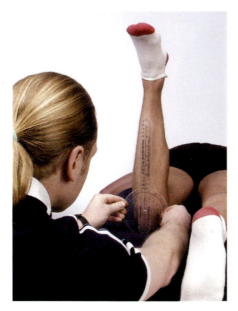

Measuring hip rotation:
start position

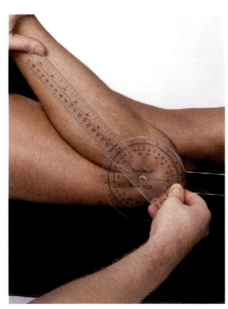

Measuring knee flexion:
end position

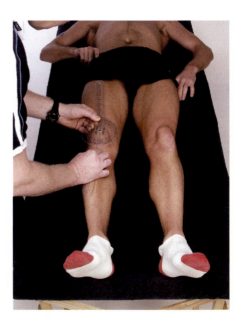

Measuring Q angle

LEG LENGTH DISCREPANCIES

Leg length discrepancy (LLD) is often a primary factor in postural, biomechanical and injury problems. A marked, long-standing discrepancy in leg lengths can easily lead towards pelvic tilt, scoliosis, back pain or uneven gait. If repetitive activities are regularly performed, such as running, then the individual becomes more susceptible to overuse injuries. Discrepancies of less than around 12 mm are usually asymptomatic for the majority of people; certainly LLD is not uncommon. Individuals who train regularly, especially running athletes, may however, experience symptoms with only a discrepancy of 5 mm. An LLD is normally described as being true, apparent, or a combination of the two.

A true LLD is where there is a real shortening of one leg. It may be due to congenital asymmetry, pathology or trauma. The actual bones (femur and tibia) of the limb are significantly shorter. Remember that there are a variety of ways in which a bone could be shorter than its contra-lateral partner. There could be differences in the degree of valgus at the hip, the femoral anteversion, the genu valgus of the knee, excessive torsion of the femur or tibia, or a straightforward shortening of the shaft. A severe fracture can leave the individual with LLD, as can a selection of musculo-skeletal pathological disorders.

To measure true leg length, the subject should be supine, with their pelvis level. Measure each leg from ASIS to medial malleolus, and compare. Try to keep both legs in the same position, and use the same reference points. If shortening is discovered, it is usual to take further measurements, so as to ascertain where the shortening lies. Measuring from ASIS to greater trochanter helps assess the degree of coxa valgus or varus. Measuring from greater trochanter to lateral joint line of distal femur assesses the femoral shaft. Measuring from medial joint line of proximal tibia to medial malleolus assesses the tibial shaft. Alternatively, visual inspection from lateral view, with subject supine, knees together and flexed to 90°, should reveal any shortening in the comparison of each limb.

An apparent LLD is a functional rather than actual shortening, where one leg appears shorter than the other. This can easily result from a pelvic imbalance, where there is an anatomical asymmetry between the two innominate bones, a misshapen sacrum, a sacro-iliac dysfunction, a pelvic tilt or rotation, or a scoliosis. A hip or knee contracture (chronic soft-tissue shortening) often follows on with worsening arthritis. A unilateral pes planus or cavus, or other structural problem can demonstrate that the foot may also play a role in an LLD.

To measure for apparent leg discrepancy, which is a measurement of each side of the lower body, rather than purely of each leg, the subject is, again, supine. The therapist should position the subject's legs as much as is possible in line with the trunk, allow for any tilting of the pelvis or contracture of muscles (because that is probably the cause of the discrepancy). Take a measurement from either the xiphoid process or umbilicus (both are centralized reference points) to the medial malleolus.

TIP
Treatment for LLD obviously depends upon what is causing it. Commonly, the client is recommended a combination of orthotic devices or shoe modifications, physical therapy treatment, and a home exercise programme to help address musculo-skeletal imbalance.

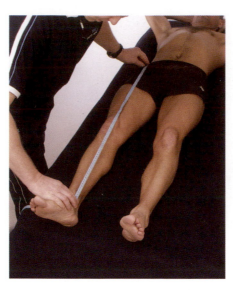

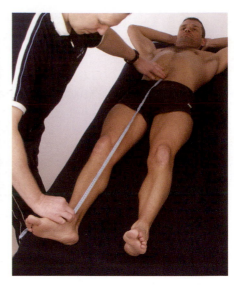

Measuring true leg length

Measuring for apparent leg length discrepancy

GAIT ANALYSIS

Gait analysis is a complex but worthwhile procedure. During normal (ideal) gait, there is a continuous, harmonious, flowing sequence of biomechanical events. These movements occur throughout most of the body's major joints and kinematic chains. Any one of the vast array of biomechanical abnormalities or injury problems can lead to an inefficient gait pattern. Once a compromised or compensated gait pattern has become manifest, it will often worsen and exacerbate the causative factors. Athletes are particularly prone to progressive worsening of such situations, owing to the repetitive nature of most training regimes. The continual biomechanical stresses that occur during walking and running, especially where malalignments are evident, or where compensatory movements occur to avoid pain, mean that gait analysis is an important part of the identification and rectification of such problems. It is normal to evaluate posture, leg lengths and joint ranges of motion prior to assessing gait, so that the therapist has an idea of what to expect.

Obviously, during gait, which the majority of healthy people manage without too much conscious effort, a great deal of neurological controlling activity occurs, which is especially concerned with the firing of the rapidly responding involved muscles. Even when reacting to the challenge of an uneven terrain or the competition of a race, the body's systems normally function incredibly efficiently, and it is quite amazing how capable we are at producing such smooth reactive motion. Remember that visual, vestibular and proprioceptive senses are continually incoming to help produce and refine whichever movements are required. Muscles work both concentrically and eccentrically to produce the control required during locomotion.

There are a variety of methods to analyse gait. Simple observation, on a treadmill, preferably with a video recorder, which allows for anterior,

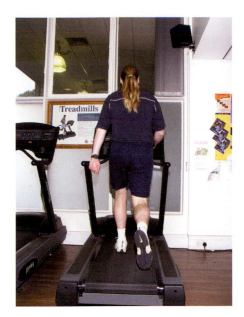

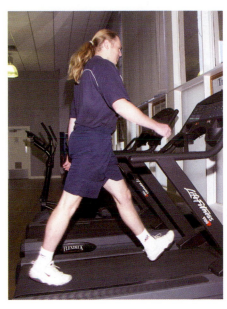

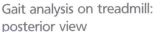

Gait analysis on treadmill: posterior view

Gait analysis on treadmill: lateral view

posterior and lateral views of the motion to be slowed down and repeatedly viewed, is the easiest method. However, this method is limited to the therapist's individual competence in observational analysis. Computer analysis, with electrodes placed upon the functioning limbs, is the norm in the sports science lab, possibly combined with force plates, which measure the ground reaction forces.

Gait analysis should be performed with the subject in shorts and both in trainers and in bare feet. If the subject is using **orthotics** (whether prescriptive or over the counter) to assist in gait efficiency, then they should be observed walking both with and without. The therapist should position themselves to view clearly anterior, posterior and both lateral aspects.

If pain, restriction or a true or apparent LLD is identified, then the cause, extent, severity and aggravating and relieving factors should be noted.

Painful (antalgic) gait is normally easy to observe. The rhythm of the gait is affected, with the subject taking the weight off the affected limb as quickly as is possible. A mild pain may show itself only as a shortening of the stride on the affected limb. A stiff leg gait occurs when either the hip or knee are very limited in their movements. The affected limb tends to swing (circumduct) outward when moving forwards. During gait with LLD, the subject will dip down when weight bears on the shortened leg. A Trendelenburg gait is where one hip is weak or painful, which shows with a characteristic lateral pelvic tilting down towards the affected side. The well-known Trendelenburg sign can also be sometimes observed during standing postural assessment when asking the subject to raise one leg. Normally, the pelvis will rise on the unsupported side. The subject may also need to shift their upper body weight awkwardly over towards the weight-bearing side.

Observe the feet for painful pressure areas, corns, calluses or blisters. Also look for biomechanical abnormalities such as pes planus, pes cavus, hallux valgus, varus or valgus heels. The client's footwear, especially their daily

TABLE 4.1 The two basic phases of gait

Stance phase (60% of total gait, at normal walking speed)	Swing phase (40% of total gait, at normal walking speed)
Contact (heel-strike) Initial contact with the ground	**Acceleration** (initial swing) The limb begins to advance
Mid-stance (foot-flat) Single-leg support, with body directly over weight-bearing leg	**Swing through** (mid-swing) The non-weight-bearing limb is advanced to where it passes directly underneath the body
Propulsion (toe-off) Pushing off from the ground	**Deceleration** (terminal swing) Controlled slowing of swing in preparation for heel-strike contact

TIP

A selection of problematic gaits has been classified as follows:

- osteogenic: due to bone abnormality
- arthrogenic: due to joint stiffness or laxity
- myogenic: due to weakness or pathology of muscle
- neurogenic: due to organic disorder of the nervous system
- psychogenic: due to functional disorder of the nervous system
- prosthetic: due to wearing an artificial limb.

TIP

A leg length discrepancy, increasing age and slower gait tend to cause a reduction in both step and stride length.

shoes and trainers can be analysed for, firstly their suitability, and secondly for signs of uneven wear. Normally, wear is fairly even but is greatest at the tip of the shoe and the heel, both towards the lateral aspect.

Children especially should be monitored for any early signs of biomechanical abnormalities, as they can so often be rectified if attended to with, for example, orthotic inserts or other shoe modifications.

Gait analysis should ideally compare the subject's actual gait pattern with what is considered to be normal, i.e. observe for deviations from the norm. Be aware that restricted movement in one region will usually produce compensatory increased movement at other regions in the kinematic chain.

There are two separate and fundamental phases within the gait cycle: stance and swing. Try to study the positioning of the subject's functioning body parts during the three components of each phase. Step length is normally considered to be the distance between the heel-strike of one foot and the heel-strike of the contra-lateral foot. Stride length is normally considered to be the distance between the successive heel-strikes of one foot, which could also be described as being two steps.

The full cycle of gait (gait cycle) consists of one full step by each of the legs, that is, each leg completes both stance and swing. During gait, there is a period where both feet are in contact with the floor: this is called double-stance. The period of double-stance progressively decreases as speed increases. During the analysis of running gait, there are seen to be many altered components, including the float phase, where there is no contact with the ground.

Stride width is the distance between the two feet. It is normally measured from the mid-points of the two heels during each of their contact phases, and tends to be around 7 cm. An individual with poor balance may increase their stride width so as to have a wider base of support. It tends to be wider during slow gait, and narrower during faster gait. Foot angle is the degree of out-turning (or, abnormal in-turning) of the foot. It is influenced by the degree of hip rotation, femoral or tibial torsion, soft-tissue tightness around the foot and the tarsal alignments, and is normally about 25°.

BIOMECHANICAL COMPONENTS, IN RELATIVE SEQUENCE, FORMING EACH PHASE OF GAIT

STANCE PHASE

Contact
Initially, there is a position of double-stance, where the heel of stance leg and toes of opposite limb are both on the ground.
The foot is slightly supinated, mainly through the subtalar joint.
The lower limb is adducted under the body, which tilts the foot so that contact with ground occurs on the lateral border of heel or mid-foot.
The ankle joint is close to neutral (90°).
Hip is flexed to about 30°.
Knee is initially in near full extension.
The pelvis moves laterally over the leg (with closed-chain adduction of the limb).
Pronation and plantarflexion begins.
Lower leg internally rotates.
Tibialis anterior eccentrically controls any foot slap.
Tibialis posterior eccentrically decelerates pronation.
Knee begins to flex to about 20°.
Hip begins to extend and internally rotate.
Hip abductors eccentrically control lateral pelvic movement.

Mid-stance
The body continues to progress over the weight-bearing limb.
Hip continues to extend.
Tibialis posterior initiates supination, so as to cause decreased mid-foot mobility.
Limb begins to externally rotate.
Hip abduction develops.
Calf eccentrically controls dorsiflexion and the general forward motion of the body.

Propulsion
The body continues to move forward over the limb, in readiness for swing phase.
Plantarflexors cause the heel to rise.
Knee extends.
Hip becomes hyperextended, internally rotated and adducted.
Supination continues.
Body weight moves from lateral to medial midfoot, which is the more powerful lever for propulsion.
Toe-off marks the end of stance and the beginning of swing.

SWING PHASE

Acceleration
Hip flexes and externally rotates, so as to allow the leg to clear the ground.
Knee flexes and externally rotates.
Pelvis rotates anteriorly.
Pelvis tilts down laterally (on swinging limb) as weight-bearing is taken on stance limb.
Dorsiflexion and pronation occurs so as to allow forefoot ground clearance.

Swing through
Swinging limb passes the stance limb.
Hip continues to flex to around 30°.

Deceleration
Hip remains in flexion.
Knee begins to extend.
Ankle moves to neutral, until dorsiflexors eccentrically control degree of plantarflexion at heel strike.
Supination begins.
Deceleration of swinging limb occurs, and foot is stabilized in preparation for next heel strike.

Reciprocal arm swinging occurs during gait. This is where the arms move in the same forward and backward motion as their opposite leg. For example, at heel strike on the left leg, the contra-lateral (right) arm swings forward. This action helps us to maintain balance and gives extra power to the body during power walking and running. During each phase of gait, the shoulders tend to stay fairly level, and the trunk tends to stay fairly upright and vertical.

Gait abnormalities can be treated in a variety of ways. Obviously, the treatment of choice depends upon the nature of the presenting problem. Shoe modifications include widened or thickened soles or uppers, orthotic motion control inserts, heel wedges and ankle supports or braces.

Gait training is crucial for the rehabilitation of a host of conditions, including: severe accident or injury; stroke; cardiac problems; severe neurological disorders. Therapist-assisted walking, whether with parallel bars, on crutches, on a treadmill or on a walking frame, forms just part of the remedial plan, which may also include proprioceptive, flexibility, strength and endurance exercises.

Relatively minor biomechanical abnormalities, such as an over-pronating foot or a high-arched foot, are often quite asymptomatic. However, sometimes these conditions are left unattended to, and sportspeople can be particularly vulnerable to injuries such as Achilles tendonitis or plantar fasciitis. When this is the case, both the cause and the symptoms need to be sorted in order to prevent chronic worsening.

MANUAL MUSCLE TESTS

Manual muscle tests are tests where the subject performs active contractions of specific muscle groups against the therapist's (manual) resistance, usually with the tested muscles placed in a mid-range position. Normally, isometric contractions are performed, but isotonic contractions can also be assessed as these provide further information specifically associated with the functional range of motion. The contractions are normally held for about five seconds, and repeated a few times to determine weakening.

Successful muscle testing occurs as the therapist's awareness of muscle origins, insertions and actions improves. Knowledge of the main myotomes helps when assessing for neurological impairments. Any weakness, and possibly associated atrophy, discovered in the muscles of a particular myotome can be an indication of a problem at the relevant spinal segment.

Manual muscle testing assesses the apparent strength (or weakness) of muscles. It also provides other useful diagnostic information, such as whether or not the subject reports pain on resisted contractions. The strength of contraction can be graded using a simple scale, such as: 0 for no contraction (zero); 1 for slight contraction (poor); 3 for weak contraction (fair); 4 for normal contraction (good); 5 for strong contraction (very good). During such tests the involved muscle group should ideally be palpated and observed at the same time. The therapist should always compare the involved muscle groups with their contra-lateral counterparts.

TIP

A myotome is a group of muscles innervated by a single nerve root (i.e. from a spinal nerve at a particular level). Most muscles receive their innervation from more than one spinal nerve root segment. Therefore, each spinal nerve supplies more than one muscle, and each muscle is supplied by more than one spinal nerve segment.

TIP

Spinal segments and myotomes:

- C1/2: neck flexion
- C3: neck lateral flexion
- C4: shoulder elevation
- C5: shoulder abduction
- C6: elbow flexion and wrist extension
- C7: elbow extension and wrist flexion
- C8: ulnar deviation, thumb extension and finger flexion
- T1: finger abduction and adduction
- L1/2: hip flexion and adduction
- L3: knee extension
- L4: dorsiflexion
- L5: hallux extension
- S1: plantarflexion, eversion, hip extension and knee flexion
- S2: knee flexion and hallux flexion.

Quite commonly, neurological impingement, either at a nerve root or anywhere along the distribution of a spinal nerve, can lead to progressive weakening of the muscle groups that are supplied by the affected nerve. Often there are other neurological signs and symptoms in conjunction with a specific pattern of muscle weakness, such as back pain, radiating pain (as in sciatica), numbness or pins and needles. Remember that weak muscles can quickly become atrophied muscles. In these cases, further testing should be performed to assess the level and severity of neurological impairment, and it is normal to refer to a trained medical professional to deal with such a condition, as inappropriate care can easily lead to exacerbation.

Examples of manual muscle testing techniques

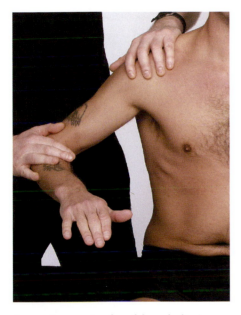

Assessing main shoulder abductors (deltoid group)

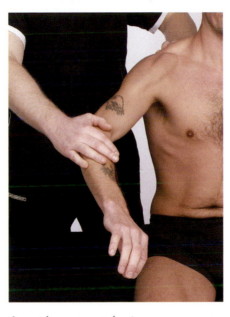

Assessing supraspinatus

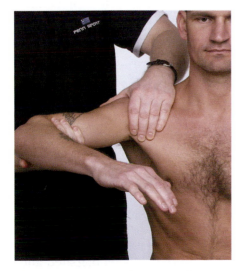

Assessing shoulder horizontal adductors

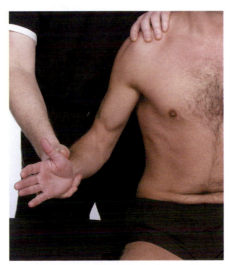

Assessing shoulder lateral and medial rotators

TIP

Manual muscle tests assess contractile tissues (muscles). **Ligament stress tests** assess inert (non-contractile) tissues (ligaments). Therefore, these two types of test help the therapist to differentiate between muscles and ligaments when assessing common soft-tissue injury problems.

TIP

Typical responses from manual muscle testing:

- strong and painless = normal
- strong but painful = minor trauma within the muscle (1st degree strain) or tendon (tendonitis)
- weak and painful = severe trauma such as 2nd degree strain or fracture
- weak but painless = neurological impairment or 3rd degree strain (complete rupture).

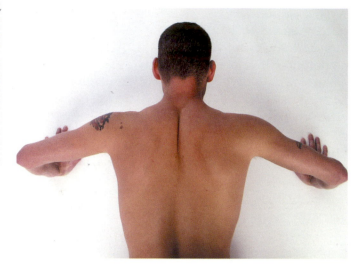

Assessing for 'winging' of the scapula. The serratus arterior muscle, which protracts and stablizes the scapula, can be assessed for neurological impairment (weakness) by having the subject perform a press-up position, either against a wall or on the floor. 'Winging' is where the medial border of the scapula is raised up from the thorax

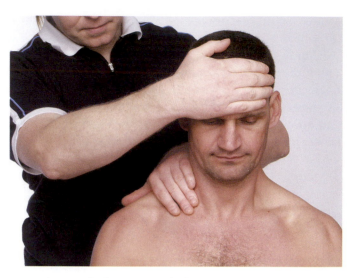

Assessing neck flexors. Neck flexion is performed in the main by bilateral sternocleidomastoid and scalene action

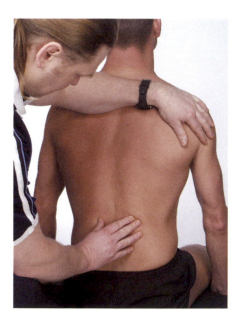

Assessing trunk extensors. The erector spinal group, together with bilateral quadratus lumborum, are the main muscles responsible for extension and hyperflexion of the trunk

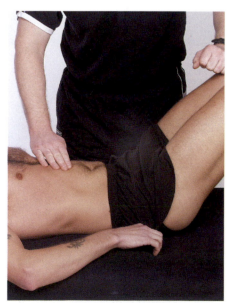

Assessing trunk flexors. The main trunk flexors are the rectus abdominus and oblique muscles

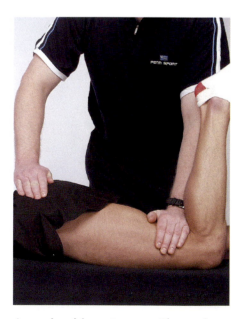

Assessing hip extensors. The main extensors of the hip are the gluteus maximus and hamstrings

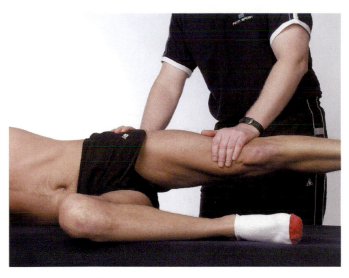

Assessing hip abductors. The main abductors are gluteus medius and minimus, and tensor fascia lata

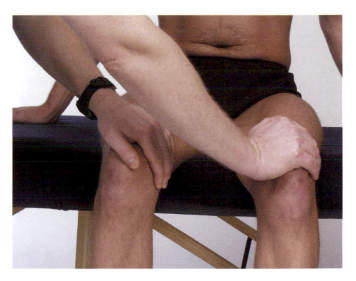

Assessing hip adductors. Hip adduction is performed by five adductor muscles (pectineus, brevis, longus, magnus and gracilis) each originating on the pubic bone

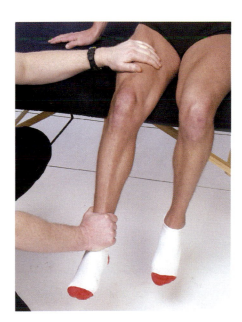

Assessing knee extensors. The main extensors are the quadriceps group

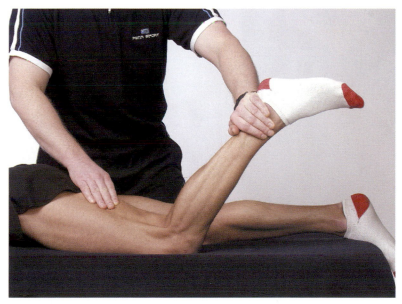

Assessing knee flexors. The main knee flexors are the hamstrings, assisted by gastrocnemius

LIGAMENT STRESS TESTS

Ligament stress tests are simply tests that place a longitudinal stress along the length of a ligament. Ligaments are non-contractile, supportive and relatively taut and strong connective tissues. They stabilize joints and attach to adjacent articulating bones. They help to keep a joint's movement within its correct plane of motion, and also often form part of the synovial capsule. When a joint is forcibly impacted, twisted or stretched, beyond its normal positioning, it is the ligaments that are often torn. Like muscle strains, ligament sprains are classified as being minor partial tearing (1st degree), more severe partial tearing (2nd degree) or complete rupture (3rd degree). It is common for a ligament injury to result in swelling and bruising, and for functional movements to become very painful. There may be an associated dislocation or subluxation, and often other structures are injured during the same incident (e.g. muscles or tendons; cartilage; bone; nerves).

During a ligament stress test, the therapist is looking for excessive laxity of the joint or a painful response from the subject. Obviously, other tests are necessarily performed in conjunction, such as careful palpation around the joint and especially over the insertion sites of the affected ligaments.

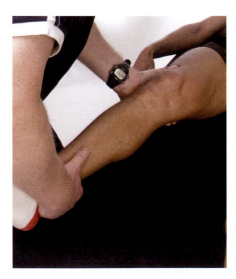
Assessing knee medial collateral ligaments

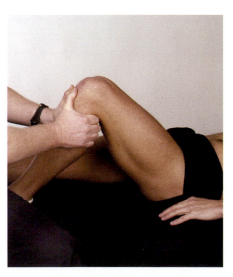
Assessing knee posterior cruciate ligament

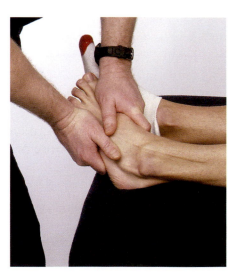
Assessing lateral ankle ligaments

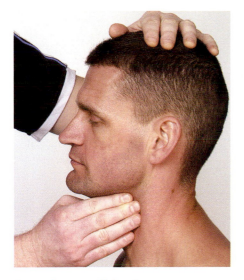 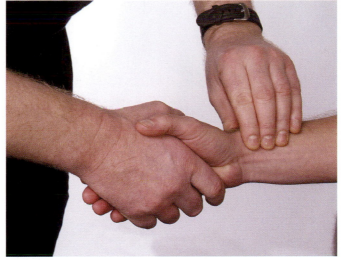

Assessing carotid pulse   Assessing radial pulse

CIRCULATORY TESTS

There are many different circulatory tests. Blood pressure measurements along with resting, exercising and recovery heart rate monitoring are discussed in other chapters.

Assessment of arterial pulses is important for several reasons. In a first aid situation, it can be imperative that the therapist is able to locate and assess the main pulse sites. Similarly, during exercise testing, the therapist will need to be able to take a pulse reading. Sometimes, peripheral pulses need to be assessed so as to locate the presence and location of circulatory impairment.

Pressure from the therapist's palpating fingers should not be too heavy. The pulse should be assessed for rate and regularity. Progressively weakening or absent pulses can be considered medical emergencies, if associated with serious injury, such as fracture or dislocation. Normally, exercise, injury and shock produce an increase in pulse rate.

NEUROLOGICAL TESTS

Testing for sensation can be difficult, as it relies greatly upon subjective responses. Knowledge of dermatomes and their mapping on the body can provide useful diagnostic information relating to problems of spinal nerve supply. As discussed in chapter 2, dermatomes are specific strips of skin supplied by spinal sensory nerve roots, and each dermatome region of the body relates to a specific spinal segment. Aching and pain, paraesthesia (pins and needles) or anaesthesia (numbness) in a particular dermatome, are all possible symptoms of a problematic nerve supply.

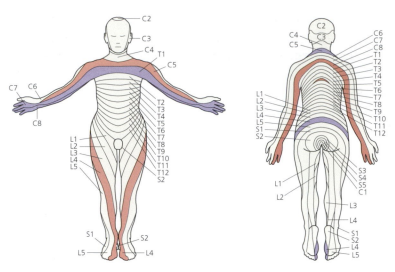

Dermatome map: anterior view   Dermatome map: posterior view

The deep tendon reflexes also relate to specific spinal segments and the involved sensory and motor fibres. A **reflex test** involves tapping a particular tendon briskly with a reflex hammer and observing the quality of the reflex. The reflexes are taken on both sides of the body and compared. They are graded as being absent, diminished, normal or exaggerated. An abnormal reflex helps the therapist to localize impairment.

Lower (or peripheral) motor neurons, serving the skeletal muscles, originate at the spinal cord, and when injured, the related tendon reflex tends to diminish or become absent. Upper (or central) motor neurons originate in the cerebrum, relay impulses to the spinal cord, and when dysfunctional, their related tendon reflex tends to exaggerate in its briskness.

The commonly tested tendon reflexes are perhaps best remembered by the numerical sequence relating to their particular spinal level (i.e. S1, L2, 3, 4, C5, 6, 7). Usually, the tendon is on a slight stretch, the subject is relaxed, and the tendon is struck gently a few times so as to elicit a response.

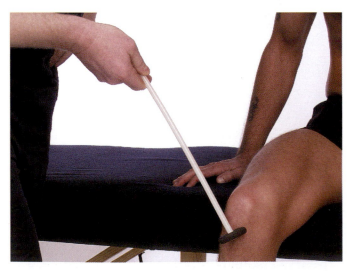

Assessing the patellar tendon reflex (knee jerk), which relates to L2/3/4

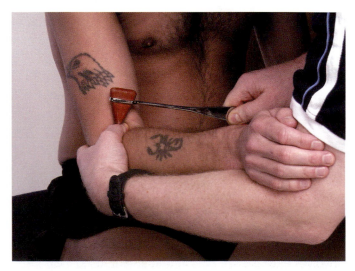

Assessing the biceps tendon reflex which relates to C5/6

Sometimes, it is the therapist's thumb, which is placed upon the tendon and then struck, as with the biceps reflex. It is not always easy eliciting a response, and it should be remembered that some people, quite normally, have diminished or exaggerated reflexes, and that the young and the elderly tend to show reduced responses.

REGIONAL INTEGRITY TESTS

Further physical tests are normally performed so as to specifically assess particular tissues and structures. It is unfortunately beyond the scope of this book to describe all commonly used assessment techniques, but the figures demonstrate a small selection of tests which can help to provide additional diagnostic clues.

Always be aware that an injury problem or medical condition may require more advanced medical assessment. Remember that pain can often be referred from viscera, or be as a result of infection or disease. Other reasons to be vigilant include: obvious deformity, such as dislocation; joint instability; significant loss of motion; abnormal reflexes; abnormal cutaneous sensations; severe unrelenting pain; paralysis, or inability to move a body part; extreme weakness in a myotome; any injury with questionable severity or nature. Most of the time, however, physical assessment merely points the therapist towards whichever exercise or treatment strategies are most appropriate to benefit their client.

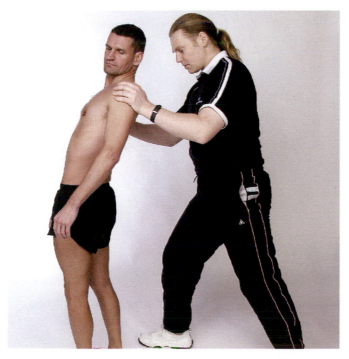

Assessing forspinal dysfunction: the 'Quadrant' test involves extension, rotation and lateral flexion to the painful side. A positive result reproduces the pain, and can be suggestive of the invertebral foramen narrowing

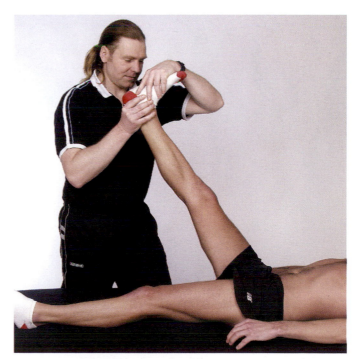

Straight leg raise test. Passive SLR, with dorsiflexion assesses for sciatic nerve irritation. A positve result is where symptoms (pain in leg or back, or very limited RoM) are reproduced

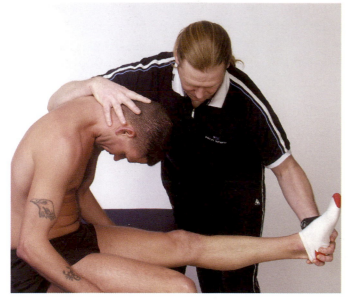

Slump' test. Another test of nerve irritation. A positive test (which reproduces the pattern of pain) is possibly indicative of tension on spinal nerve roots

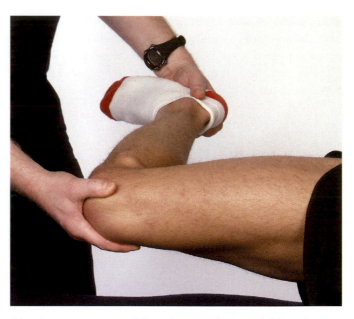

Ober's test: start position. A test of ilio-tibial band tightness

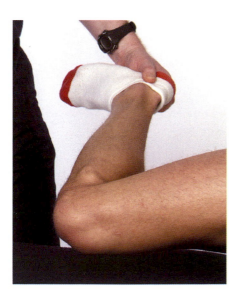

Ober's test: end position. Normal tension allows hip adduction to occur when the leg is dropped

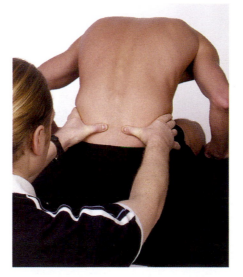

Assessing for sacro-iliac dysfunction. While palpating sacro-iliac joints, the client slowly bends forwards into flexion. Movement of one sacro-iliac joint before the other can suggest dysfunction

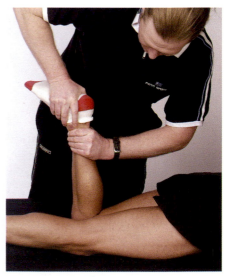

Assessing for meniscal problems: 'Apley's grind' test. A positive result is where compression down into the joint, plus tibial rotation, produces pain in and around the joint

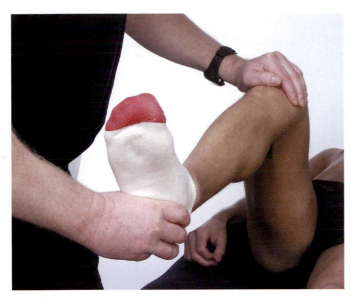

Assessing knee function. The knee and hip joints are carefully articulated, while observing and palpating for abnormalities

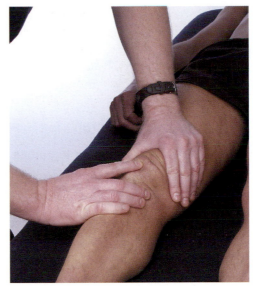

Assessing knee function. The 'fluctuation' test. The therapist 'milks' down superiorly any tissue excess fluid towards the knee with one hand. A positive result (i.e. definite effusion) is where the other hand palpates an increased bulging or pressure

CHAPTER SUMMARY

Biomechanics is the study of posture, movement and physical functioning. Being able to assess the musculo-skeletal (biomechanical) system is crucial to providing sports therapy. Physical assessment, which is combined with knowledge of the history of the client and all observations made during the initial consultation, points the sports therapist towards whichever exercise or treatment strategies are most appropriate in order to gain most benefit for their client. Basic objectives might include: assessing and evaluating current condition; analysing posture, body shape, joint movements and gait; being able to recommend specific actions; evaluating and monitoring the effectiveness of treatment, exercise and advice; helping to improve functional performance; presenting information to other health-care practitioners. A selection of methods and techniques are employed which analyse such aspects as: height and weight, postural alignments, body contours and circumferences, muscle tone and strength, RoM, leg lengths, gait and functional activities.

Other important physical tests, such as the measurement of body fat, lung function and blood pressure are discussed in chapter 13.

WEBSITE

Visit the companion website at www.thomsonlearning.co.uk/ healthandfitness/ward where you will find the answers to these questions for you to check your progress through the book.

Knowledge Review

1   Why is the study of biomechanics so important to the sports therapist?

2   What is meant by the following terms: (i) diagnosis; (ii) prognosis; (iii) sign; (iv) symptom; (v) somatype?

3   List ten items of equipment used by the sports therapist for physical assessment.

4   What are the basic objectives of a physical assessment?

5   What techniques are commonly employed by the sports therapist during physical assessment?

6   Describe BMI and WHR, and discuss the positives and negatives of each.

7   Why is careful palpation such an important skill for the sports therapist to develop?

8   List ten possible causes of postural problems.

9   Describe the ideal plumb alignment in the lateral, posterior and anterior views.

10   List ten common postural deviations.

11   Describe the correct principles for assessing ranges of movement at joints.

12   Describe the normal gait sequence.

13   What are manual muscle tests, and what information can they provide?

14   Explain how ligaments are assessed.

15   Why can basic neurological tests be useful in physical assessment for sports therapy?

chapter 5

SPORTS INJURY OVERVIEW

Learning Objectives

After reading this chapter you should be able to:

- recognize common causes of sports injuries
- grasp the main principles of injury prevention
- understand basic classifications of injury
- develop knowledge of common sports injuries
- develop knowledge of basic first aid procedures
- develop strategies for injury rehabilitation

This chapter should develop your confidence in attending to common sporting injuries. Physically active people, especially sportspeople, are always going to have some vulnerability to injury. People suffer new injuries or aggravate old ones, and many simply have to manage their injury problems on a regular basis. Injuries are encountered on the field, in training and competition, in the fitness studio, and during normal daily activities. The busy sports therapy clinic will, every week, provide treatment and advice for various and numerous injuries.

It is important to recognize that an athlete can be the champion of their sport at whatever level they perform, or just as applicably, be the part-time enthusiast who plays when they can, because they can. Whether a fitness obsessive or reluctant exerciser, unfortunately, any individual can suffer injury.

All the best in preparation, from careful training and correct equipment to the actual tactics on the day, cannot guarantee injury-free performance. However, if the athlete is properly fit for the activities they are involved in, and knows how to prepare, in terms of warm-up, apparel and mental approach, then risks are minimized.

The warning signs that something is not quite right, such as an unusually tight muscle, a sharp pain on movement, a localized swelling around a joint, or an obvious contour deformity, for example, should be attended to immediately. Minor sports injuries so often lead to more serious (participation-threatening) problems, simply because insufficient care and attention are paid to them in the athlete's normal approach to sport and training.

The scientific knowledge base for exercise and therapeutic intervention has grown steadily in recent years. As the knowledge base in these fields has widened, and existing methods re-evaluated, and newer techniques researched and integrated, the very practice of fitness and sports training and injury management demonstrates an even greater consideration and adherence to evidence-based principles. This is due both to the growth in the number of people now studying these subjects, and to the quality and diversity of the work they are undertaking, and to the continual professional development (CPD) that is available to those already in practice. Certainly now, there are more sports therapists implementing carefully designed training regimes and, equally, more individuals are exercising, both regularly and effectively. Sports science and sports therapy are now integral to what we all do, but our injuries result for a variety of reasons.

This book can offer only an overview and guide to injury assessment and management. If in practice, you are presented with a suspected serious injury or pathology, medical condition or pain of undiagnosed nature, it is imperative that medical advice is sought. The most appropriate and effective treatment strategies result from having the right person for the job in hand. It is the sports therapist's role to work under the advice of medically qualified people, and to apply their own therapeutic expertise when the time is right.

Sports injury management incorporates four main subject areas:

- Understanding the causes of injury (aetiology).
- Providing injury assessment and diagnosis.
- Performing injury treatment and rehabilitation (acute, post-acute and chronic).
- Implementing strategies for injury prevention (the attempted avoidance of injury or reoccurrence of injury).

AETIOLOGY: INTRINSIC AND EXTRINSIC FACTORS IN THE CAUSES OF SPORTS INJURY

There are two basic types of causes of injury: intrinsic and extrinsic. Intrinsic causes of injury are those of an, individual, anatomical or pathological nature. Individuals can be more prone to injury by their inherent 'make-up'. Good quality training and preparation can, however, alter these constituents.

Obviously the age, sex and physical fitness of the individual are factors. Low endurance, poor strength, flexibility and agility can all predispose to injury. Certainly, people should really be fit for the sports that they want to play. Anatomical malalignments, postural deviations and associated muscle imbalances and joint abnormalities are strong intrinsic factors in injury causation. Body composition, too, should ideally be suited to the activities

TIP ✔

The four main areas of sports injury management are:

- aetiology (causes)
- assessment and diagnosis
- treatment and rehabilitation
- prevention.

TIP ✔

The aetiology of injuries is important to the prevention of their reoccurrence.

TIP ✔

Intrinsic injury: resulting from, individual, anatomical or pathological factors.
Extrinsic injury: resulting from external factors, such as training errors, inappropriate equipment and the nature of competition.

undertaken. The previous injuries that an individual has suffered often results in increased susceptibility to further related problems. Similarly, everyone has their own medical history, and it should be remembered that many health complaints can be easily exacerbated by inappropriate or excessive exercise activity: arthritis, asthma or coronary heart disease, for example. Guidance is the key, and this should be offered liberally by the sports therapist.

Extrinsic causes of injury are those derived from more external factors. The training parameters placed upon the individual, whether by their instructor or coach, or self-inflicted, should not be poorly designed. Sudden changes in training, such as rapid increases in intensity, frequency or duration can easily lead to problems. Equipment for the sport should not be ill-fitting, unsuitable or worn-out. All protective equipment has to be sufficient. The environmental condition surrounding the activity on the day is a classic extrinsic factor. The other main extrinsic factor is the nature of the game. Competition demands extreme effort from both the individual and their opponents, which is especially evident in contact sports. Additionally, it is difficult to prepare for the impact from a projectile, such as a hard ball, other than having protective clothing, continual awareness of all activities, and generating a responsible atmosphere.

> **TIP** ✔
> Training and preparation errors are often the root cause of injuries.

INJURY PREVENTION

It is an inescapable fact that exercise and, in particular, sports are potentially very hazardous activities. There are many important safety factors that must be recommended both in the general preparation for exercise, and during the exercise session itself. An awareness of the potential hazards enables the coach, instructor or therapist to enjoy their teaching of exercise safe in the knowledge that they are prepared for most eventualities and can avoid many of the problems before they occur.

> **TIP** ✔
> Remember that prevention is always preferable to cure!

Be aware that training and actual competition are different. Training does not necessarily need to be performed with extreme or maximal effort, and should be carefully planned to achieve its various objectives. Competition, however, is about winning, and serious injuries and acute medical emergencies are not that uncommon, especially during events. Exercise-related death does occur, albeit very rarely. Most fatalities occurring during sports tend to be due to either traumatic accidents or underlying **cardio-vascular** disorders. When organizing any form of exercise, whether in a group situation, gym or on the field, competitive or not, there are many considerations to take into account.

> **TIP** ✔
> Injury prevention should be at the forefront when preparing and advising players. Each sport has its own fitness needs, skills requirements, protective equipment and particular potential for injuries.

Safety factors in the prevention of injuries

Older age groups

Because exercise is, everywhere, strongly recommended to help offset problematic ageing, more and more middle-aged and elderly people are taking up regular fitness training. Some will be completely new to such exertions, others well experienced, but with older age comes normal reductions in functional abilities. Be aware that older age groups are more likely to have relatively reduced flexibility, strength, endurance, co-ordination and balance. They are more likely to suffer arthritis or certain cardio-vascular disorders. Older people can injure more easily, and they recover more slowly.

Children

Children are not little adults. They can be very prone to sports-related injuries if their sports are not well coached. Musculo-skeletal immaturity dictates that all intense strength-based, training and competitive activities should be monitored and graded. Try to keep activities broad-based, and varied rather than sport-specific during early development. Matching according to sizes rather than ages is preferable. Children are also at a greater risk of heat injury than adults. Remember that children lack (some) of the experience and awareness of adults.

Gender

Women tend to be more vulnerable to biomechanically related injuries. Women are naturally physically weaker and smaller than men, which means that most sports are performed separately. Women tend to have the most biomechanical disadvantages: wider hips with increased femoral angle and genu valgus; wider Q angle; narrower shoulders; wider carrying angle of the elbow; breasts. Sports bras provide the necessary support and movement to avoid breast discomfort. Women also have to contend with the menstrual cycle, which for some can be problematic. Heavy periods, painful periods (dysmenorrhoea), typically with abdominal cramps, or absent periods (amenorrhoea) can all have implications for exercise. Pregnancy is not normally a reason to stop participation in exercise, although the type, intensity and positionings must be considered, and obviously any signs of problems (bleeding; low abdominal pain; back pain) mean exercise must be stopped immediately.

Men, on the other hand, are generally less prone to such intrinsic injuries, but they do traditionally demonstrate a greater natural tendency towards 'macho' (risk-laden) behaviour, which can bring its own potential for problems.

Medical conditions

Any affecting medical disorder can be aggravated by inappropriate exercise. Common problems include: asthma; hyper- or hypotension; heart problems; arthritis; recent operations; diabetes; epilepsy. Individuals should be screened for medical conditions and the medications they take. Medical consent to participation and careful monitoring of performance is essential.

Injury history

Ideally, the fitness instructor knows of their participants' main injury problems, and makes exercise concessions for them. The sports coach or trainer probably gets to know his or her athletes' problems and provides assistance with their rehabilitation. Either way, old injuries can easily be aggravated. If exercisers have injuries, recommend they that seek proper attention (sports therapy, physiotherapy, osteopathy, podiatry, orthopaedic consultation, etc.). Remember that training with injuries may make the injuries worse. Compensatory postures, movements and gait quickly lead to new injury problems.

Awareness of the de-training effects often incurred during the healing and rehabilitation of injuries

Injuries can often limit normal fitness training, which leaves the individual prone to regional (and general) weakening, atrophy, lost power and reduced endurance.

Current fitness levels

Every exerciser has their own level of fitness. Whatever the fitness level, it is the instructor's responsibility to instruct while adhering to the correct scientific principles of exercise training. Doing too much too soon (more than one is accustomed to) or too often is a recipe for injury. Overload, in terms of increasing the intensity, duration or frequency of exercise, should be applied gradually (progressively) so as to allow the body to adapt safely and successfully to an improved level of fitness.

Postural and other biomechanical problems

Any significant structural malalignment has the potential to affect the efficiency of performance, and should be attended to. It will be best to combine remedial with general training.

The structure of the exercise on the day

Whether a fitness class, training session or big match, all exercisers should take part in a thorough warm-up to prepare for the activities that are to follow. On competition days, this can include pre-event massage. Thorough cool-down eases the recovery process as well as gradually returning the body to its resting state.

Nutrition

A healthy balanced diet is very important for health and performance. Adequate hydration, generally and before, and during and after exertions is crucial. Dietary specifics are often incorporated into sports training regimes. Also, obviously, individuals should not exercise soon after consuming a heavy meal (allow two to three hours).

Under the influence

The trainer should be aware to the possibility of any participants being under the influence of alcohol or recreational drugs.

Avoid any particular exercises that cause pain

There is nothing better than pain to act as a warning sign to problems. It is generally considered bad practice to train through any pain greater than normal exercise discomfort. There are often alternative exercises available, which avoid overly stressing problem muscles or joints. Get pains checked.

Great care with controversial exercises

Some exercises are considered controversial because they can be harmful, such as the 'hurdler's stretch' (overstresses the medial ligaments of the knee during extreme flexion), head circling (can cause excess wear at C1/2) or the 'plough' (extreme neck flexion). Poor positioning in exercise is a big factor in injury causation. Knees, necks and backs are particularly vulnerable. In functional training, for some sports, it is acceptable to replicate the movements of the game, some of which could in other circumstances be considered controversial (some martial arts, for example). Generally, it is also recommended to avoid particular exercises that are not well controlled, because there will be less effective improvements in strength or co-ordination.

Provide exercise variations for beginning, intermediate and advanced participants

One key to being a successful exercise instructor is developing an ability to offer, demonstrate and coach easy exercise alternatives. Do not be afraid to make useful considered suggestions.

Encourage fitness testing

If new exercisers take a simple test of fitness before their exercise programme is formulated, then the instructor has a much better understanding of how to help plan their exercise, with less chance of overstressing the body. In the competitive field, athletes returning from injury should undergo a different type of fitness test (a functional fitness test) which ultimately assesses their ability to begin competing again.

The exercise environment

If indoors, make sure the area is suitable for the activity and the number of participants. It should also be free from clutter, spillages and obstructions. Fitness studios benefit from being well lit and having sprung-wood flooring and large mirrors. If outdoors, the weather is always an influence, and athletes or players should prepare accordingly. The ground surface particularly needs consideration, and playing fields should be checked for debris. Whether indoors or out, there must be first aid provisions.

The exercise equipment

All forms of exercise and sport require at least minimal equipment. Specialist clothing is desirable for many activities. Risks are reduced by wearing the appropriate clothing, which may be supportive and protective and/or environment-responsive, especially footwear. Equipment clearly includes the bats, balls, racquets, nets, sticks and other items integral to the game. These should be the correct type, and be regularly inspected, maintained and replaced when necessary. Remember that, ideally, a tennis racquet is, for example, individually prepared for the person who is going to use it (i.e. handle size, overall weight and string tension). By encouraging the right equipment for the job in hand, the trainer is reducing the potential for injury.

Avoid unnecessary or excessive repetition during exercise

Overuse injuries occur quite easily. Muscle fatigue can lead to strain. Tendonitis and other repetitive strain injuries can develop quite quickly under inappropriate or unaccustomed repetitive loading, but may take a long time to resolve. Repetition, especially when weight-bearing, causes undue stresses to joints, also muscle imbalance can develop. Obviously, such a discipline as distance running has repetition at its heart, and distance runners have their own collection of commonly suffered injuries to show for it (shin splints, ilio-tibial band (ITB) syndrome (runner's knee), stress fractures, Achilles tendonitis, etc.). Encourage rest and recovery days.

Awareness of exercising heart rates

It is better for all if exercisers are encouraged to develop an awareness of how hard they are working (the Borg scale of **perceived exertion** is a useful point of reference – see chapter 12). Heart rate monitors are often built into aerobic stations in gyms. Portable monitors (strap around chest and watch-like receiver) are commonly used by keen runners and cyclists. Manual pulse tests are easily performed, by anyone, at any time. Chapter 12 discusses how to work out a maximal heart rate. To achieve safe aerobic benefits, for beginner and intermediate exercisers, it is recommended to work out within the aerobic zone of 50–80 per cent of maximum. Heart rate monitoring enables safer and effective training to take place, and it can be easier to monitor the effects of periodic increases in exercise intensity. The cardio-vascular system is also less likely to be overstressed.

Continual observation and coaching of the participants

It almost goes without saying that the instructor should be watchful and helpful when running exercise sessions. Check for poor technique, signs of fatigue or other problems, but try not to intimidate. Be aware that people respond differently. Do not push people too hard.

Be aware of the signs that exercise should stop

This is obviously vital. Acute exercise problems can and do occur. Anything from a muscle strain to a myocardial infarction (heart attack) can occur during vigorous exercise. Be vigilant for signs of laboured breathing, loss of co-ordination, dizziness, chest pain, nausea, particular muscle or joint pain.

Be aware of the signs of over-exertion

There should ideally always be adequate rest and recovery from exertions. Training exercise should not be so frequent or intense so as to cause excessive **delayed onset muscle soreness** (DOMS) or other unwanted symptoms. Regular over-exertion can lead to suffering undue fatigue during exercise and poor ability to recover from training. Heart rates may stay elevated after cool-downs. Poor sleep can ensue, together with a weakening immune function (making the individual more susceptible to coughs and colds). Women can experience amenorrhoea. Overuse injuries increase in incidence. Exercise addiction, where training adversely affects health, is certainly a growing problem.

Avoid exercise when unwell

People should be encouraged not to undertake strenuous exercise when feeling unwell or displaying symptoms of ill-health. It is usually rest that the body requires. The body is quite well equipped to deal with such minor health complaints as the common cold, and should be allowed to do so. Asthma and hay fever sufferers can go through difficult periods relating to the environmental atmosphere. People with diabetes, arthritis, cardiac problems and multiple sclerosis all have their good days and bad days.

Sport-specific skill training

Organized competitive sport participation requires the development of certain skills, strengths and techniques. Sport skills training is normally built into a core fitness training regime. Depending on the sport, skills training is normally partly made up of activities that replicate those used in the game. Additional methods include specific agility, co-ordination and reaction work, strength, power, endurance, stability and flexibility training, as appropriate, to the most applicable regions.

Benefits of cross-training

By varying the types of exercise performed regularly, the individual is reducing their potential for overuse injury, and maintaining, or even improving, aspects of their fitness at the same time. A typical example of cross-training is the distance runner who cycles or swims on non-running days. Aerobic endurance is still developed, the body is still thoroughly worked, but the knees and ankles, hips and back, are given a relative rest from impacting. For general fitness development this type of training, combined with other recommended exercise, is best. Varying activities also helps keep us motivated. The widening variety of available exercise classes now allows individuals to enjoy the differing benefits that the various classes offer well (e.g. spinning, Pilates, yoga, body pump).

Adherence to rules

Rules are there to control events. Sport is competitive and therefore rules are a requirement. Rules encourage fair play, and therefore reduce the possibility of injury. There are also the rules in non-competitive situations, in the gym for example. The sports therapist or trainer should keep in mind the rules of the situation and try to make sure they are kept to.

Pre-season training

Athletes, cyclists, footballers, rugby players, cricketers, hockey players, gymnasts and tennis players should all prepare for competitive seasons with all-year conditioning, applying the principles of periodization training, and specific pre-season work. Pre-season fitness training usually intensifies over a period of two to four weeks prior to first competitive action.

Sports psychology

Sports psychology is designed to maximize performance by way of the incorporation of specifically adapted psychological principles. Ideally, competitors are focused, mentally prepared and confident in their sports. Wherever the athlete is inappropriately anxious, frustrated, under stress or demotivated, whether as a direct result of their performances, injuries or for other personal reasons, sports psychology may help to improve the situation.

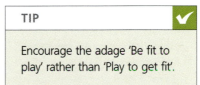

TIP ✔

Encourage the adage 'Be fit to play' rather than 'Play to get fit'.

Encourage players to take sports therapy

Sports massage and regular hands-on attention generally detect and attend to possible problems before they become a problem. Therapy is also a great way to recover from extreme exertion, and generally leads to improved performance.

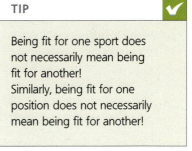

TIP ✔

Being fit for one sport does not necessarily mean being fit for another!
Similarly, being fit for one position does not necessarily mean being fit for another!

CLASSIFICATION OF INJURIES

Injuries can be trivial or more serious, and they can be classified in a variety of ways. As previously discussed, injuries can be described as being intrinsic or extrinsic. They can also be classified according to the type of tissue that is injured, for example, soft, hard and special tissue injuries. They can be classified according to the type of insult inflicted upon the tissues, that is direct or indirect, such as with the direct impact of a hard tackle, or the indirect forces exerted during the overloading of a hamstring muscle in an explosive sprint. Injuries can be from one traumatic incident or as a result of overuse (repetitive stress). Injuries are usually described in relation to their stage of healing, i.e. acute, sub-acute or chronic. More simply, injuries are also described as being mild, moderate or severe. Furthermore, injuries are described as being regional (i.e. pertaining to a particular body region, for example, rotator cuff tendonitis is a shoulder injury), sport-related (i.e. injuries common to a particular sport, such as knee cartilage injuries in football) and age-related (for example, Osgood-Schlatter's disease, which is an injury problem affecting the insertion site of the patellar tendon at the tibial tuberosity in growing children, particularly boys, who play a lot of football).

TIP

Cramp, a common problem associated with muscle fatigue during sports, is typified as a spontaneous, prolonged and painful contraction of a muscle or muscle group. Most commonly affecting the hamstring, calf and foot muscles, the individual may be predisposed by their nutritional status (especially mineral salt imbalance, and insufficient carbohydrate loading). Other factors include whether they are dehydrated in hot weather, have muscle damage, tight muscles or impaired circulation. There is neurological involvement. Treatment normally involves gentle stretching and massage, and identification and correction of any predisposing factors.

TIP

Stitch is the sharp pain that comes on in the side of the upper abdomen, usually during running or fast walking activities. It is normally of short duration, and is often associated with having eaten or drunk prior to exercise, which can result in strain on the supportive ligaments of the abdominal organs, extra effort for the abdominal muscles, and a need for increased blood flow to and from the digestive organs. Stitch is sometimes experienced by exercisers who are not so well conditioned, and as their fitness improves, becomes much less of a problem. Relief may be obtained by easing off, supporting the abdomen with their hands, leaning in flexion towards the discomfort, leaving more air in the lungs on each out breath or by lying supine with hips and knees flexed.

Some sports and activity-related problems are perhaps not best categorized as being injuries, such as overtraining syndrome, but they are still problems none the less. These also include such conditions as cramp or stitch. Therapists should also have some awareness of how some medical conditions can, in some circumstances, be adversely affected by exercise, for example asthma (including exercise-induced), hypertension and arthritic conditions.

Direct injury

These are extrinsic injuries, usually involving a forceful impact with an opponent or implement (such as a hockey stick or ball). Often produces a contusion, but haematoma, nerve damage, dislocation, sprain, strain, fracture or open wound are all possible.

Indirect injury

These are intrinsic injuries, resulting from excessive forces generated within. Commonly, it is the major muscles that span two joints, such as the hamstrings, quadriceps and gastrocnemius, that are strained during explosive activity. Ligament sprains and meniscus tears can also result from unaccustomed, ill-prepared or excessive movements.

Acute injury

This classification of injury is defined by the early onset and short duration of the particular signs and symptoms following the trauma. The injury could involve any one or more of the body's tissues. Typically, the athlete is aware of how the injury occurred, and with acute sporting injury the common signs and symptoms can include immediate pain, tenderness, swelling, contour deformity or bleeding. An injury is normally described as being acute until the initial signs of inflammation have reduced, and the healing process has begun, which is normally after 48 to 72 hours.

Sub-acute injury

Sometimes referred to as post-acute injury, this classification is more related to the time-scale of repair, and typically, a sub-acute injury is the state of injury two to three days or a week after initial trauma. Obviously, the severity of the injury and the acute treatment provided affect the rate of healing and the quality of repair, but the sub-acute injury is where the inflammation has begun to reduce, and where there are gradual improvements in symptoms and function. The rehabilitation process begins here.

Chronic injury

These injuries usually have a gradual onset, resulting most commonly from repetitive minor insults, the cumulative effects often being the cause of a long-standing problem. Chronic problems often develop when minor

COMMON SOFT-TISSUE INJURIES

Skin: cut; abrasion; laceration; puncture wound; contusion; blister; callus; burn; sunburn.

Muscle: strains (1st, 2nd, 3rd degree); contusion, inter/intra-muscular haematoma; compartment syndrome; cramp; DOMS (delayed onset muscle soreness).

Tendon: strains (1st, 2nd, 3rd degree); tendonitis; tendinosis; tenosynovitis.

Ligament: sprains (1st, 2nd, 3rd degree).

Bursae: bursitis (infective or traumatic).

Fibro-cartilage: tear; displacement; herniation; prolapse.

Synovium: synovitis; Baker's cyst.

COMMON HARD-TISSUE INJURIES

Bone: fracture; stress fracture; contusion.

Periosteum: periostitis; contusion.

Articular cartilage: osteochondral fracture; chondromalacia.

SPECIAL TISSUES VULNERABLE TO SPORTS INJURY

Brain

Nerves

Blood vessels

Eyes, nose, ears, throat, mouth, teeth.

Thoracic organs (lungs; heart; liver; spleen).

Abdominal organs (kidneys; stomach; small intestine; large intestine).

Pelvic organs (bladder; genitalia).

injuries are poorly managed. Unfortunately, with more severe injuries, whether from one traumatic incident or from overuse, the athlete is often left with a chronic problem. Chronic problems usually demand management and rehabilitation that may involve, in addition to physical therapy, adaptations to normal daily activities.

Injuries and tissue types

The soft-tissues of the body include skin, fascia, muscle, tendon, ligament, bursae, synovium and fibro-cartilage. These are the tissues that are commonly attended to in sports therapy. Bone, articular cartilage, and the tough, fibrous, outer membrane of bone – the **periosteum** – are considered to be the hard-tissues of the body. The special tissues of the body are the various vital organs.

Impact injury

Any impacting force, be it an opponent's elbow in the face, a cricket ball in the thigh, or a bang on the head from a fall, can result in anything from a minor bruise to fracture, concussion or worse. The various keys to preventing impact injuries include: adherence to rules, wearing adequate protection and being fit and reactive and agile for the activities being performed.

A contusion (bruise) occurs following any impact that has ruptured superficial blood vessels. In the acute stage a purplish ('black and blue') discoloration of the skin results (ecchymosis), which is local to the impacting trauma. Sub-acutely, this fades to a yellowish-green. With more severe bruising, the discoloration often tracks downwards with gravity, so that sometimes the discoloration is actually lower than the site of injury. A quadriceps contusion, common in football, is sometimes called a corked thigh or charley horse.

A haematoma can result from a subcutaneous or deeper soft-tissue injury, and especially with impact trauma, if internal bleeding cannot escape through the fascial sheaths. An inter-muscular haematoma is where the swelling and bleeding are confined to the sheaths surrounding the muscle group. In an intra-muscular haematoma the swelling and bleeding are confined to the sheath surrounding one muscle, and the haematoma is therefore more localized. Myositis ossificans is a possible, but relatively uncommon, complication of haematoma. With myositis ossificans, the bleeding within the tissues coagulates, and if it is not reabsorbed, a local bone formation process takes place around it, over a period of weeks. The resulting hardened tissue becomes in the long run either relatively asymptomatic or an ongoing chronic problem.

In addition to the body's physically protective tissues (skeleton, muscles, ligaments, skin and subcutaneous fat), other tissues are vulnerable to the trauma of impact. In particular, major nerves and their plexuses, can be compressed or overstretched causing a neuropraxia (more commonly known as a burner or stinger). Such injuries can cause immediate, but often transient, pain, paraesthesia (tingling), anaesthesia (numbness) and weakness, and the athlete may be able to continue participation if symptoms abate. Axonotmesis is a loss of function due to a more severe compression, with recovery commonly taking weeks or months. Be aware that nerve tissue can also become compressed and entrapped as a result of swelling from other, nearby soft-tissue injury.

Blood vessels are also easily injured. Blood vessels can be stretched or crushed during impact. Blood vessel injuries can be complicated by the degree of internal bleeding and intravascular clotting that occurs. Vascular spasm can also follow injury, especially with fractures. An ischaemic situation can quickly develop following blood vessel damage, where there is pain, paleness and coldness, lack of pulse and weakening of muscles. This is normally considered a medical emergency.

Obviously, concussion is always a cause for concern. Head injury is common in sport. As in any first aid assessment, a variety of signs and symptoms dictates when the casualty is in need of emergency medical attention.

Alongside all the potential local consequences of an impact injury, the therapist must also be alert to the possibility of separate injuries sustained during the same incident.

Strains

A **strain** is a tear in a muscle or tendon, the result of excess tensile stress through the tissues, and is commonly called a *pulled* or *torn* muscle. Strains are more usually indirect injuries, being caused by an overloading or overstretching of the musculo-tendinous unit. Any extreme loading of the unit, such as with a heavy lift or other powerful movement such as sudden sprint, jump or strenuous throw, can result in injury. Strains often occur in the presence of muscle fatigue, and the athlete may experience a 'snapping' sensation as the injury occurs. The overload can occur during the concentric or eccentric phases of isotonic contraction, but it is generally recognized that strong eccentric contractions are more commonly the cause of muscle injury (overloading as the muscle is lengthening); however, the majority of strains tend to occur during a normal RoM. The musculo-tendinous junction is considered to be the weakest component of the unit, and is therefore a common site for acute muscle injuries. Muscle tissue tends to heal more effectively than other soft-tissues (e.g. tendons and ligaments) because of its rich blood supply. Strains are graded according to their severity.

A first degree strain is a minor partial tear. There will be mild to moderate pain on contraction or stretch, but usually very minor functional impairments, which will be more noticeable during more intense exercise. The muscle may be appear weaker than normal, and there may also be minor muscle spasm (tightening), possibly accompanied by a mild degree of swelling and discoloration. There is usually tenderness on local palpation. Recovery is usually quick and complete if correct principles of management are applied.

A second degree strain is a more severe partial tear, resulting from a more forceful contraction or stretching. There is a more pronounced set of signs and symptoms associated with a second degree strain. Pain is moderate to strong during stretch, contraction and palpation, weakness is evident, spasm may be present in both the affected and adjacent muscles, swelling can be moderate to major, and function impaired to a great degree. There may be a palpable indent in the muscle tissue. Obviously, the greater severity of muscle damage, the longer the recovery. Second degree muscle injuries will normally heal, with good treatment and progressive remedial exercise, in three to six weeks. The therapist should emphasize awareness to the possibility of aggravation of the injury by too early return to full training or competition.

A third degree muscle strain is a complete rupture, where there is a complete or virtual lack of continuity in the affected muscle. This injury is the result of a very forceful contraction or overstretching. Typical signs and symptoms include: severe pain as the injury occurs, which commonly reduces soon afterwards; significant weakness and loss of function; marked swelling; muscle spasm in adjacent muscles; complete loss of strength on specific resistance testing; palpable fibre 'bunching' (with 'bump and hollow' deformity), and local and diffuse pain. This grade of injury usually necessitates either a surgical repair, or at least a few weeks of cast immobilization, prior to a comprehensive rehabilitation programme. Return to full fitness often takes two to three months or longer.

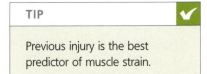

TIP

Previous injury is the best predictor of muscle strain.

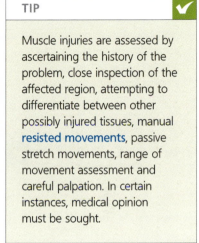

TIP

Muscle injuries are assessed by ascertaining the history of the problem, close inspection of the affected region, attempting to differentiate between other possibly injured tissues, manual **resisted movements**, passive stretch movements, range of movement assessment and careful palpation. In certain instances, medical opinion must be sought.

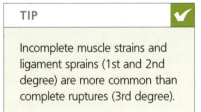

TIP

Incomplete muscle strains and ligament sprains (1st and 2nd degree) are more common than complete ruptures (3rd degree).

TIP

Ligaments are assessed by ascertaining the history of the problem, close inspection of the affected region, attempting to differentiate between other possibly injured tissues, ligament stress tests, and careful palpation. In certain instances, especially where fracture may also be suspected, medical opinion should be sought.

TIP

Commonly injured ligaments include those at: the acromio-clavicular (AC) and sterno-clavicular (SC) joints of the shoulder girdle; the medial and lateral collateral ligaments of the elbow; the dorsal, volar and collateral ligaments of the wrist; the collateral ligaments of the fingers; the medial and lateral collateral ligaments of the knee; the anterior and posterior cruciate ligaments within the knee joint; the anterior and posterior tibio-fibular ligaments of the ankle; the lateral collateral ligaments of the ankle; the deltoid ligaments of the medial ankle.

Sprains

A sprain is a tearing, partial or complete, of a ligament. Sprains, like strains, are graded according to their severity. Ligaments, which are composed predominantly of collagen fibres, possess a great deal of tensile strength, which they require to perform their job as stabilizers of joints. Ligaments also help to encourage a normal range of motion, and prevent unwanted movements. They are non-contractile, but have a degree of longitudinal pliability, which allows a modicum of stretch to safely occur. However, when ligaments are stretched beyond their normal pliable length, they will not recoil, and will remain slightly stretched, possibly leading to a laxity and reduced stability in the affected joint. This effect has been described as a plastic deformation of the fibres. If the ligament is stressed beyond its range of plastic deformity, which is at the extreme of its range of movement, it will tear. Ligaments can tear at or near to their attachments into bone or anywhere along their length. Severe sprains are often associated with dislocation or fracture.

A first degree sprain is a minor partial tearing of fibres. There will be minimal fibre damage, local pain and tenderness, and minimal loss of function. The joint should still retain its stability and have no obvious deformity, aside from possible minimal swelling and associated muscle spasm. Recovery is normally quick (two to three weeks) given appropriate therapeutic management.

A second degree sprain is a more severe partial tearing of ligament fibres. There may be pain at rest, pain on weight-bearing, and pain during stress testing. There is likely to be considerable swelling and loss of function. Return to fitness is usual within three to six weeks.

A third degree sprain is a complete rupture, where there is a complete or virtual lack of continuity in the fibres of the affected ligament. There will be severe pain at the time of injury, but later the pain may be less than that of a second degree sprain. There will also be severe loss of joint function, associated muscle spasm and marked instability. A complete rupture will often lead to a rapid swelling around the joint. This grade of sprain demands surgical repair or at least cast immobilization, prior to a comprehensive rehabilitation programme. Return to full fitness commonly takes three to four months or longer.

Fractures

A **fracture** is a complete or partial break of a bone, commonly resulting from a direct impact such as an awkward or heavy fall, or a badly timed tackle. Fractures require a considerable recovery time, from three to five weeks for a finger or toe, and up to 15 to 20 weeks for a femoral or tibial break. The fractures sustained by children tend to heal more quickly than those of adults. For competitive sportspeople severe fractures can be career threatening but, in the main, fractures can be recovered from very successfully. If fracture is at all suspected, then the individual must be referred for X-ray.

The signs and symptoms suggestive of a fracture are:

- history of fall or other forceful impact
- swelling, bruising and possibly bleeding
- local tenderness and pain
- reduced pain on gentle distraction of the bones
- increased pain on gentle compression of the bones
- localized pain on gentle percussion of superficial bony landmarks
- restricted movement
- deformity.

There are a variety of classifications of fracture. They can be open (where the bone pierces the skin), or closed. A simple fracture is a relatively clean break with little damage to surrounding tissues. A compound fracture is where there is substantial damage to the surrounding tissues. A displaced fracture is one where the bone ends lack continuity. When the affected bone or bones are shattered or broken into more than two pieces, it is known as a comminuted fracture. A transverse fracture is where the fracture line runs horizontally through the bone. A spiral fracture is where the fracture line runs in a rotational direction longitudinally through the bone. A greenstick fracture is an incomplete break, and is often seen in children, owing to the relative softness of the bone. An avulsion fracture is where the attachment site of a tendon or ligament is pulled away from the bone. A stress fracture is a hairline or micro-fracture. These fractures result from repetitive physical stress, rather than an isolated forceful incident, and are therefore classed as overuse injuries.

Commonly, undisplaced, simple fractures are initially treated with cast immobilization. More severe fractures may also be internally directly screwed or plated. Internal or external fixation is a common orthopaedic procedure for the more complicated breaks. Having an externally fixed stability frame holding the healing bones and joints in place allows for earlier patient mobility and concurrent rehabilitation.

Certain pathologies affecting the density, strength and resilience of bone, such as osteoporosis, make the sufferer far more prone to fracture, and therefore measures should be taken to prevent such occurrences. Children have a vulnerability to growth plate fractures, and these injuries can have a strong negative impact upon their physical development, leading to biomechanical problems, if not properly managed.

There are several potential complications to consider when presented with a fracture. Acute compartment syndrome can occur due to the swelling resulting from the injury, which may in extreme cases require emergency surgical release of the affected fascia (fasciotomy). Infection is a more likely secondary consequence of an open fracture. Deep vein thrombosis (DVT) sometimes occurs because of insufficient early stage rehabilitation (i.e. mobility and contractile work). The quality of the union of the fractured bone presents major problems if there is malunion or non-union.

Overuse injuries

Aside from the typical contusions, strains and sprains occurring regularly during physical activities, probably the most common sports injuries are those resulting from repetitive physical stress. The people most prone to overuse injuries are those who train very hard, frequently. Overuse injuries sometimes arise purely from one or two overexertive training sessions, and often occur early in the season. Of course any physical activity, if performed without appropriate preparation and the necessary level of fitness, can soon cause problems, because the affected structures are not yet ready to perform the work asked of them, and this is especially so for those who are beginning an exercise regime or who are returning after a period of relative inactivity.

Endurance athletes, such as those involved in distance running, race-walking and cycling, are particularly vulnerable because the nature of their sport demands an arduous training regime of repetitive motions, which are continually performed for lengthy periods of time. Similarly, aerobic class instructors are prone to overuse injury because they need to put in a lot of practice to get their routines prepared, often on top of an already busy physical working (class teaching) schedule.

Any competitive athlete or exerciser is prone to overuse problems because, in the effort to improve fitness and performance, there are almost unavoidable physical stresses placed upon the main functioning parts of the body. Therefore, the front-crawl swimmer is prone to shoulder problems (swimmer's shoulder), the tennis player is prone to lateral epicondylitis (tennis elbow), the golfer to medial epicondylitis (golfer's elbow), the jumper to patellar tendonitis (jumper's knee), and the runner to ilio-tibial band friction syndrome (runner's knee).

With overuse injuries, ascertaining and, if possible, rectifying the cause are the major parts of the treatment. Most overuse injuries begin as a minor inflammatory reaction in the affected tissues, and, obviously, the injury itself requires appropriate acute, sub-acute or chronic treatment. The initial treatment nearly always involves relative rest from all aggravating activities, while maintaining fitness with alternative exercises, combined with a course of clinical therapy.

In addition to the nature of the affected individual's chosen sports and training methods, the therapist will be looking for other related causes of the problem. Some of the first areas to explore are their posture, biomechanics and body composition. If there is any significant, predisposing, structural malalignment (especially of the affected limbs), leg length discrepancy, muscle imbalance, restricted mobility or inappropriate body composition for the activities they perform, then these must be attended to as part of the first courses of action.

The next line of assessment involves examination of their training routine and looking for striking errors (e.g. excessive intensity, frequency or duration; sudden changes to training; lack of variation; insufficient rest and recovery; insufficient warm-up). The environment in which they exercise requires attention, remembering that training regularly on hard, unyielding surfaces, such as tarmac or concrete, can soon lead to impacting injury problems such as stress fractures or periostitis. Similarly, are the equipment, footwear and clothing appropriate for both the individual and the activity? Psychological factors are also sometimes involved in the cause of overuse injuries, and if this is suspected then referral for counselling might be appropriate.

The signs and symptoms of overuse injuries tend to come on gradually, initially beginning as a slight discomfort, and perhaps, at first, aching a little after activities and easing off after warm-up. If symptoms are ignored they will more often than not exacerbate. Soon, the problem that began as a minor discomfort becomes so uncomfortable that not only sports, but also normal daily activities, are very compromised.

A stress fracture, as previously mentioned, is a hairline crack in the bone. It is most common in runners, but stress fractures are also very much a problem for throwers, footballers, ballet dancers, cricketers and other athletes. Most major bones are potential victims of stress fracture, especially the femur, tibia, fibula, tarsals, metatarsals, pubis and vertebrae, which are all weight-bearing bones. Tibial stress fractures are more prevalent in individuals with pes cavus, and fibular stress fractures are more prevalent in those who overpronate. In sports where upper body strength is very important, such as racquet sports, baseball or rowing, stress fractures are not uncommon in the bones of the arm, the scapula or even the ribs.

Stress fractures are usually defined as being either the result of abnormal stresses (overuse) placed on normal bone (fatigue stress fracture), or because of normal stresses placed on abnormal bone (insufficiency stress fractures). A stress fracture, like the majority of overuse injuries, will typically reveal itself insidiously, initially by a mild aching accompanied by localized tenderness. As the injury develops, the aching worsens and the tenderness becomes distinct and strong. Stress fractures do not always show up well on X-ray, indeed signs and symptoms may be present for weeks before radiographic evidence reveals the nature of the problem. If a stress fracture is strongly suspected, but the X-ray is negative, then other investigations should be performed, the main procedures being: bone scan; magnetic resonance imaging (MRI); computed tomography (CT) scan. Once the diagnosis has been confirmed, and a management protocol instigated, stress fractures can take anything from around six to eight weeks to six months to heal properly.

Stress fractures of the lower leg are sometimes diagnostically confused with shin splints (periostitis), as the two injuries share many similarities. Periostitis is simply an inflammation of the periosteum. The most common site for this problem is at the medial, distal tibia (medial tibial stress syndrome), which is commonly referred to as shin splints. **Overtraining** (excessive hill training, for example) and the presence of biomechanical malalignment (especially overpronation) are the main causes of this familiar problem. The typical symptoms are local pain and tenderness, and deep aching and stiffness after activity, There may be palpable thickening and nodules in the affected region. Management usually requires relative rest, anti-inflammatory treatment, biomechanical correction and massage therapy to tight or thickened muscle fibres.

Articular (hyaline) cartilage is very resilient, and is designed to withstand physical stress, but it is not indestructible. Arthritis is inflammation of a joint. Joints take a lot of physical stress during repetitive activities, especially those that are of high intensity. Chondromalacia is basically a degeneration of cartilage, and is a common knee problem (chondromalacia patella), particularly when predisposing factors are present (excessive Q angle; imbalanced quadriceps muscles; a frequently dislocating patella). By exposing weight-bearing joints to continually excessive physical insults, with the associated chronic inflammation, the individual is at a greater risk to developing the symptoms of osteoarthritis earlier in life. Clearly, the best prevention for this undesirable outcome, is to vary training routines and to attend to problems as they arise.

Synovitis and capsulitis are further inflammatory reactions to excessive physical stresses, or trauma, to the synovium or joint capsule of synovial joints. These conditions affect more commonly the ankle, metatarsal-phalangeal joints, the knee and hip. Occasionally, the same symptoms are observed as one of the early warning signs of rheumatoid arthritis, and are typified by localized painful swelling or effusion at the joint.

Osteochonditis dissecans is the condition of loose bodies (fragments) of bone and cartilage in the affected joint, which have been broken away during physical loading. These fragments can cause discomfort and joint effusion, and may even cause the joint to lock in position. Osteochonditis dissecans is more common in adolescents, and the main joints that are affected are the knee and ankle. If massage, mobilization or exercise does not help the problem, then **arthroscopy** (key-hole joint-cleansing operation) may be required.

When muscles are exposed to long-term repetitive loading, which causes micro-trauma to the fibres, they can undergo an inflammatory process which results in fibrosis (thickening) and adhesion formation. The end result of such a problem is possibly localized pain, reduced suppleness, and increased susceptibility to strains. Normal management or prevention of this situation is by regular stretching and massage therapy.

DOMS is a sports-related phenomenon that is not so well understood in terms of its aetiology. It has been postulated that the aching and soreness that sometimes develop a day or two after strenuous physical activities can be due to a combination of the normal adaptation of tissues to the demands placed upon them, the accumulation of metabolic products (lactic acid; exudates; enzymatic efflux; tissue debris), micro-trauma in the affected tissues, muscle spasm (which may house some damaged fibres), or increased compartmental pressure. The treatment of DOMS should involve thorough cool-downs, massage and hydrotherapy, alongside proper sports conditioning.

Compartment syndrome is quite common. This condition commonly involves, in reaction to intense training, an increase in muscle bulk, which puts pressure on the surrounding compartmental (fascial) sheath, which can accommodate only so much muscle growth or fluid accumulation. Typically, the compartments of the calf are affected, restricting both blood flow and nerve conduction, which leads to deep-seated aching, paraesthesia or anaesthesia. Conservative attention, by way of massage techniques, to the fascia so as to increase its elasticity, and to the muscles so as to decongest and relax them, can be very beneficial. If this approach fails then fasciotomy may be required.

Tendons are particularly vulnerable to overuse injury. Tendonitis is the inflammation of a tendon, and until quite recently was the term used to describe chronic tendon problems. However, the term of choice for chronic degeneration of tendon fibres is tendinosis, as the term tendonitis suggests that inflammation is present, which is often not the case with long-standing tendon problems.

Tendons are tough, resilient connective tissues attaching muscle to bone. They do not possess a great deal of elasticity (leaving that to their muscles), and when repeatedly stretched are vulnerable to micro-tearing. Because of their relatively poor blood supply and the very nature of the damage, they can be slow to heal. Repeated overloading of a tendon can cause the cross-linking structure of its collagen fibres to break apart, and the development of a chronic degenerative situation, with associated pain, tenderness and significantly reduced tensile strength. Pain from this condition is often worse after a period of rest, and may ease off during activity. The repair and rebuilding of the damaged collagen is a gradual process, and the rehabilitation can be long term, involving modified activities, progressive strength and flexibility work, heat, electrical therapy and deep massage.

Tenosynovitis is categorized as an inflammation of the synovial sheath that surrounds some tendons. The role of the sheath is to help provide smooth easy movement of the tendon underneath its supporting retinaculum. This condition is also sometimes referred to as tenovaginitis or paratendonitis. Typical signs and symptoms of this overuse problem are a thickening of the tendon, fibrous adhesions inside the sheath, and crepitus on movement. The main affected tendons are at the wrist and ankle.

Bursitis is simply the inflammation of a bursa, which can result from mechanical irritation, infection or arthritis. In sports, the repetitive movement of a tendon across its underlying bursa can easily irritate the fluid-filled pouch and cause it to become inflamed. Similarly, a fall, repeated falls, or repeated compression (e.g. 'housemaid's knee' or 'student's elbow') onto a bursa can also cause it to become inflamed. The symptoms are pain on movement, a smooth distinct swelling, sometimes reddened and warm to the touch. Where there are distinct biomechanical factors or particularly tight tendons, the bursa can easily become affected. The normal course of action is avoidance of all aggravating activities, anti-inflammatory treatment, and massage and stretching of tightened structures. In more persistent cases, sterile aspiration may be necessary.

Skin problems

Skin is a major organ. It protects, provides insulation, helps regulate body temperature and has excretory functions. It is, however, very prone to infection, irritation from mechanical, thermal and chemical trauma, allergic reactions and exacerbations of existing conditions. Dermatology is the area of medicine concerned with the diagnosis and treatment of specific skin disorders.

Obviously, being the body's initial external protector, skin is frequently injured, and cuts, abrasions and bruises occur all the time. Whenever skin is damaged, underlying tissues such as the muscles, ligaments, nerves and blood vessels may also be affected. It is important, also, to be alert to the possibility of infection with open wounds.

Skin is particularly vulnerable to fungal, bacterial and viral infections, especially in the sporting environment, where close contact occurs and

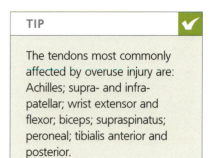

TIP

The tendons most commonly affected by overuse injury are: Achilles; supra- and infra-patellar; wrist extensor and flexor; biceps; supraspinatus; peroneal; tibialis anterior and posterior.

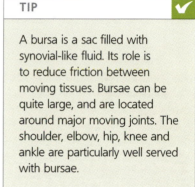

TIP

A bursa is a sac filled with synovial-like fluid. Its role is to reduce friction between moving tissues. Bursae can be quite large, and are located around major moving joints. The shoulder, elbow, hip, knee and ankle are particularly well served with bursae.

TIP

Most skin infections require an immediate appropriate response, i.e. prescriptive medication, avoiding contact with others, and close monitoring of symptoms.

where the necessary attention to hygiene can be found lacking. Skin infections are so often highly contagious, being spread by direct contact or indirectly by contact with such contaminated articles as towels and clothing.

The most common fungal infections are ringworm (tinea corporis) and athlete's foot (tinea pedis). Bacterial infections include boils (furuncles and carbuncles), impetigo and folliculitis. Viral infections affecting the skin, common to sports environments, include common verrucae (warts), which are often seen on the hands, and plantar verrucae, which occur on the soles of the feet, herpes simplex (e.g. 'Scrum pox') and molluscum contagiosum.

The most common sports-related allergic skin problem is irritant dermatitis (skin inflammation), which may be caused by hyper-sensitivity to a variety of substances and products, including items of equipment, rubber in shoes, adhesive tape, cold and heat preparations, and deodorant sprays. In such cases, a dermatologist should be sought for tests and advice, and the individual should avoid known irritants.

Of course, the athlete or exerciser is prone to such conditions as blisters and chafing (intertrigo), which occur at the sites of repetitive friction during movement. The feet and hands are the main sites of blisters, which result from ill-fitting (or new) footwear, and by performing unaccustomed, longer-duration tasks. Blisters can be avoided, to a degree, by making sure the equipment is correct for the user, by wearing in new training shoes gradually, wearing cotton socks (or even two pairs) and applying petroleum jelly at sites of friction. Foot powders, adhesive tape or 'second skin' pads can also be applied over potential sites to protect from excessive irritation. If blisters do occur, initially infection should be prevented by an application of antiseptic wash and covered with adhesive plaster (avoiding creases in the tape). If larger, painful, fluid-filled blisters form then, ideally, activities are halted until recovery occurs. Additionally, a piece of foam, with a hole cut out, can be placed over the blister to reduce the pressure on it. If necessary, blisters can be punctured and drained with a sterile needle, covered with antibiotic ointment, and then dressed, but this is not normally ideal because of the possibility of infection. If a blister needs to be drained, try to keep its roof intact for protection and to encourage callus formation.

Chafing is where the skin softens, in the presence of heat and moisture, and becomes rubbed raw. It can be more of a problem, especially between the thighs, for overweight individuals. Jogger's nipple is localized chafing of the nipple caused by friction from tight, sweaty or coarse running vests, and is more common in men, as women tend to have the protection of a bra. This problem can also be experienced in distance cycling, rowing and aerobics classes. Petroleum jelly, barrier cream, sticking plasters or even a nipple guard applied before activity is the best form of prevention.

More extreme environmental temperatures can have an adverse effect upon the skin. Prickly heat (miliaria) is not uncommon in athletes because it is related to excessive perspiration. Certain sports require a great deal of clothing, such as American football or fencing, which leads to excessive sweating, and some individuals have a natural tendency to sweat profusely.

Sunburn is best prevented by wearing appropriate factor sunscreen and clothing protection. If possible, avoid exercise during the middle of the day in very hot conditions, as there is also the risk of heat exhaustion, heat stroke and heat cramps.

Most skin problems can be prevented by being steadfast in hygiene, which especially includes showering and changing from damp clothing soon after exercise, and not sharing towels, etc. Sports equipment gets used by many people and should be cleaned regularly. Therapists should be observant to the possibility of allergic reactions, and should be able to discreetly ask participants and clients if they suffer from any particular allergies. Especially in team situations, athletes should be encouraged to make it known to those concerned if they are suffering from any infective skin conditions.

STAGES OF SOFT-TISSUE INJURY HEALING: THE INFLAMMATION AND HEALING PROCESS

There are three basic and generalized phases of response to injury, each affected by the severity of injury, the tissues predominantly involved, and the therapeutic interventions applied during each phase.

Acute inflammatory phase

Inflammation is the sequence of reactions which take place in the body in response to injury. Inflammation can result not just from physical injury, but also from thermal injury, electrical injury, chemical injury, infection or immune reactions. Considered a defence reaction, and very much part of the healing process, soft-tissue inflammation resulting from sports injuries can be caused by pressure, friction, repeated load, overload, repeated stretch, over-stretch, or impact trauma.

There are five classic signs and symptoms of soft-tissue inflammation: redness; swelling; warmth; pain and tenderness; impaired function. The redness and warmth are due to the increase in circulation (hyperaemia) that typically occurs a few minutes after suffering the injury. Swelling occurs for a variety of reasons: there may be bleeding from ruptured capillaries;

THE THREE STAGES OF SOFT-TISSUE INJURY HEALING

1 Acute inflammatory phase (the acute stage). This phase is the body's initial reaction to injury. Typically producing redness, swelling, warmth and pain, resulting in impaired function, it lasts for the first three to five days following the trauma.

2 Cellular proliferation phase (the early repair stage). This phase of healing, where new tissue is laid down at the injury site, typically lasts for around two to five weeks, following on from the inflammatory phase.

3 Remodelling phase (the consolidation or maturation stage). This final phase, where the new tissue gains its strength through structural organization, usually continues for several months.

vasodilation of the blood vessels running through the area; increased permeability of the vessels; flooding of fluid into the interstitial spaces surrounding the injured area. The area is painful and tender both because of the increase in tissue pressure, and because of the sudden stimulation of specific pain receptors. The pain and the swelling inhibit normal movements and functioning.

One of the main objectives at this stage is to control the inflammation. An excessive period of inflammation is not conducive to ideal repair. Prolonged increased vascular activity and the resultant swelling in and around the damaged tissues impede the rate of early repair, and increases the amount of secondary hypoxic death of previously undamaged cells adjacent to the injury site. In the acute stage, the well-known acronym **RICES** (Rest, Ice, Compression, Elevation, Support), reminds us simply of how to approach many of the musculo-skeletal injuries we have to attend to. Other interventions may be necessary: immobilization; hospitalization; medication.

Immediately after the injury has occurred there is a degree of cell necrosis (death) in the affected tissues. This is followed by the acute vascular response. Vasoconstriction occurs initially, owing to the instant release of hormones, as a protective mechanism, and this lasts for just a few minutes. The vasodilation and increased vessel wall permeability follow, which are due to the release of histamine and other chemicals. This response can last for an hour or so. There follows a leakage of plasma (rich in electrolytes and proteins) from post-capillary venules, a leakage of lymph (lymphatics are also ruptured in the injury), platelet gathering (clot formation) and haemostasis (variety of mechanisms to stem bleeding), and leucocyte margination (a variety of white blood cells gather and adhere to the walls of the affected vessels, and are important in the protection and clean-up operation). The combined result of all this activity is a localized oedema, with a degree of secondary hypoxic death. Phagocytosis (the ingesting and disposing of tissue debris) is a crucial part of the process, and is performed primarily by the macrophage cells (which are themselves converted leucocytes). Phagocytosis typically completes the acute stage, and the next phase of healing begins.

Cellular proliferation phase

This stage of soft-tissue healing is when the first structural repair work begins, with the development of a network of new capillaries and lymphatics, which means that the injury site now has improved circulation and drainage. There then follows a proliferation of fibroblasts at the injury site. Fibroblasts are specialized cells that develop in the connective tissues, and they are responsible for the production of the new ground substance of repair and for the precursors of collagen, elastic fibres and reticular fibres. Collagen is the main structural component of skin, tendon, ligament, bone, cartilage and scar tissue. Typically, by the fourth or fifth day, a weak mesh of fibrous connective tissue has been laid down at the injury site. At this stage, the newly formed tissue is fragile, vascular and vulnerable to re-injury. Over the following three or four weeks, the capillary network reduces and the new tissue gradually strengthens in its structure, with the formation of cross-

TIP ✔

Having just suffered an injury, the individual may be quite concerned as to the seriousness of the problem. They will be hoping for a quick recovery, with minimum discomfort. Sportspeople especially, are very physically active, and if the pain of an injury stops them from being as active, or worse threatens their future participation in sport, it can be very frustrating, even devastating. From the sports therapist they require an educated assessment of the problem, and appropriate treatment, or at least good advice.

links between the collagen fibres. The strength that develops in the tissue during this phase of healing allows for carefully controlled rehabilitation exercise and treatment to be instigated. At this stage, mobility exercise within a safe and pain-free range is usually combined with early graded strength work. As the injury is still in early repair, excessive stress to the tissue should be avoided.

Remodelling and maturation phase

The repairing (scar) tissue contains relatively unorganized collagen fibres, and the union between the damaged structures is still moderately fragile. The fibres of collagen are initially randomly arranged (in a haphazard formation), but over time and with careful rehabilitation they become aligned along the lines of external stress that are placed upon them during both normal activities and rehabilitation exercises. This is the consolidation or remodelling phase, and as the scar tissue matures, it gradually becomes more avascular with poor elasticity. The rehabilitation at this stage normally becomes gradually more aggressive, in terms of mobility, flexibility, strength, proprioception and power, which are all crucial to the long-term functionality of the repaired tissue.

FACTORS AFFECTING THE HEALING OF INJURIES

The rate and quality of the healing of damaged tissues depend upon a variety of factors. Obviously, the size, severity, tissue type and location of the injury directly influence the degree of physiological response and, in addition to the nature of the injury, the individual's normal state of health, whether it is conducive to speedy repair, or whether it is compromised in some way, also has a significant effect upon the resulting outcome. There are many medical conditions that can have a detrimental effect on an individual's capacity to heal, and these need to be identified during consultation. The healing of injuries is also affected by the individual's age (younger people tend to heal more quickly than old), and their general metabolic and nutritional status. It should also be borne in mind that clients often present with more than one injury, or with other ongoing problems, which the therapist must work around and take care not to aggravate. Sometimes, because there are several problems to contend with, the therapeutic approach does become more limited, for example, the client may not be able to assume preferred treatment positions, or there may be specific contra-indications to certain techniques. Such instances usually require a thoughtful plan of action, utilizing methods that can be safely employed, combined with a sensitive and sensible explanation for the client. Therapists should really see these more complicated cases as a challenge that provides the opportunity to gain valuable experience and increased confidence.

TIP

Following injury, the acute inflammatory response either leads on to a complete repair, with the injured tissue being replaced, ideally with similar tissue, or more likely, with scar tissue. The unfortunate alternative outcome, when the affected tissues are poor to heal and subjected to continued physical stress, is chronic inflammation, where tissues remain swollen and painful, and where a degeneration process ensues.

If the acutely injured individual has not paid a visit to the casualty department or minor injuries clinic at their local hospital, then it is often the GP who is their first port of call. The patient may, at this point, require referral for more specialist assessment. Unfortunately, a wait of weeks or even months is not unusual for an appointment with an orthopaedic consultant or even physiotherapist, and the patient may choose to seek out private treatment in the short term. For minor sports injuries the doctor may prescribe anti-inflammatory medications or pain relief. The doctor or practice nurse may dress or strap an acute injury, and may also aspirate an inflamed bursa. Some GPs and physiotherapists will offer corticosteroid injections (often combined with an anaesthetic agent) for certain injuries and problems such as tendonitis, tenosynovitis, synovitis, bursitis, chronic strain and osteoarthritis. Doctors trained in joint manipulation or acupuncture may also offer these procedures if appropriate, but this is less common.

Prescriptive medications are those recommended by a doctor or consultant. Over the counter (OTC) drugs are those perhaps recommended by a doctor, physiotherapist or pharmacist, but not specifically prescribed. Both prescriptive or OTC drugs should be taken with care and awareness of their effect, benefits and potential adverse effects. Therapists must be able to glean from their client which medications they take regularly, occasionally and currently, and for how long and also whether they suffer any adverse effects from taking them.

The sports therapist can sometimes be presented with clients who have had recent surgical treatment for their injury. Surgery for sports injuries is often viewed as a last resort, but it is frequently performed. Treatment by conservative methods (physical therapy) is usually considered preferable to the cost, inconvenience, discomfort and inherent prognostic risk of invasive surgical intervention. Arthroscopy (key-hole surgery) is one of the most commonly used surgical techniques for sports injuries. This technique usually involves two small punctures into the affected joint – one for the arthroscope (a miniature telescopic camera) and the other for inserting a selection of instruments for cleansing, flushing, trimming or extracting pieces of the joint. Arthroscopy has become widely available during the past 20 years or so, and is generally regarded as a great advancement in surgical technique. It is usually performed under local anaesthetic, causes minimal tissue trauma, and normally allows earlier post-operative participation in rehabilitation and return to activities.

Any form of surgical intervention should be followed up with a post-operative assessment from the specialists concerned, and probably with at least some form of physiotherapy, be it guided exercise or actual treatment.

Some clients will have already received a course of physiotherapy prior to attending for sports therapy. Whether following on from hospital or physiotherapy treatment, post-medical rehabilitation can be an important part of the sports therapist's work. Ideally, there will be a formal liaison between the practitioners involved, at least in the form of a report detailing the individual's diagnosis and previous rehabilitation. Any uncertainties regarding their recent history should be clarified by way of communication between the sports therapist, client, and GP or physiotherapist.

TIP

Medical agents in the pharmaceutical treatment of sports injuries may be applied in a variety of ways: orally; topically (agent applied to the skin in the form of rubs, liniments, creams and sprays); locally acting injection; generally acting injection; phonophoresis (analgesic or anti-inflammatory agent applied through the skin by ultrasound).

Treatment methods and modalities for soft-tissue injuries

For the treatment and management of the majority of minor sports-related injuries, the following treatment tools and techniques will suffice:

- **cold packs**/ice cup/cold spray
- taping and strapping
- progressive and specific remedial massage techniques
- progressive and specific remedial exercises
- electro-therapy (**electrical muscle stimulation/transcutaneous electronic nerve stimulation**/Audiosonic/**G5 machine**/percussor/ultrasound)
- thermal therapy (infra-red/paraffin wax bath/**hot packs**/contrast baths)
- nutritional recommendations.

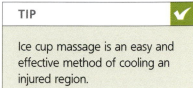

TIP

Ice cup massage is an easy and effective method of cooling an injured region.

The way in which an injury is treated depends upon the severity and time-scale of the problem. Whether the injury receives optimum treatment and attention is a big factor in whether the injury becomes a chronic problem. In the vast majority of minor cases, the acute approach is attended to with basic rest and cooling. Crucial to the long-term outcome is not only how the sports therapist attends to the presenting symptoms of the client at each visit, but also what they identify as the causes of their problems (the aetiology of injuries is very important to the prevention of their recurrence).

The sports therapist has quite a selection of methods that can be used at each stage to enhance the healing process. The strapping up of injured joints reduces the possibility of aggravating the injury by limiting unwanted movements, and therefore allows the early repair tissue to be laid down. Strapping can also be used later in the recovery process by providing support and protection during remedial exercise and also during functional return. (See chapter 11.)

There are a variety of **remedial massage** techniques, most of which have the flexibility to be applied with differing intensities. This basically means that massage techniques can be applied to improve the healing of most injuries, and in each phase, remembering that the main contra-indication is direct treatment over an acute injury site. Audiosonic massage is useful in early stage treatment, but strong electrical massage is probably best reserved for the remodelling phase. Ultrasound has a similar flexibility in that it too can be used, in many instances, in each stage of the healing process. Electrical muscle stimulation (EMS) is particularly indicated to passively exercise muscles without causing stress to injured joints, and therefore is very useful in both the proliferation and remodelling phases of repair. Heat therapy is a majorly important intervention, increasing local circulations, relaxing muscle tightness and calming pain messages. Heat is used during the middle and later phases of healing. The main use for transcutaneous electronic nerve stimulation (TENS) is the modification of pain, and so it can often be a useful adjunct when managing more chronically painful problems.

The methods and modalities used for the treatment of injuries by sports therapists vary among individuals, and depend upon the level of training undertaken by the therapist and the resources available to them. It is normal

---

KEY OBJECTIVES FOR THE EFFECTIVE MANAGEMENT OF INJURIES

Early stage

Protection against further damage.

Limitation of any bleeding and swelling.

Medical attention if necessary.

Reassurance and advice.

Reduction of pain.

Prevention of stiffness.

Encouragement of optimal repair.

Maintenance of fitness, if possible, through alternative, non-aggravating exercises.

Intermediate stage

Gradual re-education of movement.

Restoration of proprioceptive mechanisms.

Increase mobility of joint and soft-tissue.

Increase power of muscles.

Maintenance of aerobic fitness.

Late and functional stages

Optimal repair and scar tissue formation.

Gradual restoration of confidence in using affected part.

Gradual restoration of function and return to activities of daily living (ADL).

Progressive overload of intensity, frequency and duration of training.

Improvements to training (education/structure of regime/skills coaching).

Perform return to fitness test prior to competitive level action.

Prevention of recurrence of the injury by generating increased awareness in the athlete.

TIP

The crucial thing for therapists to remember is that sporting injuries require appropriate management. If inappropriate management is instigated, problems can easily worsen. Before applying any modality, or recommending any exercise, be sure that it is the right thing to do.

---

for the sports therapist to use a combined approach, where, for example, electrical and thermal therapy is combined with massage, remedial exercise and specific advice. The therapist may also have additional qualifications and skills, perhaps in osteopathy, homeopathy, naturopathy or acupuncture, which can be incorporated into their practice.

The student therapist should continually develop their confidence in attending to injuries by getting as much practical experience as they can, preferably working with others as part of a team, not being afraid to ask the right questions, and delving deep into their reference books and course notes. In the course of time, most injuries that lend themselves to sports therapy will respond well. Therapists should follow the processes of consultation, assessment of the problem and resulting treatment and recommendations with a certain confidence that will come from having studied and practised hard. To provide safe and effective injury treatment, the therapist will always be aware of the potential dangers of treatment, and of having an appreciation of the potential contra-indications to their treatments. Keeping alert to any warning signs that something is not quite right with the injury, or their treatment of it, is part of the therapist's protection against causing any undue harm. Similarly, having a suspicion that the presenting injury would benefit from having someone else attend to it means that the therapist is the person who should recommend this.

INJURY COMPLICATIONS

The more common complications of sports injuries can be related to a poor initial diagnosis, inadequate or inappropriate treatments during the early stages of healing, or insufficient care and attention given to the injury by the athlete.

COMPLICATIONS OF INJURY	
Common complications	**More severe complications**
A slow resolution of symptoms.	Chronic inflammation.
Ongoing pain and discomfort.	Chronic pain.
Frustration, anxiety, depression.	Infection.
Biomechanical problems.	Delayed, non-union or malunion of fractures.
Excessive scarring.	Deformity.
Excessive adhesion formation.	Early onset or worsening osteoarthritis.
Joint laxity.	Soft-tissue shortening and contracture.
Restricted joint mobility.	Irreparable nerve damage.
Weakness.	Unresolved paralysis.
Reduced proprioception.	Myositis ossificans.
Increased vulnerability to further problems.	Reflex sympathetic dystrophy (RSD).
	Enforced retirement from sports.
	Enforced changes to work activities.

COMMON SPORTS INJURY PROBLEMS

As previously discussed, sports injuries fall into a variety of categories. It is not within the scope of this book to be able to fully describe all kinds of sports injuries and how they are best attended to with treatment and rehabilitation. It is recommended that if you would like to increase your depth of understanding of sports injury management, then you should consider studying at higher levels, and certainly look to other specific sources of information (see the bibliography and recommended reading).

Obviously, each injury is unique, as is each affected body region, different tissue types and the actual severity of the problem. Whether the athlete has injured muscles or ligaments in their arm or their leg does not always make a great difference to the fundamental strategy of treatment that the therapist should formulate. They should look at the underlying cause of the problem, the severity of the injury, the tissues that are mainly affected, the current stage of healing, the resulting effect of the injury on the athlete's functional abilities and then what the first course of action should be. Acute soft-tissue injuries usually require rest from aggravating activities and probably cold treatment, often combined with compression and elevation. Once inflammation has subsided, early rehabilitation can begin in the form of hands-on treatment, modalities and, commonly, safe-range mobility work and early strength and proprioceptive work. Support, in terms of taping or strapping, may be appropriate during both remedial exercise and activities of daily living, alongside clear guidance from the therapist. Obviously, the region that is affected does have an influence on the treatment strategy, but a muscle is a muscle, and a ligament is a ligament, and they can often be treated in similar ways wherever they are.

Successful therapeutic outcome for sports injuries should result from:

- knowing the body's musculo-skeletal anatomy
- knowing the history of the client, their sport and their presenting injury
- knowing how to assess the different tissues at each region (manual muscle tests; ligament stress tests; nerve tests; special tests)
- selecting the most appropriate therapeutic techniques for each treatment session
- encouraging and explaining to the injured athlete how to best help themselves.

Most sports, whether team games or individual pursuits, are classified as either contact sports (e.g. rugby and karate), non-contact sports (e.g. badminton and golf) or essentially non-contact, but where some physical contact can occur (e.g. netball and cricket). Physically harmful contact can potentially occur in most activities, for example, in a running or cycling race with fellow competitors, or in a game of volleyball with a fellow team member.

COMMON SPORTS-RELATED INJURIES

This list is not comprehensive, but it does include many of the more prevalent injuries in certain sports. Sports therapists may work with teams or individual athletes, and it is in their interest to get to know well the most common problems associated with the sport, and the best strategies to prevent and treat them.

Aerobics/exercise classes: calf strains; ankle sprains; Achilles tendonitis; plantar fascitis; tibial periostitis; femoral tibial and metatarsal stress fractures; patellar tendonitis. A slip or a fall can result in a variety of injuries. Fitness instructors who teach many classes are particularly vulnerable to overuse injuries, as are over-enthusiastic participants.

Badminton/squash/tennis: lateral or medial epicondylitis (tennis elbow); shoulder strains, sprains, impingements, bursitis and tendonitis; calf strains (tennis leg); upper extremity nerve entrapment; abdominal muscle strains; ankle and knee sprains; back and knee pain. Emphasis must be placed upon good technique and appropriate equipment. In squash there is a greater chance of impacting injury with the opponent or court wall. Collisions can occur in doubles games in badminton or tennis. Amateur racquet sports players sometimes need reminding to fitness train in preparation for their sport.

Basketball: calf strain; ankle sprain; upper extremity strains, sprains and tendonitis; abdominal and back muscle strains; tibial and navicular stress fractures.

Boxing: contusions; facial cuts; cranial and facial fractures; concussion; cervical strains and sprains; rib fractures; wrist strains and sprains; metacarpal-phalangeal synovitis; chronic brain injury. In training bouts and competition the even matching of opponents is very important.

Cricket: contusions; haematoma; shoulder strains, sprains, impingements and bursitis; upper extremity avulsion and stress fractures; lumbar stress fractures; back strains; wrist and hand strains and sprains. Different playing positions in cricket present different types of injury.

Cycling: neck, back and knee pain; lower extremity strains and sprains; ulnar neuropathy (handlebar palsy); carpal tunnel syndrome; ilio-tibial band friction syndrome; chafing. Cycling accidents can result in all manner of injuries. Correct set-up of the bike is crucial in the avoidance of overuse injuries.

Discus/javelin/shot-put/hammer: upper extremity strains, sprains, impingements, bursitis and tendonitis; ulnar neuritis; avulsion fractures of the elbow; back strain; knee pain. Emphasis must be on good technique and appropriate equipment.

Distance running: thigh and calf strains; Achilles tendonitis; ilio-tibial band friction syndrome; patellar tendonitis; patello-femoral syndrome; tibial periostitis; femoral, tibial and metatarsal stress fractures; sesamoiditis; plantar fascitis; ankle sprains; back pain. Distance running involves a great deal of repetitive pounding. It is crucial to correct any biomechanical problems, to choose appropriate running surfaces, and to wear suitable running shoes.

Football: head, facial and dental injuries; contusions, especially quadriceps; skin abrasions; ankle sprains; knee collateral and cruciate sprains; meniscus tears; thigh strains and haematoma; groin strains; osteitis pubis; hernia; thigh and calf cramps; compartment syndrome; neck and back pain; chondromalacia patella; anterior ankle tenosynovitis; osteochondritis; Osgood Schlatter's disease. Direct impact from an opponent can result in a variety of injuries. Goalkeepers are vulnerable to a selection of additional injuries. Amateur footballers sometimes need reminding to fitness train in preparation for their games.

Golf: back strain; intervertebral disc herniation; medial or lateral epicondylitis; shoulder strains, impingements and tendonitis; wrist strains, sprains and tenosynovitis (de Quervain's disease). Emphasis must be placed upon good swing technique to avoid injuries. Be particularly aware of the possibility of being struck by either a golf club during a swing, or by a flying ball.

Gymnastics: shoulder and wrist impingements, dislocations, strains and sprains; lumbar stress fractures; spondylolysis; osteochondritis of the elbow. Awkward falls can cause all manner of injuries. Children and adolescents are particularly vulnerable to gymnastic injuries, and their training routine must be carefully managed.

Jumping: hamstring, quadriceps and calf strains; patello-femoral syndrome (jumper's knee); infra-patellar tendonitis; tibial periostitis; tibial stress fractures; Achilles tendonitis. The high jump may pose greater incidence of neck and back injuries. The long and triple jump present similar commonly suffered injuries as those seen in sprinting.

Martial arts: contusions; facial cuts; facial fractures; concussion; cervical strains and sprains; quadriceps haematoma. In both training and competition, even matching of opponents is very important. There are a selection of different martial art disciplines, each having their own potential for particular injuries.

Rowing: back and thigh strains; back and knee pain; upper extremity strains; wrist tendonitis; rib stress fractures. Additional dangers include drowning or collision with motor boats.

Rugby: head, facial and dental injury; shoulder strains; sprains and dislocations; neuropraxia of brachial plexus; clavicular fractures; hip and thigh contusions; neck and back pain; groin and thigh strains; ankle sprains; metacarpal-phalangeal sprains. Rugby is a particularly close contact sport, typically with many relatively heavy and well-built players, which can present problems for some of the opposition players, particularly the backs.

Sprinting: hamstring, quadriceps and calf strains; patello-femoral syndrome; infra-patellar tendonitis; tibial periostitis; tibial stress fractures; Achilles tendonitis; plantar fascitis; compartment syndrome; bursitis of hip and knee.

Swimming: shoulder strains, impingements and bursitis; neck, back and knee pain. Good technique is crucial to avoiding overuse injury.

Volleyball: patellar tendonitis; patello-femoral syndrome; chondromalacia patella; ilio-tibial friction syndrome; ankle sprains; Achilles tendonitis; shoulder impingement; rotator cuff strains; metatarsal stress fractures; wrist and hand strains and sprains.

Weight-training: muscle strains; shoulder and elbow tendonitis; shoulder bursitis; intervertebral disc herniation. Good technique, appropriate weights, repetitions and sets are crucial to the avoidance of both acute and overuse injuries. Maintenance of a safe exercising environment is very important. Regular weight-trainers should beware of causing muscle and postural imbalances.

In the sports therapy clinic, the therapist will attend to many different types of injuries, and not all of sporting origin. Tradespeople, musicians, computer operators, truck drivers, factory workers and even sports therapists all have a certain potential for suffering both acute and overuse injuries. Repetitive stresses, poor working postures, awkward working positions, unprepared heavy lifting, and mental and emotional stress leave the worker vulnerable to physical problems.

FIRST AID FOR SPORT

TIP

The main aims of first-aid are:

- to preserve life
- to protect the casualty from further harm
- to relieve pain
- to call for medical assistance.

Being able to provide first aid is always going to be a part of the sports therapist's role. Any health and fitness professional or sports therapist will be expected to know basic first aid. They must take a well-recognized first aid qualification, one that preferably has a particular emphasis on sports medicine. The qualification should be updated as and when required, usually every three years, with refresher, upskilling and assessment courses.

The sports therapist may, during their day-to-day activities, be the person responsible for attending to the common on-field injuries and problems, such as cuts and abrasions, strains and sprains or fainting. Occasionally, there are more serious situations to contend with. A heavy fall can easily dislocate a shoulder or cause a fracture. A hard tackle can badly twist a knee and tear the ligaments and cartilage. A clash of heads can result in a great deal of bleeding and cause concussion.

With head injuries, it is sensible to assume that there may also be neck and spinal injury. Often, with head injuries, there will not be obvious major structural damage, even when a serious injury is suspected. Concussion is a common sports injury, and certainly, head injuries, however apparently minor, should always be treated with care, and the individual should be closely monitored. Signs and symptoms of concussion, which may appear over a period of hours, include visual disturbances, nausea, dizziness, headache, behavioural changes, balance problems and amnesia. Always get medical assessment for head injuries that give any cause for concern.

TIP

Once an emergency has become evident, appropriate action must be taken, in a calm but speedy and efficient manner.

In the gym, as in anywhere, there is always a danger of a medical emergency occurring. Even though clients are normally prescribed appropriate exercise programmes, and also screened for their health and fitness prior to their participation, there is never any guarantee that they will not suffer from any health problem either during or after their exercise. Therefore, therapists should be able to recognize signs of such problems as someone having a heart attack, having an epileptic seizure or going into shock. Once the situation has become evident, appropriate action must be taken, in a calm but quick and efficient manner.

One well-known acronym that may help the sports therapist when responding to injuries at sports events is SALTAPS (See, Ask, Look, Touch, Active movements, Passive movements and Strength tests). By following the procedural approach that SALTAPS offers, the therapist should be able to assess whether a player is fit to continue on the field of play. Obviously, there are other more specific assessment techniques to call upon, and

ON-FIELD ASSESSMENT TECHNIQUES: SALTAPS

See the injury occur.

Ask the player what has happened, and where it hurts.

Look at the injured area. Bleeding, swelling or deformity may suggest a severe injury. It may be that, at this point, a decision is taken to take the player off the field of play and get medical assistance.

Touch the affected region to palpate for pain, tenderness, abnormal skin sensations or anatomic deformity. Again, further verbal communication is important to establish the severity of the injury. Further participation may be decided against. At this stage, in a competitive situation, the player may be expected to be moved to the sidelines, and the therapist may either provide assistance, or ask for a stretcher to be brought on.

Active movements can be attempted if previous tests allow. The therapist should observe for restricted movements and whether they cause pain. Grade 1 injuries will be painful, but a near full range of movement will be performed. Grade 2 injuries will be restricted and painful. Grade 3 injuries will be painful and little or no movement possible. If nothing serious is suspected at this stage, then the next stage of assessment can follow.

Passive movements are performed by the therapist without the player's assistance. This can involve joint range of motion assessments and ligament stress tests. Again, if the problem still does not yet appear to warrant that no further participation takes place, then the on-field assessment can continue.

Strength tests help to evaluate the functional performance of the affected muscles. All available movements should be resisted by the therapist. This can be followed by getting the player into a standing position and observing their ability to walk, jog forwards and backwards, side-step, stop and start, jump, and perform a short sprint. If the player can perform all movements relatively comfortably, then they can probably continue.

questions to ask, but using a memory jogger such as SALTAPS helps to reduce the panic that may occur when faced with an injury at the moment it occurs.

Bear in mind that, sometimes, minor side-line attention may be required, such as dressing a wound or taping a joint, before the player can resume their participation. Also, be aware that it is a big responsibility to make the decision on an injury, and whether continued participation is acceptable. If there is any doubt as to the severity or nature of the injury, then the player really must be provided with a more exacting medical assessment. Do remember that as sports injuries occur during exertion, where there is increased circulation moving through the working muscles, there is likely to be a greater degree of internal (and/or external) bleeding than if the individual was not exercising.

Basic on-field approaches:

- Minor injury (e.g. cut; abrasion; cramp; contusion; strain): first aid attention and if all concerned are confident that it is okay to continue, then return to game.

- Moderate injury (e.g. contusion; strain; sprain): first aid attention, removal from field, further assessment and treatment, and possibly referral for medical attention.

TIP	

Strategies and priorities for first aid do change from time to time, and this book is no substitute for an up-to-date medically recognized training course. Studying, practising and qualifying in the fundamental techniques of first aid should be considered an absolute must for all sports therapists.

TIP	

The proficient first-aider will be able to contend with all manner of incidents, to their level of training, at the scene. Initial good management of a suspected sprain or strain, dislocation or fracture, shock, choking incident, asthma attack, epileptic seizure or heart attack can be crucial to the resulting outcome.

FUNDAMENTAL PRINCIPLES OF EMERGENCY FIRST AID

1. Quickly assess the general situation and make the area safe for yourself and others.
2. Keep calm. Tap and ask, clearly and loudly, if the casualty is okay. Inform them that you are there to help, and that you are a qualified first-aider.
3. Call for emergency medical help if there is any likelihood that it is needed.
4. Perform a primary survey (ABC: airway; breathing; circulation), and provide appropriate treatment (e.g. rescue breathing; cardio-pulmonary resuscitation (CPR); recovery position) if necessary. If available, use protection such as latex gloves or resuscitation mask.
5. Check for and control any serious bleeding (e.g. elevate limbs; direct pressure over the wound; pressure point proximal to the wound).
6. Do not move the casualty unless they are in immediate danger.
7. Check for signs of shock, and provide appropriate treatment.
8. Stay with the casualty and continue to provide treatment and reassurance until assistance arrives.
9. Performing a quick top to toe assessment is important, so as to check that nothing has been missed.
10. Clean the incident area if unsafe or contaminated.
11. If the incident occurs at a place of work (or sports centre), the details must be recorded.
12. First aid kits need replenishing after use.

- Severe injury (e.g. strain; sprain; dislocation; fracture; concussion; spinal injury; collapse; heart attack): first aid and immediate expert medical attention.

Questions to ask at the scene:

- What happened?
- Did you feel anything unusual at the time of injury?
- What position were you in?
- How did you land or fall?
- Where does it hurt now?
- Does it hurt when you move?
- Does it hurt anywhere else?
- Do you feel any other sensations?
- Have you ever injured this area before?
- Do you have any medical conditions?

Questioning techniques that help to assess the injured player's mental functioning can be useful:

- What day is it today?
- Who are your opponents today?
- What is the score?
- Where are you in the league at the moment?

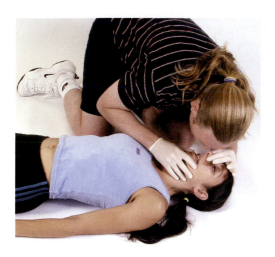

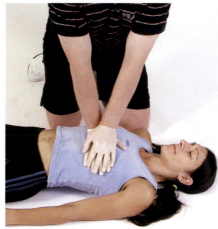

Recovery breathing   External chest compressions

Probably the most essential skills for the first-aider are the primary assessment techniques, rescue breathing and cardio-pulmonary resuscitation (CPR). The best way of remembering the primary assessment procedures is to think of ABC. At the scene of an incident the patient will either be conscious or unconscious. They should be checked for a clear **Airway** (inspect mouth). Their **Breathing** must be assessed next (look and listen closely, and feel). **Circulation** is checked by feeling for carotid pulse. No breathing and/or no pulse is an absolute medical emergency. Emergency medical services should be called immediately, preferably by the help of a bystander, or if alone, by the first-aider.

Recovery breathing (mouth to mouth resuscitation/ventilation; expired air resuscitation) can be performed while holding the patient's nose, with their chin slightly lifted and their head slightly tilted. In a cycle lasting about six seconds, give two breaths for about two seconds each, enough to cause an observable rise in their chest. This cycle is followed by regular reassessment of breathing (coughing; movement) and pulse, and repeated until breathing resumes.

When there is definitely no pulse, CPR must be performed. This combines recovery breathing with external chest compressions. It is normally recommended to give two recovery breaths followed by 15 chest compressions (at the rate of about 100 per minute), and reassessment. This cycle should be repeated until breathing and pulse return. Rhythmic chest compressions should be performed through the heel of the hand, directly down onto the middle of the lower half of the sternum (not focused over the ribs, xiphoid process or upper abdomen).

Being able to place a person in the recovery position is a relatively easy but very important skill to learn. The recovery position helps the unconscious patient who is breathing and uninjured to maintain an open airway (keeping the tongue from the back of the throat), and allows any fluid or vomit to drain easily. Each individual incident will require an assessment of whether the recovery position is appropriate, and whether adjustments need to be made, especially where the patient has suspected spinal or internal injuries. The person should be closely monitored, and circulation to the lower arm should not be restricted.

TIP	

All first aid techniques, and especially recovery breathing and CPR, should be refined to suit the presenting situation. For example, infants, children, adults, the elderly and the disabled will ideally be attended to with an individually appropriate response, the specifics of which should be learned on a course of first aid training.

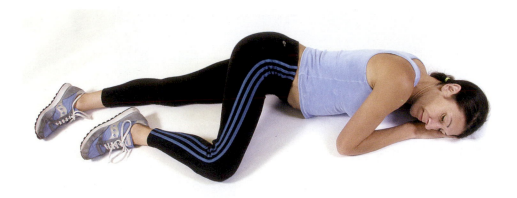

Typical recovery position

Shock is often a complication of injury. This condition is normally taken to mean that, for various reasons, an insufficient blood supply is reaching the vital organs. A heart attack, severe bleeding, loss of other fluids (severe diarrhoea, vomiting or burning, for example) or strong nervous stimulation (such as an emotional reaction to an incident – fear, anxiety, pain) are all common causes of shock. Of course, the first aid treatment for shock depends on the reason for it, but it will usually involve firstly attending to the cause, offering reassurance, preventing the patient from getting cold and positioning them correctly.

Fractures are common injuries. As with any incident, the first-aider must assess the scene and prioritize the initial treatment. Any fracture is potentially complicated, but suspected fractures of the skull and spine warrant particularly careful attention. Certainly do not move a casualty unnecessarily, and do not attempt to forcibly straighten or relocate a joint. Only in certain situations may a collar be very carefully placed around the neck by the first-aider. Limb fractures often require support and/or immobilization.

Fainting, where there is a temporary reduction in blood flow to the brain, can occur at any time, particularly in those with hypotension or on some medications. It can also occur if the person is in a hot atmosphere, has been standing up for a long period, not eaten food or drunken sufficient fluids for a few hours, or has had an emotional reaction to an incident. Fainting is also sometimes seen in the clinical situation, and is more likely when someone receives their treatment while sitting up or standing. The typical signs and symptoms of fainting are: feeling light-headed and/or sweaty, looking pale and possibly passing out. The person may not completely lose consciousness, but the normal response to this situation will be for the first-aider to assist the person to lie down, loosen their clothing, raise their legs to about 45° and reassure them. Alternatively, the person may be positioned sitting up, but with their head between their knees. Fainting episodes are normally resolved almost as quickly as they occur; however, if the person becomes and remains unconsciousness, then emergency action (ABC) must be taken.

The conscientious sports therapist will keep up to date with important procedures and make sure they are prepared for most eventualities, and part of this obviously means keeping a well-stocked first aid kit.

CONTENTS OF A BASIC FIRST AID KIT FOR SPORTS

A guidance leaflet giving general guidance on first aid

Assorted sterile adhesive dressings

Triangular bandages

Crepe bandages

Safety pins

Assorted sterile unmedicated wound dressings

Disposable latex gloves

Individually wrapped moist antiseptic wipes

Eye wash and sterile eye pads

Scissors

Tweezers

Assorted plasters

Micropore tape

Disposable apron

Cold chemical pack

At sports centres and events it is good practice to have ice or cold packs readily available

Emergency foil blankets

Recovery blanket

FROM FIRST AID, THROUGH TREATMENT AND REHABILITATION, TO A RETURN TO SPORT

The first part of any effective management of an injury clearly begins with the appropriate acute response, and continues with a series of progressively intensifying treatments and rehabilitation exercises. Remember that each injury is different, in terms of severity and stage of healing, and should be attended to with an appreciation of what is in the injured athlete's best interests. Remember that, in injury rehabilitation, setbacks can occur, often for no fault of the sports therapist or the athlete. No one should feel personally responsible for any recurrence of an injury or for slow progress.

RICES is a common method of dealing with acute injuries. It helps to control and reduce swelling and pain. With strains, sprains and contusions the therapist (or player) should ice over and around the injury often during the day (10–20 minutes, every 2 hours). Do not apply ice directly to the skin (see chapter 10 for guidance on applying cryotherapy). The injured area is normally compressed with elastic tape, bandage or support, though not so as to impede essential circulation. Remove compression during elevation and for sleeping. When elevated, the limb should be supported and raised, if possible, to a level above the heart. Elevation combined with compression may inhibit venous and lymphatic return, and therefore the two should be performed separately. Acute injuries are normally best supported, during daily activities, with a sling, taping, support, splint, crutches or walking stick, depending on the area affected.

To provide useful sports injury management the sports therapist should be well trained and practised and have at their disposal some good quality tools of the trade. They should learn from their practical experiences, share and discuss ideas and knowledge with fellow practitioners, and also keep abreast of developments in their field by reading up on the latest research.

TIP	
For many acute soft-tissue injuries, remember the acronym RICES: Rest; Ice; Compression; Elevation; Support.	

TIP	
Thermal therapy is indicated in the mid and later stages of injury rehabilitation.	

TIP	
Stretching is an important part of injury rehabilitation.	

TIP	
Deep tissue massage is indicated in the mid and later stages of injury rehabilitaiton.	

TIP	
Upper body training can be carefully stepped-up in the presence of lower body injury.	

TIP

It is important to provide protection (support) for acutely and sub-acutely injured ankle ligaments.

TIP

Early strength training normally involves isometric work.

TIP

Proprioceptive training is an important aspect of many rehabilitation programmes. An example of this is single-leg, closed-chain balancing on a wobble board.

TIP

A lateral epicondylitis support strap can be very helpful in the early stages of managing tennis elbow.

TREATMENT AND REHABILITATION: MILD TO MODERATE HAMSTRING STRAIN

Early stage

Assessment of the problem. If injury is suspected as being severe, then assessment techniques should not aggravate the condition, and medical referral will be appropriate.

RICES for 24–48 hours.

Sub-acute stage

Review of injury, and more detailed assessment. Especially look for causative factors.

Continue RICES as necessary (particularly cryotherapy and support).

Weight-bearing if comfortable.

Massage above injury site.

Modalities may possibly include pulsed ultrasound and TENS.

Mobility of hip, torso and knee (active knee flexion and extension, after local ice application), all depending upon severity and presence of inflammation, and all within comfortable (pain-free) RoM.

Begin treatment of any possible underlying causative factors, such as problems at the lumbar or hip regions.

In injury allows, develop alternative exercise programme to maintain fitness (e.g. upper body and contra-lateral limb strength, flexibility and endurance work), without stressing the injured region.

Later stages

Continual review of progress of injury and management strategy.

Introduction of thermal therapy (e.g. hot packs; infra-red).

Remedial massage techniques (deeper stroking and kneading, cross-fibre frictions, soft-tissue release, positional release, neuro-muscular and muscle energy techniques).

Electro-massage (audiosonic, G5 and percussor).

Pulsed and continuous ultrasound.

Hydrotherapy (jacuzzi; steam; sauna; pool exercise).

EMS.

Remedial exercises (stretching; isometrics; proprioception, co-ordination and balance training; concentric and eccentric isotonics).

Functional training (cardio-vascular work; plyometrics; speed work; skill work; core stability).

Fitness test.

Return to full training and competition.

CHAPTER SUMMARY

This chapter has looked at the big subject of sports injuries. A sports therapist is expected to be able to understand injury prevention, assessment, treatment and rehabilitation. Into this comes knowledge of how injuries occur and minimizing the risk. Injuries are classified in various ways, and it is important to understand about different types of injuries. The inflammation and healing processes very much guide how injuries need to be treated. A variety of factors influence the healing of injuries. First aid skills are always essential in the sporting environment.

Knowledge Review

1   What are the main areas of focus in the field of sports injuries?

2   What is the difference between intrinsic and extrinsic injuries? Provide an example of each.

3   List ten important factors in the prevention of sports injuries.

4   Describe the typical signs and symptoms of (i) a 2nd degree muscle strain and (ii) a 3rd degree ligament sprain.

5   What is DOMS, and why might it occur?

6   Briefly describe the three stages of soft-tissue injury healing.

7   What factors influence the healing of injuries?

8   List ten possible injury complications.

9   List some common injuries that occur in distance running, tennis and swimming.

10 What are the main aims of first aid?

11 Describe the fundamental principles involved in the immediate first aid response to an emergency.

12 What questions should be asked of an injured player on-field?

13 Describe a basic strategy for managing a mild calf strain, from the acute stage through to a return to sport.

WEBSITE

Visit the companion website at www.thomsonlearning.co.uk/ healthandfitness/ward where you will find the answers to these questions for you to check your progress through the book.

chapter 6

NUTRITION

Learning Objectives

After reading this chapter you should be able to:

- understand the role in health and exercise of six categories of nutrients: carbohydrates, fats, protein, vitamins, minerals and water
- know the elements of a healthy diet
- understand nutrition strategies in performance
- understand weight control
- appreciate health issues for athletes

PRINCIPLES OF NUTRITION

Nutrients maintain life. Attention to the quality and variety of foods we eat is vital to ensure we have all the nutrients required for health. In sport and exercise, intense effort and energy expenditure place unusual demands on the diet of athletes. Some athletes find it difficult simply to eat enough calories to meet their energy needs, let alone ensure they have all the nutrients required for optimum performance.

Nutrition science is a complex and specialized field. This chapter will help you understand the principles of good nutrition in general and for athletes. Its specific application in the promotion of optimum health and performance, however, requires detailed study and is the role of a registered nutritionist.

You should be wary of giving even general advice to some categories of people: children and teenagers, those on a medically prescribed diet or undergoing medical treatment, very overweight and underweight individuals, those with identified food allergies or intolerances, pregnant women, people with gastro-intestinal disorders, or people who regularly take over-the-counter medication.

Nutrients are the absorbable components in food. There are six kinds of **essential** nutrients: carbohydrates, fats, protein, vitamins, minerals and water. They fall into three groups:

- macronutrients
- micronutrients
- water.

MACRONUTRIENTS: THE FUEL SOURCES

Carbohydrates, fats (also known as lipids and oils) and protein are known as macronutrients because the body needs each in large amounts every day. The body runs on energy supplied by the macronutrients in the form of glucose and glycogen. The specific conditions under which each macronutrient is used as fuel have been described in chapter 2. You may wish to refer back to that chapter.

Energy is the body's capacity for doing work. The diet should meet an individual's total energy needs. Individual requirements depend on three factors:

- The basal metabolic rate (BMR) is the energy required merely to maintain the body's systems and regulate temperature. It is measured in the morning after an overnight fast, while the individual rests in bed. BMR is higher when body weight is heavier, higher in men than women, and tends to decrease with age.
- Processing food in the body uses up energy, accounting for about 6–10 per cent total energy expenditure in men, about 6–7 per cent in women.
- The energy expended in physical activity.

The energy value of food is expressed in **calories**. A **calorie** is the measure of energy value in food. One calorie is the heat needed to raise the temperature of one gram of water by one degree Celsius. Energy values in food are usually described in terms of kilocalories (kcal): the heat required to heat one kilogram of water by one degree Celsius.

Carbohydrates (CHO)

Carbohydrate foods are the starches, sugars and cellulose found in grains, pulses, fruit and vegetables. Carbohydrates are our primary energy source: they are converted to glucose for immediate use and **glycogen** as reserve energy. Glucose is used to produce the body's currency of energy, ATP (adenosine triphosphate). Each gram of carbohydrate yields 4 kcal of energy.

Types of carbohydrate

Carbohydrate molecules are all made from carbon (C), hydrogen (H) and oxygen (O), and can exist alone and in pairs, known as simple sugars, or in chains, known as starches or complex carbohydrate.

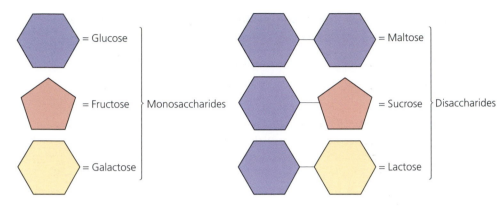

Carbohydrate molecules

- Monosaccharides such as glucose, fructose and galactose are the simplest form of carbohydrate.

- Disaccharides are pairs of monosaccharide units joined together. Sucrose is the most common. Others are maltose and lactose, found in milk.

- **Poly**saccharides are long chains of glucose molecules numbering from several to hundreds or even thousands. Starch, cellulose and glycogen are all polysaccharides. There are two starch types: amylose (a long single chain of glucose molecules) and amylopectin (containing many branched chains of glucose molecules). A starchy food has a mixture of the two types in different ratios.

Digestion of carbohydrates

Carbohydrate foods are broken down in the digestive tract by digestive enzymes to their simplest mono-forms, then taken to the liver or absorbed into the circulation. Glucose can be used directly, but fructose and galactose must be changed into glucose by the liver for use in the body.

After eating, the hormone **insulin** is released from the pancreas and escorts excess glucose from the circulation into cells. Any glucose not used for immediate energy is converted to glycogen in a process called **glycogenesis**. Glycogen is stored in both the liver and muscles. When these storage sites are full, excess glucose is converted to fat, and stored in adipose tissue as triglycerides.

Glycogen is used for energy when free glucose in the circulation has been used up. Glycogen is converted back to energy in **glycogenolysis**. Glycogen stores are limited, providing about 500 g or 2000 kcal of energy. About 80 per cent of our glycogen is stored in skeletal muscle.

Carbohydrates and blood sugar

How quickly the body absorbs carbohydrate depends on two factors:

- The amount of work needed to break the carbohydrate down to its simplest parts.

MACRONUTRIENTS: THE FUEL SOURCES

- Whether it can then be used directly in the circulation (like glucose), or must first be converted to glucose in the liver (like fructose).

This affects blood sugar levels in an important way.

For general health, stable blood sugar is important. Rapidly absorbed carbohydrates increase blood sugar levels quickly, which can be followed by a sharp drop, as a result of action by insulin. Fluctuating blood sugar and elevated insulin levels are a common denominator in many health problems, including type II diabetes, heart disease and obesity. Clearly for most people, slowly absorbed carbohydrate foods have health advantages over rapidly absorbed types. But fast absorbed carbohydrates can be useful for athletes in certain situations.

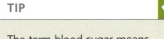

> **TIP** ✔
>
> The term blood sugar means the same as blood glucose.

All carbohydrates are not equal

Until recently, blood sugar response was thought to depend on whether carbohydrates were simple or complex. The theory was that, because of their large molecular size, starches such as rice and potato would be slowly digested and absorbed, causing a slow gradual rise in blood sugar. Simple sugars were all thought to be absorbed rapidly, causing fluctuations in blood sugar. But in recent years, the actual effect on blood sugar levels of different foods has been measured.

The **glycaemic index** (GI) measures the degree to which carbohydrates in different foods raise blood sugar levels, compared with pure glucose. Foods with high GI scores (i.e. that raise blood sugar quickly) include:

- potatoes and bread
- many kinds of rice
- highly refined bakery and confectionery goods
- baked beans.

Good choices for steady blood sugar levels include:

- pasta
- porridge
- lentils and some legumes
- nuts, including peanuts
- apples and oranges.

> **TIP** ✔
>
> Swap white potato for sweet potato – it has a lower GI and more nutrients.

The GI of carbohydrate is difficult to predict. Many factors have an influence, including: the ratio of starch types (amylose takes longer to digest than amylopectin); whether and how food is cooked; whether it is refined. The presence of fibre, fat and acid all slow digestion, reducing the impact on blood sugar.

The GI provides useful information, but is still a crude yardstick. Blood sugar response to a meal depends on many factors. Micronutrients are often bound to carbohydrate in food, so eating a wide variety is important.

> **TIP** ✔
>
> Vinegar or lemon juice can lower the glycaemic and insulin response of accompanying food. So enjoy a side salad with vinaigrette dressing with a meal.

Fibre

Fibre is the indigestible part of plant foods, so does not provide energy. Its role in health is its ability to bulk up the contents of our intestines,

TABLE 6.1 Good dietary sources of fibre

Food items	Fibre (g)
One apple or pear	4.0
Broccoli (100 g)	3.5
Cereals, bran (45 g)	3–4
One banana	3.0
Cereals, other than bran (35 g)	2.5–2.8
Two prunes, dried	2.4
Carrots (100 g)	2.4
Brussels sprouts (100 g)	2.3
Cabbage (100 g)	2.1
Half a baked potato	1.9
Beans, runner (100 g)	1.9
Cauliflower (100 g)	1.6
One small orange	1.6
Rice, brown (cooked) (60 g)	1.6
One small tomato	1.5
Bread, wholemeal (one slice)	1.3
Onions (100 g)	1.2
Ten cherries	1.1
Half a grapefruit or pineapple	0.8
Meat/fish/eggs/dairy	0

and provide food for the 'good' bacteria in our guts. The presence of fibre in food slows absorption, promoting steady blood sugar levels. More fibre in the diet is related to a lower risk of many diseases, like heart disease, some cancers, and bowel diseases. You should aim for 15–30 g per day: the average adult UK diet provides 12.4 g daily.

Carbohydrate requirements

Carbohydrates should provide around 50 per cent of a healthy diet. A wide variety of carbohydrates should be eaten, mostly as unrefined, fibre-rich fruits, vegetables, grains, lentils and legumes, nuts and seeds. The recommended intake of five portions of fruit and vegetables daily is an absolute minimum.

Carbohydrate use in exercise

In sport and exercise, eating enough carbohydrate to fuel performance is vital. Increasing dietary carbohydrates can significantly improve endurance. During heavy training or periods of high energy expenditure, carbohydrate requirements can rise to 55–70 per cent (about 400–600 g).

The body burns a mixture of fat and glycogen in exercise. The ratio of carbohydrates to other macronutrients depends on which energy system is being used. Glucose is the preferred muscle fuel, particularly as exercise intensity increases.

During high-intensity **anaerobic training**, glycogen (with creatine phosphate) is used very fast and may be depleted after 30–45 minutes. Longer duration, low-to-moderate aerobic exercise uses a mixture of fuels from both carbohydrates and fat. Glycogen is the fuel that runs out first. The effect of glycogen depletion during exercise is known as 'hitting the wall': extreme fatigue, dizziness and hunger.

Both fast and slow-releasing carbohydrates have a role in the athlete's diet. Mostly, low GI carbohydrates should be preferred to encourage blood sugar stability. But during events that last longer than an hour, high GI carbohydrates have a role in providing short-term energy. In the hour or two following exercise fast-releasing carbohydrates quickly replenish glycogen stores in both muscle and liver. Glycogen depletion is linked to slower rates of muscle regeneration. Sports drinks can be an easy way of ingesting these carbohydrates.

> **TIP**
>
> With less than 24 hours between exercise sessions, fast glycogen replenishment is particularly important. High GI carbohydrates are needed: if you like jelly beans, now is the time to eat them!

Carbohydrate loading

The size of glycogen stores varies among individuals; training can increase muscle glycogen capacity. Endurance athletes, such as long-distance runners and cyclists, may use carbohydrate loading to maximize their glycogen stores before an event. Glycogen depletion used to precede increased carbohydrate intake and tapered exercise in carbohydrate loading. Research suggests this is unhelpful. Now athletes are advised to taper training intensity a week before the event. A normal mixed diet with about 55 per cent of carbohydrate calories is eaten until the last three days. Then activity is further reduced, and the ratio of dietary carbohydrate increased to about 70 per cent. Protein, minerals and vitamins needs must be met.

Lipids/fats

Fats (or lipids) have had a bad press recently. Fat consumption has been associated with health problems such as obesity, heart disease and cancer. But fats are not all the same. Some fats are absolutely vital for good health, others are less useful, and some we should avoid altogether.

Uses of fat

All types of fat provide 9 kcal of energy in 1 g of fat. The many roles of fat in the body include:

- concentrated energy
- supply of up to 70 per cent of energy in rest
- energy storage in adipose tissue
- cell membrane structure
- protective padding and support for vital organs

- insulation for temperature maintenance
- production of vital hormone-like substances called prostaglandins
- means of absorption for fat-soluble vitamins.

Triglycerides are the main type of fat in food. A triglyceride has one molecule of glycerol and three fatty acids. Each fatty acid is a chain of carbon atoms, varying in length from 4 to 24 carbon atoms. In digestion, fats are broken down by bile and digestive enzymes to their smallest components, glycerol and fatty acids. Any not used immediately are reassembled as triglycerides and stored in adipose tissue and the liver.

Fat provides concentrated energy. Unlike glycogen stores, fat stores hold an almost inexhaustible energy supply. Even very lean athletes have large fat stores, holding more than 40 000 kcal of stored fat in the body. But adipose tissue fat stores are not as readily available for energy use as carbohydrate. Fat needs oxygen for it to be broken down for energy, so its importance as an energy source depends on the activity type. Fat-burning is most efficient during low-to-moderate intensity, longer-duration exercise. So energy from fat is very important in endurance sports such as marathon running, but less important in power sports such as sprinting where glycogen is the primary fuel. The ability to burn fat at higher intensities increases with aerobic fitness (V_{O_2}max).

Carbohydrate contributes to the fuel mix even when triglyceride use is high. So 'hitting the wall' occurs with plenty of energy available in fat stores.

Saturated and unsaturated fats

The chemical composition of fats has implications for health. Fatty acids can be saturated or unsaturated. Each carbon atom in the fatty acid chain has four arms. If each carbon is attached to its neighbour by one arm and each free arm is attached to a hydrogen atom, the fatty acid is saturated. If one or more carbons in the chain is attached to its neighbour by two arms (a double bond), and hydrogen atoms are therefore not attached to every free arm, the fatty acid is unsaturated.

Saturated fats

Fats from animal sources, such as dairy foods and meats, are high in saturated fatty acids. Most saturated fats are solid at room temperature. Dietary saturated fats are associated with health problems, such as heart disease, hypertension, some cancers and inflammatory processes.

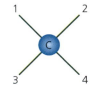

Four arms on a carbon

Four arms on a carbon

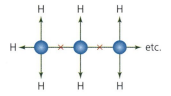

Carbons and hydrogen chain

Carbons and hydrogen chain

Polyunsaturated fats

Unsaturated fats are more liquid at room temperature. Monounsaturated fats such as oleic acid (high in olive oil, avocados and some nuts) have one double bond. Polyunsaturated fats, found in most vegetable oils, have more than one double bond. They are damaged by heating or oxygen exposure so should be used with care in food preparation. Polyunsaturated fats are the source of some specific types of fatty acids essential for good health.

Essential fatty acids (EFAs)

Many fatty acids exist but only two are essential, that is, they are required for growth and health and must be obtained from the diet because the body cannot make them:

- Omega 6 fatty acids come from linoleic acid. Food sources include unsaturated vegetable oils, nuts and seeds, chicken, turkey, lamb and pork.

- Omega 3 fatty acids come from alpha-linolenic acid. Excellent sources of omega 3s are oily fish (e.g. sardines, mackerel, tuna, salmon, and herrings) and some vegetable oils such as canola, flaxseed and walnut. Omega 3 fats in particular have been found to reduce the risk of heart disease and to lower blood pressure. Many of us get less than we need of this fatty acid.

The exact requirement for EFAs has not been established, but balance seems important. Most of us should eat more omega 3 fat-rich foods.

Hydrogenation and trans-fats

Polyunsaturated oils are vulnerable to rancidity and damage, and are liquid at room temperature. Hydrogenation is a process that adds hydrogen to unsaturated fats, increasing their saturation and thus their shelf life and solidity. In this form they can be used in food manufacture. These modified fatty acids are known as trans-fats. Many processed foods, such as margarine, cakes, biscuits and cookies, contain hydrogenated or partially hydrogenated fats. Accumulating evidence implicates them in health problems, particularly cardio-vascular damage, and they are best avoided.

Protein and amino acids

Protein is needed throughout the body, for the growth, maintenance and repair of cells, including muscle cells. It is the major component of hormones, DNA, antibodies, enzymes, muscle and other body tissues. Protein represents about 74 per cent of the dry weight of most body cells. Protein is a large molecule, comprising between 10 and 100 amino acid molecules. Protein in the body is built from these amino acid sub-units.

Dietary protein is broken down in the digestive system, by hydrochloric acid in the stomach and digestive enzymes, into its constituent amino acids. These are then:

- taken into cells to build the specific new proteins required
- taken to the liver to make plasma proteins
- used as energy – 1 g of protein provides 4 kcal of energy
- or stored as glycogen and fat. The body has no protein stores: all are functional.

Amino acids

Amino acids, rather than proteins, are the important nutrients. Of the 20 or so amino acids used to make proteins in the body, 8 or 9 are essential. These must come from the diet because our bodies cannot make them. All essential amino acids must be available to enable the body to build or repair muscle. If just one is missing, proteins cannot be made. Complete proteins are foods that include all essential amino acids. Most animal products, such as lean meat, fish, eggs and cheese, are complete proteins.

Incomplete proteins usually lack one or more of the essential amino acids. Most plant sources of protein are incomplete. Fortunately the same amino acid is not missing in all, so all essential amino acids can be obtained by eating a variety of plant foods such as grains, beans, vegetables, fruits, nuts and seeds.

> **TIP**
>
> Classic combinations of plant foods containing all essential amino acids are: rice and peas; peanut butter sandwich; beans on toast.

Use of protein as energy

Despite the availability of fat stored in even lean bodies, the body breaks down protein to use as energy, known as catabolism, in some circumstances, for example, when glycogen is depleted, during intensive power exercise or long endurance events.

The body has no protein stores, so if no protein is fed, muscle protein is broken down. When amino acids are used for energy, they cannot be used for building and repairing muscle tissue and other functions.

Protein requirements for health and exercise

About 15–20 per cent of total energy intake should come from protein. Most non-athletes need 1 g per kilogram of body weight. More protein is required in illness, growth, tissue repair, pregnancy, training and performance.

Exercise duration and intensity affect protein requirements. Exercising for several hours can result in a loss of muscle mass. Current research for endurance athletes suggests the following protein requirements:

- Moderate training (about one hour a day): 1.2–1.5 g per kg body weight.
- Moderately hard: 1.5–1.9 g per kg body weight.
- Heavy, long, hard training: about 1.9 g per kg body weight.

> **TIP**
>
> Research suggests that optimal amino acid levels are achieved by eating some protein-rich food at each meal and snack.

Increased protein is required to build muscle mass. After exercise, intake of protein with carbohydrate helps repair of muscle damage.

Protein content

The protein content of even lean 'high-protein' foods may not be what it seems, as shown in Table 6.2.

TABLE 6.2 Protein content of food

Food	Amount and type	Protein content
Beef/lamb/pork	100 g lean cooked	~30 g
Ham/bacon	100 g lean cooked	~23–27 g
Chicken	100 g lean cooked	~24–30 g
Fish	100 g, flesh only, cooked	~20–26 g
Tofu	100 g, steamed	~8 g
	100 g, steamed, fried	~23 g
Red kidney beans	100 g, dried, boiled	~8.4 g
Lentils	100 g, dried boiled	~8.8 g

Values taken from *The Composition of Foods*, by McCance and Widdowson, published by The Royal Society of Chemistry.

MICRONUTRIENTS

Although micronutrients do not provide energy and we need them in relatively small quantities, they are essential for health.

Vitamins

Vitamins are a group of unrelated organic compounds. Some vitamin K and B6 can be produced by intestinal flora but others must be obtained from the diet. Vitamins can be classified as fat-soluble or water-soluble.

Fat-soluble vitamins

The fat-soluble vitamins A, D, E and K are absorbed from the digestive tract bound to lipid. They can be stored in the body's fatty tissue, so excess intake can cause toxicity. Care should be taken if supplements are used.

Water-soluble vitamins

Water-soluble vitamins, the B vitamins and vitamin C, are not stored by the body. Excess is excreted in urine, so the risk of toxicity is lower. The B vitamins were once thought to be a single vitamin but more than a dozen B-complex vitamins have now been identified. They have different functions, but work synergistically, so should be supplied together.

TABLE 6.3 Fat-soluble vitamins

Vitamin	Sources include	Functions include	Symptoms of deficiency include
A (retinol)	Fish liver oils, liver, eggs and dairy, green and yellow fruit and vegetables	Vision, skin (inner and outer), bone and tooth growth, antioxidant	Poor night vision, skin disorders, eye problems, increased infection risk
D (cholecalciferol, ergosterol)	The 'sunshine vitamin',* fish liver oils, oily fish, eggs	Calcium absorption, normal growth, bones and teeth, antioxidant	Rickets, bone loss, joint problems
E (alpha-tocopherol)	Cold-pressed vegetable oils, wholegrains, nuts, dark green leafy vegetables, egg yolk	Fat-protective antioxidant, cardio-vascular system, reduces oxygen needs of muscles, enhances vitamins A and C activity	Anaemia, sterility
K (phylloquinone)	Alfalfa, liver, cabbage family, watercress, kale, legumes, cereals, fruit, meat	Blood clotting, bone health	Excess bleeding, blood clotting abnormalities

*Vitamin D is formed from substances in the skin exposed to ultraviolet light.

TABLE 6.4 Water-soluble vitamins

Vitamin	Food sources include	Functions include	Symptoms of deficiency include
B complex (B1: thiamin; B2: riboflavin; B3: niacin; B5: pantothenic acid; B6: pyridoxine; folic acid; B12: cyanocobalamin; biotin)	Brewer's yeast, unrefined wholegrains, liver, green leafy vegetables, fish, poultry, eggs, meat, nuts, beans) B12 is available only from foods of animal origin, except possibly *Spirulina* algae. Calcium is required for its absorption	Individual functions but general oxidation of food and production of energy; converting carbohydrates into glucose; metabolism of fats and proteins; red blood cell production; nervous system function	Wide range because group has so many functions: fatigue; GI problems; neuromuscular dysfunction; beri-beri; pellagra
C	Berries, guavas, broccoli, sweet peppers, citrus	Growth and tissue repair; collagen synthesis; gum health; antioxidant; protects other nutrients; may be cancer-protective; immune function; aids iron absorption; activates folic acid	Anaemia; scurvy; poor wound healing; gum problems; frequent colds and infections; easy bruising

Free radicals and antioxidants

Free radicals cause us considerable damage. Body cells are composed of atoms, which contain electrons. When all the electrons in an atom are in pairs, the atom is stable. A free radical atom contains an unpaired electron and is very unstable. It tries to regain stability by stealing an electron from another atom. Oxygen is usually the unstable atom, so free radicals are also called oxidants and free radical damage known as oxidative stress.

Free radicals are produced internally as part of metabolism, but our free radical load is substantially increased by external sources, such as radiation, smoking, burnt food or damaged oils. Free radicals are a factor in various types of cancer, cardio-vascular disease and many age-related diseases. Long-term aerobic activity, including running and bicycling, can increase production of free radicals. Exercise-related effects of free radicals include muscle cell membrane damage and increased protein breakdown. Free radical damage may contribute to muscle inflammation and soreness, and accelerate fatigue.

Antioxidants are our free radical defences. An antioxidant protects cells against free radical attack, by supplying the missing electron or removing the extra one, resulting in stability. In the body, many kinds of antioxidants protect us, including internally produced antioxidant enzymes, and antioxidant nutrients in our diet. The antioxidant nutrients most capable of fighting free radicals include vitamin A and its precursor beta-carotene, vitamin C, vitamin E and the mineral selenium.

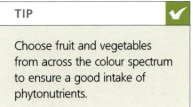

TIP

Antioxidant nutrients function as a team, so we need a good supply of all of them.

Phytochemicals

Some extracts from plants called flavonoids and isoflavones have been found to reduce free radical-related and inflammatory disease. Examples are grapeseed extract, pine bark extract and lycopene in tomatoes. Many different flavonoids and functions have been identified.

TIP

Choose fruit and vegetables from across the colour spectrum to ensure a good intake of phytonutrients.

Minerals

Minerals are inorganic substances essential for normal cellular functions. Minerals are present in high concentrations in skeletons and teeth, and throughout the body dissolved in the body's fluids. They exist as ions or combined with various organic compounds. Of about 60 minerals in the human body, 21 are considered essential.

Macro, or major, minerals are required in amounts of more than 100 mg daily: calcium, magnesium, sodium, potassium and phosphorus. No less essential are the trace minerals, needed in amounts of less than 100 mg a day: boron, chromium, copper, iron, manganese, molybdenum, selenium, sulphur and zinc.

Calcium

The body's most abundant mineral, calcium has many functions, aside from in bones and teeth. They include roles in muscle action, blood clotting, and transmission of nerve impulses. Good dietary sources include dairy foods, tinned sardines and salmon with bones, broccoli, green leafy vegetables and seafood.

Inadequate calcium intake lowers bone density and increases risk of bone fractures. Osteoporosis, a disease with low bone density, is common among older women. The hormone oestrogen is protective, so reduced levels at menopause are a contributory factor. A good supply of essential nutrients (such as calcium, magnesium, vitamin C, D, K, manganese and boron) is needed, together with regular weight-bearing exercise.

Female triad

Some female athletes who train intensively and strive for low body fat are at risk of three health problems, known as the female athlete triad:

- Disordered eating and/or use of practices such as excess exercise, saunas, self-induced vomiting, fat-free diets or diet pills, enemas, laxatives and **diuretics**.
- Irregular or absence of menstruation, triggered by low body fat, which removes oestrogen's protective effect on bone.
- Reduced bone mass, increased stress fracture risk and osteoporosis.

Activity levels should be reduced and total energy intake increased, so body weight increases. Good levels of calcium and other bone nutrients must be ensured.

Magnesium

Magnesium is needed in about 300 enzymes regulating metabolic processes. It is required for bone health and, proper function of the neuromuscular system, and helps maintain blood pressure. Only small amounts are lost in sweat. Dietary sources include legumes, nuts, whole grains, mushrooms, bananas, vegetables and seafood.

Iron

Iron is closely associated with the body's transport and storage of oxygen. Most body iron is combined with haemoglobin in red blood cells, increasing blood's oxygen-carrying capacity about 65 times. In muscle myoglobin, iron helps store and transport oxygen. Food sources include meat, poultry, oily fish, liver, eggs, green leafy vegetables, beans, lentils, dried fruit and nuts.

TIP	

Consumption of foods rich in vitamin C increases iron uptake. So drink a glass of orange juice with your boiled egg for breakfast.

Physically active young women can be at risk of iron insufficiency, and vegetarians have increased risk. In studies, female vegetarian runners had poorer iron status than counterparts eating the same amount of iron but from mostly animal sources. Vegetables contain up to 60 per cent less iron (and other depleted mineral levels) than 50 years ago. Iron supplementation should, however, be avoided unless a deficiency exists.

Sodium, potassium and chlorine

The electrolyte minerals sodium, potassium and chlorine (in the form of chloride) remain dissolved in the body as electrically charged particles called ions. They are key players in:

- conduction of the body's electrical energy
- regulation of water flow between cells and bloodstream

- muscle contraction and relaxation
- fluid balance.

Good sources of potassium include dried fruits, molasses, raw salad vegetables, potatoes and nuts.

Sodium helps nutrients into cells, and is added to food in cooking, refining and processing. Rich sources include yeast extract, bacon, sauces, ham, many cheeses and bread. Chlorine is closely associated with sodium, so is available in sodium-rich foods.

Sodium and chlorine deficiency usually only occurs in dehydration after profuse sweating during prolonged exercise without adequate fluid, or in hyponatremia (see below). Sports drinks can help.

Vitamins and minerals in exercise

Most vitamins have some function relevant to exercise, but only the B complex vitamins and vitamins C and E have been studied for performance benefits. Benefits of supplementation with some of the B complex vitamins were found, but only with a pre-existing (even marginal) deficiency. Research on vitamin C supplementation found performance may not benefit without pre-existing deficiency. However, its antioxidant action can help combat free radical damage, so may help muscle recovery. It also offers protection against upper respiratory tract infections, i.e. colds and coughs. Vitamin E is an important antioxidant but no clear performance benefits have emerged.

The case for supplementation

Nutritional requirements are highly individual, depending on age, size, levels of activity and **metabolism**. Needs are increased in the very active, illness, pregnancy, smokers and heavy drinkers, or with certain medications. Dieters, vegans, convenience food eaters and individuals with gastro-intestinal problems that affect absorption may have a low nutrient intake.

Intensively grown foods have reduced levels of nutrients. Processed 'convenience' food is of low nutritional quality. Storage and transport further decrease the nutritional value of many plant foods.

In 1985 the Bateman Report found that more than 85 per cent of people who generally thought they ate a well-balanced diet failed to meet even the most basic recommended levels of all essential nutrients. There is no evidence today's diet is any better. Furthermore, training requirements often leave athletes limited time to prepare food properly.

Supplementation, on the other hand, can be expensive and complicated. Supplementing individual nutrients can create imbalances; toxicity can be a concern; and athletes must be sure they are not taking a banned substance. A good multivitamin and mineral formulation by a respected manufacturer can be a safe choice. Check with the manufacturer that the supplement will not contravene any regulatory body requirements. Or seek advice from a registered nutritionist.

WATER

Water constitutes between 45 and 70 per cent of our body composition depending on our fat levels (fat contains less water than lean tissue). Water is found throughout the body. Blood is about 83 per cent water; muscle about 75 per cent; bone around 22 per cent; and fat tissue only about 10 per cent.

Water has many important functions, for example:

- It provides transport between and delivery to different tissues in the body.
- It regulates body temperature.
- It maintains blood pressure.
- It provides lubrication, for example, for the joints, eyes, brain and spinal cord.

Fluid balance

With no water stores, the body constantly seeks fluid balance. We get thirst signals when water is needed, and increased urination excretes any surplus. With too little water we become dehydrated, and without it would die more quickly than if deprived of any other nutrient. So we need plenty of water every day. A sedentary person in temperate climate needs between two and three litres of water a day. Requirements increase with activity and temperature.

Sources of water

About two-thirds of our daily water intake is in the form of liquid, absorbed with little digestive effort. Water also comes from food. All foods are a mixture of water and solids. Fruits, vegetables, cooked cereals and milk are 80–95 per cent water. Meat contains from 75 to 45 per cent, depending on how well cooked it is.

Water is bound to glycogen in a ratio of about 3:1. It becomes important in exercise when glycogen stores are broken down for energy. This water source can be increased by glycogen-increasing techniques such as carbohydrate loading.

Hyponatremia is a condition caused by drinking more water than the kidneys can excrete, diluting the body's sodium concentration. Over about nine litres of water a day can cause symptoms of headache, blurred vision, vomiting, convulsions and eventually even coma or death. In sport, hyponatremia can be a risk during ultra-endurance events. In an Ironman triathlon event, 30 per cent of athletes were affected.

TIP	

A drink containing some sodium chloride (table salt) reduces the risk of hyponatremia.

Water loss

Body water is used up in a number of ways. Rates of water loss are affected by the weather, acclimatization, activity duration and intensity, sweat rate, clothing, health, alcohol and caffeine consumption, use of medications and diuretics, and body fat.

- Water excreted as urine has been filtered through the kidneys. Alcohol and caffeine have a diuretic effect. Some foods, e.g. protein, speed up dehydration.
- Sweating is the major mode of water loss during exercise.
- Small amounts of water are lost in breathing and defecation. Water loss increases with gastro-intestinal distress symptoms such as diarrhoea and vomiting.

Managing fluid balance in exercise is critical to optimal performance.

> **TIP** ✔
>
> The colour of urine can be used to monitor to the hydration state. A pale straw colour indicates good hydration. (NB: B vitamin supplementation can make the urine deeper yellow.)

Dehydration

Body water is central to temperature control. About 80 per cent of energy generated by exercise is in the form of heat. This must be removed from the body, or the core temperature rises, with potentially tragic results. For example, over 100 footballers have died since 1980 from heat-related factors.

The adverse effects of **dehydration** happen in the following way:

- Sweating is the main mechanism for heat regulation in exercise. More than a litre an hour may be lost during prolonged exercise.
- Fluid loss increases with duration and intensity of exercise and in hotter, more humid environments, resulting in dehydration.
- Dehydration causes the body's water levels to fall, including blood plasma.
- Lower blood volume reduces cardiac output, affecting the delivery of oxygen and nutrients to contracting muscles.
- To maintain blood supply to the muscles, the circulatory system reduces blood flow to the skin.
- Heat loss is reduced and the core temperature rises.
- Performance is affected. Nausea, fatigue, confusion and collapse may result.

Studies have found that even small fluctuations in the body's water balance can adversely affect performance.

Preventing dehydration

The amount of fluid required for optimum performance is much greater than indicated by thirst. In studies, athletes voluntarily replaced only half the water lost during exercise. When force-fed with fluids exactly matching those lost, subjects performed better, with a lower heart rate and core temperature. Dehydration associated with prolonged activity can be prevented with a well-planned and practised hydration strategy:

- Before the event:
  - drink plenty of water the day before
  - drink 300–600 ml water with the pre-event meal

- drink 150–300 ml each 15 min until about an hour before the event
- drink 150–300 ml about 20 min before the event.
- During endurance exercise, drink about 150 ml every 15–20 min. Full fluid restoration is important post-exercise.
- Rehydrate fully during the 2–4 h after the event. Estimate body fluid loss by weighing before and after the event (after urination). In the hours immediately after the event, drink a litre per kilogram of body weight lost.
- Avoid diuretics such as caffeine and alcohol.

Sports drinks

Sports drinks can benefit performance by improving rehydration in events longer than an hour. An ideal rehydration drink should taste good, be absorbed rapidly, cause little or no gastro-intestinal distress, maintain body fluid balance, and offer potential to enhance performance.

Gastric emptying

Absorption depends on gastro-intestinal function. Food in the stomach mixes with gastric secretions, such as **enzymes**, hydrochloric acid and electrolytes. It then empties from stomach to small intestine in a process called gastric emptying.

This is affected by a number of stimuli:

- greater volume increases rate of emptying
- increases with cooler fluids
- decreases with increasing calorie content
- decreases with more acidic solutions
- decreases with more highly concentrated solutions.

Variables in a sports drink

Most sports drinks are carbohydrate solutions, to supply fuel for energy and fluid for rehydration.

- Carbohydrate type. Different sugar molecules have different gastric emptying rates. For example, fructose empties faster than glucose. Most commercial sports drinks contain mixtures of glucose, sucrose, fructose, high-fructose corn syrup and maltodextrins.
- Sodium may be included. It causes more water to be retained without inhibiting thirst and may support glucose absorption.
- Amino acids may be useful in post-exercise recovery.
- Carbohydrate concentration affects the rate of gastric emptying. In general, strong carbohydrate solutions remain in the stomach longer but deliver more glucose to the intestine than weak ones. Lower carbohydrate concentrations favour hydration; higher carbohydrate concentrations benefit energy. The optimum concentration depends on individual circumstances:

1 Drinks with less than 4 g carbohydrate per 100 ml empty from the stomach quickly, and favour rehydration. They are useful when fluid replacement is vital, such as in shorter duration, intensive exercise at higher temperatures.

2 Concentrations of between 4 and 8 g carbohydrate per 100 ml offer some energy and hydration benefits, especially for endurance athletes.

3 A solution of over 8 per cent carbohydrate per 100 ml delays gastric emptying, reducing the fluid available for absorption, but increasing the rate of carbohydrate delivery. These drinks may be useful in longer endurance events in cool temperatures. A high carbohydrate concentration increases the danger of dehydration and may cause some gastro-intestinal disturbance.

TIP

Voluntary drinking does not reflect hydration status so the taste of drinks is important. In one study, the addition of flavourings increased consumption of fluid by about 50 per cent during prolonged exercise.

HEALTHY EATING GUIDELINES

Most people need at least half the energy content of their diet from carbohydrate, about 15–20 per cent from protein, and no more than 30 per cent from fat. The type and source of each are important. Variety is important to ensure nutrient intake. For example, calcium and iron are both essential nutrients. Meat, fish and poultry are rich in iron but poor in calcium, with the reverse true of dairy.

Guidelines for healthy eating include:

- Reduce saturated fat by eating less butter, fatty and red meats, cheese, etc. Prefer lean poultry, fish, legumes, nuts and eggs. Avoid prepared food such as sausages, paté and pies.
- Eat more 'good' fats in foods such as olive oil, avocados, nuts and seeds. Eat 80–250 g (3–9 oz) oily fish a week (sardines, salmon, mackerel, herring and tuna).
- Grill, boil or steam food rather than frying it. Use olive and canola oils for cooking when fat is required.
- Avoid processed food and hydrogenated and partially hydrogenated trans-fats.
- Avoid refined foods.
- Reduce sugar and fast-releasing starchy foods such as bread, white rice and potatoes.
- Eat plenty of slowly absorbed grains such as oatmeal, legumes, vegetables, pasta, lentils and brown basmati rice.
- Eat lots of fresh or frozen vegetables and fresh, frozen or dried fruit.
- Include plenty of fibre.
- Eat a wide variety of foods, including fruit and vegetables across the colour spectrum.
- Drink at least two litres a day (excluding coffee and tea). Moderate your alcohol intake.

DIET IN EXERCISE

TIP

A record of at least three days' food intake in a food diary can be used to assess the athlete's diet. Food frequency questionnaires are another assessment tool. Using a predetermined food list, athletes report how often each food is eaten. The questionnaire is completed retrospectively, and is less time-consuming than the diary.

Good nutrition is crucial for athletic success. Although the athlete's diet must meet increased energy needs, generally the same healthy diet guidelines apply to the athlete as to the general population. However, the macronutrient balance may be different: some endurance athletes require a regular higher carbohydrate intake: 55–65 per cent.

Many athletes striving for a lean build eat very little fat, but research suggests very low-fat diets (5–15 per cent energy from fat) offer no health or performance benefits over a moderate fat intake. In general, endurance athletes need to maintain higher levels of fat intake than strength athletes. Athletes must experiment to find and fine tune strategies to enhance performance in competition. Strategies must be practised in training.

Pre-event nutrition

The athlete should aim to begin the event with optimal fluid and fuel status, by:

- increasing low GI carbohydrate intake in the days before the event
- eating a pre-event meal rich in slow-burning carbohydrate
- a fluid intake strategy, as described earlier.

During the event

Fluid, carbohydrate and sodium ingestion offers benefits in endurance events. Begin fluid intake early in the event and continue regularly.

Recovery after the event

Important goals include replacement of liver and muscle glycogen stores, and the replacement of fluid and electrolytes lost in sweat.

- Rapid restoration of glycogen stores is helped by immediate intake of fast-absorbing carbohydrate foods in the early hours after exercise.
- Carbohydrate-rich foods should be eaten over the next 24 hours. Small, frequent meals may help encourage intake.
- One litre of fluid is required for every kilogram of body weight lost. Sweetened drinks may encourage intake.
- Protein and other nutrients are important in post-recovery processes. Some sports drinks include protein.

TIP

Slow-absorbing carbohydrates (such as lentils) are less suitable for recovery. Choose high GI carbohydrates.

NUTRITIONAL ERGOGENIC AIDS

An **ergogenic** aid is anything that enhances performance. Some ergogenic supplements, discussed below, are supported by research evidence. Each works within a specific set of exercise situations. Some athletes are non-responders, and may experience side effects or negative outcomes.

It is vital to experiment thoroughly in training before use in important events. Some athletes should avoid supplement use: children, growing teenagers, pregnant or breastfeeding women and women attempting conception.

Caffeine

Caffeine can improve endurance by increasing use of free fatty acids as fuel in moderate-intensity exercise. Coffee is taken on an empty stomach before the event. Consumption must be moderate: caffeine is a 'banned' substance at urinary concentrations of over 12 µg/ml. Little or no effect is found in some people and habitual coffee drinkers. Side effects of tremors, headaches and increased heart rate have been reported.

Creatine

Repeated supplementary doses of creatine increase muscle creatine levels. Creatine has benefits in activities where short bouts of very intensive exercise are interspersed with short recovery periods, such as in tennis or football. Side effects of nausea, gastro-intestinal upset, headache and muscle cramping have been reported. Longer-term use is not recommended.

Protein

Muscle repair or building can only be achieved with sufficient protein. Protein supplements can be an expensive way of getting the protein that can be supplied in food. However, mixed macronutrient products, such as liquid meal supplements, can help meet the high energy needs of an athlete in heavy training, or increasing muscle mass. They can be useful in post-exercise recovery to promote simultaneously enhanced protein status and glycogen restoration.

Sodium bicarbonate

Increasing acidity in the body can result in muscle fatigue, so exercise intensity cannot be sustained. Taking sodium bicarbonate, which buffers acidity, has been found to have a positive effect on exercise performance in some people. Gastro-intestinal distress has been reported.

Antioxidants

- Antioxidant vitamin supplementation has been found to reduce muscle fatigue in some, but not all, studies.
- Supplementation with vitamin C may decrease incidence of upper respiratory tract infection after very strenuous exercise.
- Vitamin E may reduce lipid peroxidation (the oxidation of fat, as a result of free radical damage) during exercise.

WEIGHT MANAGEMENT

Body weight comprises water, lean tissue, bone and fat, but when people say they want to lose weight, they usually mean fat. We know that excess fat is associated with increased risk for many diseases, including cardio-vascular disease, type II diabetes, gall bladder disease, some cancers and arthritis. Experts predict that by 2020, half of all UK citizens will be obese. The ratio of fat to lean tissue helps determine whether an individual is overweight. Fat distribution is an important indicator of increased risk of developing chronic diseases associated with obesity. Upper-body or apple-shaped obesity presents a higher risk than lower-body or pear-shaped obesity. Body fat assessment methods and norms are discussed further in chapters 4 and 13.

Fat reduction

Many people can lose body fat by reducing energy intake and increasing energy output with a combination of healthy eating and increased aerobic activity. However, this does not work for everyone. Subtle abnormalities in ability to burn fat may be behind many states of overweight. This may be exacerbated by blood sugar-imbalancing foods that trigger insulin surges.

Follow the following guidelines for fat reduction

- Aim to lose no more than 0.25–1.0 kg per week.
- Follow the healthy diet guidelines. Include all foods necessary for health.
- Choose healthy low-GI carbohydrates. Avoid hidden sugars, and quickly absorbed (high GI) carbohydrates.
- Avoid modified fats, minimize saturated fat sources, but maintain intake of omega 3 fats.
- Eat plenty of fibre.
- Maintain protein intake. Avoid red meats.
- Drink plenty of water.
- Ensure micronutrient intake with a good multivitamin/mineral supplement.
- Do three to five sessions a week of moderate or low-intensity aerobic exercise, lasting at least 30 minutes.
- Weight train to maintain or increase lean mass. Muscle tissue has a high metabolic rate, so burns more calories.

Weight gain

When athletes set out to increase weight, the intention is usually to increase lean muscle mass, not fat. A resistance training programme must be supported by an energy-dense meal plan that contains sufficient protein to meet increased needs – up to about 2 g protein per kilogram body mass.

CHAPTER SUMMARY

In this chapter we have examined the six nutrient classes, their role in a healthy diet, and in meeting the special nutritional needs of the athlete. We have considered nutrition strategies related to performance, and ergogenic nutritional supplementation. Some nutrition-related health issues relevant in exercise have also been reviewed.

Knowledge Review

1   What nutrients are known as the macronutrients?

2   What nutrients are known as the micronutrients?

3   What is an essential nutrient?

4   What is glycogenolysis?

5   When might intake of high GI carbohydrates be useful?

6   What is a saturated fatty acid?

7   What is an incomplete protein?

8   Give examples of two antioxidant nutrients.

9   Which mineral is closely associated with transport and storage of oxygen?

10   What is the major cause of water loss in exercise?

11   How can the hydration state be monitored?

12   What are the benefits of including sodium in a sports drink?

13   Name a good source of omega 3 fat.

14   For what type of sport does creatine have potential benefit?

WEBSITE @

Visit the companion website at www.thomsonlearning.co.uk/healthandfitness/ward where you will find the answers to these questions for you to check your progress through the book.

section two

THE PRACTICE

chapter 7

SPORTS AND REMEDIAL MASSAGE TECHNIQUES

Learning Objectives

After reading this chapter you should be able to:

- recognize the environment and equipment necessary for massage therapy
- acknowledge safe and effective working practices
- understand the potential effects and benefits of sports massage
- describe and apply the various techniques and applications of sports massage
- develop knowledge of remedial massage approaches

This chapter begins the explanation of one of the fundamental techniques of sports therapy. **Sports massage** is where most sports therapists begin their therapeutic practice, and where many choose to stay. On one level, it may be considered a basic and natural art, but when performed expertly it is difficult to surpass in terms of what it can offer the athlete (and the general public). There is little to compare with massage, other than perhaps exercise, when considering just how much benefit a non-pharmacological and non-surgical therapeutic method can offer the individual. Massage is traditional, non-invasive, low-risk and **holistic** (it works to support the body's own healing processes). Although there is never enough evidence to satisfy everyone, there has been a fair amount of research published on the effectiveness of massage. Much of this, however, has focused upon the more non-specific realms of **relaxation** therapy for well-being and adjunctive care. There is gathering evidence to demonstrate how massage can be helpful for certain types of pain, and indeed, it is often mentioned in related literature how we instinctively rub ourselves when suffering a painful knock. Clearly, more well-formulated research is required into the various technical applications of massage in order to satisfy the growing need for evidence-based practice and, certainly in this field, there needs to be a great emphasis on practice-based evidence. To gain improved respect and integration, the profession must also maintain high standards of training and regulation of its many practitioners.

Massage has always been used as an aid to health, and by all manner of people. From mothers for children's ailments, to nurses in respiratory care, and to osteopaths and medical massage therapists treating all types of conditions, massage is used because it is effective. Not only is it a therapeutically useful technique, but it is also a very popular treatment (subjectively it is known that massage feels good). Another bonus is that massage can be used to treat or relieve a very wide variety of conditions – perhaps not always as the main prescriptive medicine, but as a strong adjunct. Clients turn to massage therapists for many reasons. Obviously, sports massage has developed for sportspeople, and it is universally accepted that massage can be helpful for musculo-skeletal injuries. Massage therapy is also widely used for such wide-ranging conditions as anxiety, depression, palliative cancer care, fibromyalgia, asthma, arthritis, constipation, headache, migraine, multiple sclerosis and insomnia. Whether the object is to use specific massage techniques to attend to specific dysfunctions and injuries, or whether the object is to generate a relaxation effect, the therapy is more than useful and always will be considered to be so.

EFFECTS AND BENEFITS OF SPORTS AND REMEDIAL MASSAGE

Massage or soft-tissue manipulation seems to benefit athletes therapeutically, prophylactically, mechanically, physiologically, and psychologically.

WALTER L. LARIMORE MD (IN MELLION 1994)

Massage is an essential element in sports physiotherapy.

VIVIAN GRISOGONO (IN MCLATCHIE *ET AL*. 1995)

There are many applications and benefits to sports massage. It can be used for:

- stripping out tight muscles
- loosening restricted joints
- warming up and stimulating the body before a competition
- relaxing and decongesting the body after exertion
- improving recovery between training and competition
- restoring energy when fatigued
- treating strained muscles and sprained ligaments
- helping to keep a minor injury from becoming a more serious problem
- breaking up adhesions
- releasing tight connective tissues
- improving lymphatic circulation
- increasing blood circulation
- reducing swelling
- toning muscles
- muscle balancing
- treating postural deviations

- relieving pain
- deactivating **trigger points**
- treating orthopaedic and arthritic conditions
- enhancing body awareness
- reducing stress and anxiety
- providing psychological boost
- helping to keep the athlete in peak condition
- improving performance generally
- improving performance during competition
- injury prevention
- general relaxation
- increasing well-being.

> It is well documented that massage, particularly deep massage, can be used to increase local circulation and to decrease muscle spasm and stiffness.
>
> CAROLYN KISNER AND LYNNE ALLEN COLBY (1996)

The techniques of massage affect, to varying degrees, all systems of the body either directly or indirectly. This depends upon which techniques are being employed and which objectives the therapist is endeavouring to achieve. It is important to remember, therefore, that massage techniques have both direct or mechanical effects, and indirect or reflex effects. By some, massage therapy is used as a specific complementary treatment for a wide range of medical conditions, but it must be noted that the specific use of 'applied' massage for particular pathologies is an advanced area of study, requiring a deep understanding of the mechanisms at work, both in terms of the pathology and of the massage techniques.

Massage can help relieve pain through a variety of mechanisms:

- The *pain gate theory* is often used to explain that when additional mechanical stimulation (in this case, massage) is carefully applied to a pain-sensitive region (or to other strategic positions on the body), it can, in effect, confuse or override the pain signals travelling to the brain and help block them out. This is why we instinctively rub ourselves when we feel pain.

- As a result of massage the brain can be stimulated to release **endorphins**, the body's own morphine-like painkilling chemicals, into the nervous system.

- By increasing both local and general relaxation (reducing spasm, tension and stiffness), the tissues experience an improved blood circulation, which results in increased removal of metabolic waste and improved oxygen and nutrient supply to the tissues. As the body relaxes, pain decreases.

- Psychologically, the experience of pain is known to be reduced simply by the act of therapeutic or caring touch.

For the therapist, it is crucial to be aware of all safety points relevant to the provision of massage. As discussed in chapter 3, contra-indications are those conditions that could possibly be exacerbated by particular treatments. In the case of massage, common contra-indications include acute injuries and

---

TIP

Sports massage has a selection of potential physical, physiological and psychological effects, which may directly or indirectly benefit all systems of the body, including:

- circulatory effects
- neuro-reflexive effects
- musculo-skeletal effects
- connective tissue effects
- psychological effects.

TIP

The two basic types of effect that massage can have on the body can be described as being mechanical or reflexive. Mechanical effects occur directly as a result of the stretching, stroking, pressing and kneading of the affected tissues. Reflex effects occur indirectly, still as a result of the massage techniques employed, but where a chain of reactions is set up that leads to a change in physiological functioning.

inflammation, infections, skin disorders, open wounds, burns, varicose veins, thrombosis, recent scar tissue, and a whole host of other medical conditions, from cancer to cardiac problems. That said, massage can still be a helpful therapy, either directly or indirectly, for most conditions, with the potential for benefit achieved through the very careful and well-considered application of it. It is the choice and type of techniques applied, the intensity of such techniques, and the time-scale of the treatments, all relating to the severity and healing stage of the condition, that produce the flexibility of massage therapy. Of course for any serious conditions, injuries or pains of unknown nature, medical approval must always be gained before any massage treatment is provided. This is a major responsibility for the sports therapist.

One particularly notable benefit of massage is that, because it is literally hands-on, during treatment practitioners are able to continually gather palpatory information regarding the receiver's anatomical structures, tissue qualities and adaptations and response to touch. It is normal to expect a certain amount of change in the tissues, objective and subjective, during the course of a treatment: these can include release of muscle spasm, reduction of swelling, increased joint movement, reduced pain or general relaxation. Sometimes discomfort is experienced during the treatment, which is to be expected when some of the heavier remedial techniques are employed. Occasionally, there will be an unfortunate aggravation of symptoms, but this is more likely the result of inappropriate or over-intensive technique. Following treatment, there are further adaptations to be expected. These can include, in the short term: increased relaxation, well-being and energy; reduced discomfort; increased range of movement; improved confidence, optimism and mood relating to the individual's problem; muscle stiffness in response to the deeper or more corrective techniques. Longer-term adaptations follow a similar line when a course of massage therapy is undertaken. The benefit a client experiences is dictated by whether the treatment is indeed the right or best one for them, the skill level of their therapist, and whether other treatments are used in conjunction. A multi-disciplinary approach is usually considered the best form of client care, although this is not to say that massage alone cannot offer optimal benefit in some cases.

SPORTS MASSAGE

TIP

Sports massage is the systematic manual manipulation of the soft-tissues, designed to produce specific responses in the athlete and ultimately improve their performance.

Sports massage is that specific area of massage therapy that has been developed to help improve sports performance, and it is now an accepted and integral part of the considered scientific approach to sports training, preparation, recovery and injury management. Sports massage may also be known as performance massage, athletic massage or deep tissue massage, and it would seem these days that most elite athletes at least have easy access to this therapeutic aid, whether they take advantage regularly or not. Indeed many sports clubs and fitness centres now have on-site professional massage facilities. Of course, as a therapy, it can be just as useful to non-athletes. Borrowing the standard massage techniques of effleurage, petrissage and tapotement, it is also normally combined with passive mobilizations, stretching and often with many other more remedial techniques.

There are certain differences between sports massage and general body massage. For one, sports massage has developed, over the years, to directly help athletes prepare and recover from their training and competitions, and therefore it has generally been performed on people who have good knowledge and awareness of their bodies. Athletic bodies in many disciplines, especially those that involve a great deal of strength training, tend to be fit, toned and hard, which can have implications for the therapist when attempting to access and attend to deeper structures.

REMEDIAL MASSAGE

The standard dictionary definition of the word remedial may offer such phrases as 'providing a remedy'; 'to relieve or cure'; 'to correct or put right'. Remedial massage, therefore, is that particular aspect of massage therapy that is proclaimed to relieve, improve or cure a selection of problems. There are other names that remedial massage goes by, and it may just as easily be labelled advanced, corrective, applied, therapeutic, sports, gymnastic, rehabilitation, medical or orthopaedic massage. The experienced sports massage therapist will be able to call upon many remedial techniques when working to improve function and performance, injuries, postural problems, restrictions and other conditions.

THE MASSAGE ENVIRONMENT AND EQUIPMENT

The sports therapist must create the right environment for their practice. Clinical treatment rooms should be comfortably warm, extremely clean, well-ventilated, smoke-free, sufficiently spacious, preferably private, relaxing environments, with ease of access for all. At sports events, however, there will be times where treatment takes place in a tent, a changing room, in the open air at the side of the track, or in other non-ideal locations.

In the clinic, typically useful, or essential, equipment will include: a screen or partition; treatment couch; treatment chair; couch covers; small hand towels; large bath towels; blanket; couch paper roll; pillows; bolster cushions; paper tissues; surgical spirit; eau de cologne; sports massage oils and lotions; ice; heat equipment; electrical equipment; step; stool; consultation sheets and record cards; first aid kit; storage cupboards; equipment trolley; hot and cold running water; soap and hygienic dispenser; paper towels; waste bin. The mobile on-site or at-event treatment centre obviously is adapted as best as possible to the situation, and the therapist should try to find out exactly where they will be located. Most

TIP

Sports massage is designed to help improve athletic performance. It can be adapted to:

- enhance the pre-event preparation and warm-up
- offer assistance and recovery during an event
- aid recovery immediately post-event
- provide maintenance between events
- treat sporting injuries.

TIP

There are five different practical aspects to sports massage: pre-event; during event, post-event; maintenance; remedial.

TIP

Sports massage therapists need to have great working anatomical knowledge: bony landmarks; positions and actions of muscles; surface anatomy; organ anatomy; superficial nerves and blood vessels; endangerment sites.

TIP

Remedial massage is a physical therapy method that incorporates a selection of well-documented manual techniques which have been developed to improve certain ailments and conditions, and in particular musculo-skeletal problems.

essential equipment can be made portable, and the key to successful operation is thorough preparation, good organization on the day and, beforehand, getting some practical experience of providing such a service.

MASSAGE MEDIA

> **TIP**
>
> Remember that older clients tend to have drier skin, and therefore the therapist should ensure that adequate lubrication is applied and techniques adapted to suit.

Massage media are the various types of oils, creams, balms, lotions and powders that are used to reduce surface friction during flowing moving strokes. Media are certainly not essential to practise massage, and in many instances it can be preferable to work through clothing or towels, or directly onto dry skin. Without a **massage medium**, treatment can often be more controlled (no slipping), and cleaner and easier (and more cost-effective) (also in the pre-event situation, the athlete is not left with any greasiness or residue).

The advantage of using a medium is that it makes such techniques as effleurage and petrissage easy to perform in their classical manner. Moves are glided into and smooth, flowing movements are possible. Massage oils themselves can also offer mild therapeutic benefits, such as superficially warming or cooling the muscles, stimulating the circulation, providing mild analgesia, and, especially with essential oils, can add considerably to the relaxation effect. Care should always be taken with the amount of oil that is used. Too much oil, and the client and couch is covered in it, and the therapist loses some control. Not enough oil can cause some techniques to become quite uncomfortable. Folliculitis (inflammation of the hair follicle) can easily result, especially on the legs, from inadvertently pulling on hairs when not enough lubricant is applied when performing certain techniques. Deep friction, neuromuscular and other similar techniques are much better performed with very little oil so as to maintain the appropriate level of control. It is easier to apply more oil than it is to remove excess.

Unless additionally trained, sports massage therapists are not aromatherapists, and therefore should not blend or prescribe specific oils and creams. Essential oils are potent, concentrated plant, herb, root, flower, berry or tree extracts, each with their own particular indications, precautions and contra-indications. It can be worthwhile training in this area, because both essential oils and base (carrier) oils have strong indications for particular uses in massage for certain ailments. Unless qualified in aromatherapy or herbal medicine, sports masseurs should utilize only plain base oils or pre-blended products, and adhere strictly to manufacturers' safety and application guidelines. Be aware that some clients may be sensitive to certain products, and allergies are not uncommon. When sensitivity is known, do not use the irritant products, when it is suspected a simple patch test can be performed. Use the anterior elbow crease (cubital region), wash and rinse the area and apply a small amount of the product intended for use. Allow 15–20 minutes to see if there is a reaction (itching, inflammation, rash, etc.). Prudent therapists may choose to buy specifically hypoallergenic lubricants.

In some sports, such as football and rugby, especially in the colder weather, oils and rubs are commonly used by the players before the game. These liniments and embrocations are usually particular brands or blends and are designed to help superficially warm the body, relieve aches and invigorate the body. (An argument against the use of such products is that they can actually draw blood superficially towards the skin, *away* from the working muscles.)

Base massage oils fall into three categories: vegetable (grapeseed, almond, sunflower, wheat germ, etc.); mineral (petroleum-based, tending to clog the pores and dry the skin); and pre-blended. Blended oil products for sports massage commonly include such ingredients as lavender, ginger, black pepper, chamomile, eucalyptus and tea tree oil, in relatively safe dilutions (but do still check for client sensitivity). Most oils do not tend to have a very long shelf life, and if not stored correctly can turn rancid.

Creams come in a variety of guises, and these too can be mixed with essential oils. Generally, creams are more manageable than oils, less greasy, more emollient (softening for the skin), absorb more readily, but a little less easy to dispense.

Specialist sports lotions are now available. These normally feature a blend of ingredients, and may be water or oil-based. They also tend to be less greasy and more absorbent than pure oil, and can be ideal for pre-event treatments.

Massage media can sometimes stain clothing and towelling, so should be used with care. Remember that all oils, creams, lotions and powders should be stored and dispensed hygienically and in a manner that reduces potential for contamination. Plastic squeeze bottles, pumps and shakers are the best methods.

When the therapist is about to apply an oil, cream or lotion, their hands should obviously be clean and warm, and the lubricant should be placed in their cupped hand so as to warm it prior to application. Never pour or squirt oil or cream directly onto the client – that is very poor practice.

Some clients may appreciate having the lubricant completely removed after the massage. An alcohol-based product (cologne) can do this, but be aware that alcohol is drying to the skin. Wiping the skin with a clean hot, wrung-out, hand towel removes most of the lubricant, and can be a pleasant experience for the client.

Dry lubricant powders can be useful for clients who dislike the feel of oil or cream, and for pre-event work. It may also be chosen where the client has very oily or hairy skin, or if they perspire easily. If talc is used keep it to a minimum, because of possible nasal and respiratory irritation, skin sensitivities (Control of Substances Hazardous to Health – COSHH – regulations), and because it can be quite messy.

WORKING POSTURE

Massage is performed by using the whole body, not just the hands. Each technique demands of the therapist a skilled application in specific degrees of force, power, intensity, control, direction, movement, leverage, frequency and duration. If the therapist, or client, is not positioned appropriately, then something has to give, and more often than not it is the therapist who is left with their own repetitive stress injuries.

Safe working practice for the therapist includes always keeping in mind and in practice a safe, but effective working posture. This includes setting up the couch height so that the majority of techniques can be correctly applied without having any adverse effects upon the therapist's body, especially on their back posture and the way in which hand techniques are applied (fingers, hands, wrists and elbows are very vulnerable to repetitive strain). A hydraulic couch offers greater flexibility for both therapist and client ease of movement. A typically good height to work with a couch is where fingertips just touch the couch while standing, or where the therapist's leg can easily be placed on the couch (knee flexed, semi-kneeling). This, relatively low height allows for a greater use of body weight during deeper or heavier work. Where the couch has fixed height, or where adjustments can only be performed prior to the client climbing on, then a step (like those used in step classes) can prove very useful.

The therapist needs to maximize the use of their body, for two main reasons: to avoid overuse injuries, which can easily occur, and to be able to perform strenuous work for hours at a time. It is also particularly important to protect fingers, thumbs and wrists from hypermobility. The best way of avoiding painful fingers and thumbs is to get into the good habit of reinforcing one hand with the other, and by using other tools of the body, such as: the lateral fleshy border of the forearm; the proximal aspect of the ulna border; the olecranon process of the elbow; the knuckles; the heel of the hand. Therapists must try also to avoid working themselves through pain, and any unnecessary tensing of the body (such as when hunching the shoulders). Additionally, be aware that smooth, uninhibited, relaxed breathing during the physical administration of sports massage is yet another aspect of the therapist actively protecting themselves against undue problems.

Sports massage is much like a sport in itself as it is physically demanding. Body weight can be carefully added to most techniques without the employment of great amounts of muscular effort. A dynamic working stance is strongly recommended. Knees should generally be kept from full extension, hips should be square on with the direction of moving strokes, and the feet should manoeuvre and pivot concurrently with the strokes (walk stance). A lunge position is an especially useful way of lowering the centre of gravity, and saves the back from strain. Poor habitual back posture during treatments will so easily lead to or exacerbate chronic backache. When treating facing the couch, a squat-like position (astride stance) can be used to lower the centre of gravity. The therapist should also not be afraid to, in certain instances, lean on the couch, rest one knee on the couch, place one foot on a step, kneel on the floor, or sit on a stool at either the head or foot of the couch to provide particular techniques.

A certain amount of strength, **mobility**, **flexibility**, co-ordination and endurance is, of course, essential for effective practice of sports massage, but that does not mean that the practitioner need be super strong. It is not as much about strength as it is about technique. Therapists should work on fitness for their job, and they will get fitter for their work simply by doing it.

TIP

Remember that the therapist needs to maximize the use of their body, for two main reasons: to avoid overuse injuries, which can easily occur, and to be able to perform strenuous work for hours at a time.

By utilizing the principles of appropriate fitness training for the job in hand, they will perform their work well, recover quickly from a demanding schedule and, in the long run, preserve their career. Exercises to make sports massage easier to perform include hand and arm strength and flexibility training, lower body strength work (so that the back does not become overstressed by stooping postures) and, as always, core stability so that the strength and power behind some of the techniques are less of a gruelling effort.

Sports therapists should also take sports therapy massage for themselves. This is particularly recommended (few people respond to the preacher who does not practise what he preaches!). If the therapist generates a fitness mindset and an athletic approach to every practical session, then their work should retain its enjoyability, because there is less likely to be discomfort or undue fatigue, both during or after treatment sessions.

Of course, not all massage sessions are performed on a couch: sometimes the floor is used (with an exercise mat or futon mattress), and sometimes the client is seated. However the treatment is situated, the working posture must remain good because this protects the therapist and helps makes the techniques more efficient.

CLIENT POSITIONING AND DRAPING

First of all, remember to begin the physical assessment of your client before they lie down on the couch and try to stop the client from moving about. Some clients, specifically the less mobile elderly and those with particular injuries will find it difficult to climb onto a high couch, which is where a hydraulic couch (or step) is most advantageous. Additionally some clients will struggle, because of discomfort, to assume certain treatment positions such as lying prone, supine or side-lying, let alone extreme stretch positions.

Therapists should also explain and agree which items of clothing, if any, should be removed prior to treatment. It may be that the client requires assistance with undressing or climbing onto the couch. If not, then it is usual for the therapist either to leave the room or to go behind a screen until the client is ready. Of course, the client must be instructed as to how they should position themselves on the couch, and towels, pillows or blankets should be made available for them. Many sportspeople and athletes will be accustomed to these procedures, but those new to such treatments will benefit from having things clearly explained to them as they go along.

There are a variety of client treatment positions: prone lying; supine lying; side-lying; seated upright on the couch or chair; seated inclined on the couch; or seated on a specialist treatment chair. In addition to the starting position, the client may be supported with pillows or bolsters. Variations are used: to simply perform normal treatment; to allow for client comfort or preference; and to expose specific treatment areas.

An important feature of the treatment couch is its face hole or cradle, which should be secure and comfortably padded. In the prone lying position, this keeps the client's head and neck in alignment with the rest of the body, and therefore reduces unnecessary strain and encourages a more relaxed posture. Where a face hole is not available, the client's head and chest can be supported with small rolled towels. It is recommended that treatment does not take too long in any one position, especially where the weight of the forehead and face is supported in a face hole. Be aware of and responsive to the need of the client to change position during treatment.

Pillows and bolsters (or folded or rolled up towels) are particularly useful in providing support (or drainage) for the client's head, arms, low back, hips, knees, ankles, and also for women with large breasts (add a rolled towel under the upper chest, and perhaps a pillow under the upper abdomen). Remember that the client needs to be comfortable and relaxed for the effective application of most techniques.

Draping is the appropriate covering of the client during treatment. Draping can be performed with towels or blankets, and aside from keeping the client warm and comfortable, correct draping encourages confidence and security. Clients should rarely be left with little in the way of draping. Preserving a client's modesty is essential with all clients, but especially with members of the opposite sex, children and nervous clients. Therapists must always consider keeping the amount of client embarrassment or distress during treatment to an absolute minimum. It is best practice to keep plenty of fresh towels to hand, so that there are always enough to keep the client warm and covered. Normally, only the area being worked upon at any one time is exposed, and all other areas should be covered. It can be recommended, when working on either of the hips, groin, lower sacral or gluteal areas, that an additional small towel be placed over the pubic region to help keep the client at ease, then other towels or drapes can be placed over this as required. When turning clients onto their front or back it is best to hold a large covering towel with both hands closely placed to one side of the couch. The client is then asked to turn away from you (if turning from lying on their back), or towards you (if turning from lying on their front), so that the towel stays covering them.

TREATMENT TIMING: DURATION AND FREQUENCY

TIP

Elite or professional athletes will benefit from at least one sports massage treatment per week, and ideally daily or every other day in periods of hard training and competition. Amateur athletes will benefit from weekly or fortnightly sessions.

The time allocated for an individual treatment session depends upon the particular situation and the presenting objectives. In the clinic it is usual to allow around 45 minutes to an hour for a routine maintenance session. This gives an opportunity to discuss with your client how they have been feeling, what they have been doing, in terms of activities, and provide what they need in terms of treatment. All relevant information should be documented on the client's record card.

When people come with injuries or other problems, especially for the first time, one hour is usually sufficient time to take their details, perform an assessment, provide appropriate treatment and offer relevant advice. Once the presenting problem(s) have been analysed and responded to, it is normal to recommend further treatment. This is when it can be useful to suggest two shorter treatments (30 minutes each) per week rather than one longer one, and as a rough guide, it is usual to recommend four to six twice-weekly sessions for minor sports injuries (i.e. six visits over three weeks). This frequency of treatments allows for progressive healing activity to occur and for home exercise in between sessions, and is generally regarded as offering a greater therapeutic benefit to the athlete. Obviously, if the client responds more quickly, the number of sessions can be reduced. Likewise, if progress is slow or if the condition shows no improvement or worsening, then re-evaluation must be performed and recommendations and objectives must be reviewed.

Providing individual treatment sessions for longer than an hour runs several (relatively minor) risks: the therapist may become limited as to how many clients they can fit into their working day; the client can become over-treated (unduly fatigued or injury aggravated); the therapist can become drained; clients can become accustomed to expecting long sessions; the practice can become less commercially viable.

At sports events time schedules are usually tighter. There are often more than a few people requiring attention both prior to and after the action. It is not uncommon to provide many short treatment sessions on the day, sometimes with athletes not known to you. It is not recommended to provide someone with their first ever massage just before an event; it is better to wait until afterwards. When working closely with a team or player, the emphasis will be on assisting their pre-match preparation and warm-up, and treatment will involve quick and efficient kneading, loosening, percussing and stretching major muscles, and mobilizing joints. This may take between 5 and 15 minutes per player/athlete.

After the game, because athletes tend to appreciate a post-event treatment, there is more likely to be a queue of customers, unless they have a long distance to travel. The emphasis has to be on attending to all those requiring treatment and getting a quick turn-around, because for the athlete it is not good to be standing or hanging around, perhaps in the cold, for too long after extreme exertions. Post-event treatments may take between 5 and 30 minutes, depending upon the circumstances.

MASSAGE TECHNIQUES

The most fundamental massage techniques are effleurage (general stroking), petrissage (kneading) and tapotement (percussion). To these, the sports and remedial massage therapist will often add longitudinal and transverse stroking, lymphatic drainage, deep frictions, shaking and vibrations, passive stretching, joint mobilization techniques, soft-tissue release techniques, connective tissue (myofascial) release techniques, neuromuscular techniques, positional release techniques, muscle energy techniques, as well as the various electromassage techniques. These treatment techniques are discussed in this and in following chapters.

TIP

Massage techniques should be refined and adjusted to suit the presenting requirements and objectives. The following practical components can be altered:

- choice of technique
- depth of pressure
- degree of localized movement
- direction of stroke
- speed of stroke
- repetition of stroke
- positioning of client
- duration of treatment.

TIP

Athletes whose sports involve much strength and power training will have a greater proportion of bulkier, fast twitch muscle fibres. These athletes will benefit from deeper, more concentrated work on the affected major muscle groups.

TIP

Remember that massage techniques have both direct or mechanical effects, and indirect or reflex effects.

Effleurage

TIP ✔

Effleurage palpates, relaxes, warms and decongests the body, and it helps to keep the smooth flow of a massage treatment.

Effleurage, derived from the French word *effleurer*, meaning to stroke lightly, is often the first technique used to apply massage oil, provide initial treatment contact, gently palpate the superficial tissues, relax the client and warm the muscles. It also is a technique to apply between others because it helps to keep the smooth flow of a treatment, and also helps to move on the waste products produced or dispersed from other deeper techniques. Effleurage is usually performed with the palms of the hands, either separately one hand at a time, with two hands together at the same time, reinforced one hand on top of the other or overlapping, or sometimes with the fleshy aspect of the forearm. Usually, on the completion of each stroke, the hands return to the starting position by gliding lightly back and keeping in continuous contact. During effleurage, the hands remain relaxed, avoiding hyperextension at the wrist, as they mould to the contours of the body.

The strokes of effleurage are usually graded as being superficial (light) or deep (heavier). The flow of the stroke traditionally runs distal to proximal so as to encourage enhanced venous and lymphatic circulatory flow, but may also be used across the muscle fibres, transversely. When the massage stroke directs the superficial circulations back towards the heart it is said that it is applied in a *centripetal* direction. In some instances effleurage can be applied against the flow of the circulations, more as an aid to other techniques in reducing muscle tensions. In the pre-event situation, if effleurage is used, it is usually performed more rapidly so as to stimulate the body and increase tone, rather than relax. Deeper, more specific, stroking will be discussed later in the text.

Petrissage

TIP ✔

Petrissage kneads, stretches, broadens, compresses, decongests and increases circulation through the tissues.

The word petrissage is derived from the French *petris*, meaning to knead. Kneading, wringing, picking-up, squeezing, muscle rolling, broadening, pumping and compression are all commonly used massage techniques which can fall under the category of petrissage. These are all great techniques for loosening up the soft tissues, increasing the flow of tissue fluids and local circulations, warming and relaxing the body, reducing excess

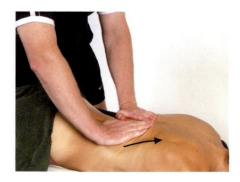
Two-handed effleurage to the back

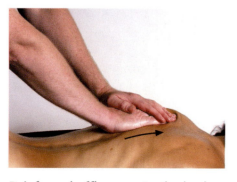
Reinforced effleurage to the back

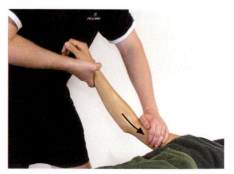
Single-handed effleurage to the upper arm

muscle tension or spasm and reducing fatigue. Of course, in the pre-event situation, the techniques are usually applied so as to invigorate, warm and tone, and therefore are applied more briskly than if relaxation and recovery are the objectives. Petrissage normally follows, and is interspersed with, effleurage – which keeps the movements smooth and flowing.

Performed with grasping hands, heels and palms, fingers and thumbs, petrissage or kneading generally is often described as being a sequential series of pressing, lifting, circular, sometimes alternate type movements. The contact with skin may be dynamic, in that the skin is constantly moved over by the hands, or alternatively the depth, pressure and speed of the technique take it through the skin so that it moves with the hand, usually either heel of hand, or thumb or fingertips, to produce a more localized kneading effect more on the muscles underneath, similar to friction techniques. Be careful to avoid excessive pressure over bony prominences and on areas where there is little in the way of body fat or muscle tissue; also avoid pinching the skin.

Petrissage techniques can be classified as follows:

- **Wringing**: tissues are compressed, sheared and lifted, typically in either an alternating circular fashion or with an alternating linear movement. Whether circular or linear, the hands normally begin the technique at opposite sides of the treated area. Palms should be moulded to the contours, with fingers together (supported by each other) and thumbs also remaining adducted.

- **Squeezing**: tissues are lifted from the underlying bone, and gently and specifically squeezed for a second or two with the pads of fingers and thumb. Can be performed singularly or with both hands at the same time, and can be repeated a few times on the same area.

- **Picking-up**: muscle tissue is grasped and lifted up from the underlying tissues by the pads of the fingers and thumb of one or both hands. This technique can be performed by one hand at a time, repeatedly and alternately lifting, squeezing and releasing the tissues, or by both hands, which combines wringing and squeezing.

- **Muscle rolling**: muscle tissue, underneath the skin and subcutaneous tissue, is lifted up and rolled through by the sliding pads of the fingers (towards) or thumbs (away).

> **TIP**
>
> One key to successful (effective) massage is the ability to feel your way through the layers of tissues and over the bony prominences, feeling for tightness, abnormality, congestion, restriction, and then providing the right amount of depth, pressure, stretch or speed of movement during each stroke. These are skills that naturally develop as experience gathers.

> **TIP**
>
> The sports masseur should try to develop a smooth flowing style which demonstrates easy transmission from one technique to another.

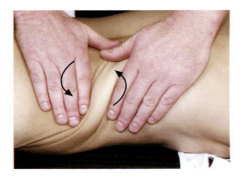
Wringing (circular strokes) to the lower back

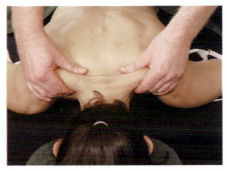
Squeezing of the upper trapezius

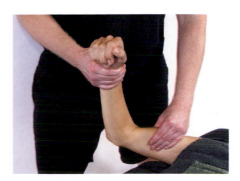
Picking-up the biceps

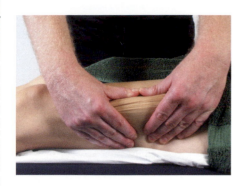

Muscle rolling on the quadriceps

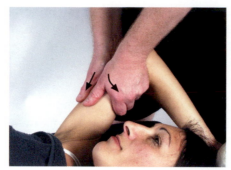

Broadening of the triceps

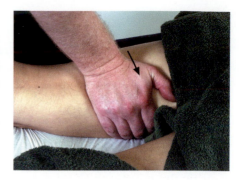

Pumping of the hamstring muscles

- **Broadening**: typically performed with the heels of the hands, which compress the belly of the treated muscle and then slide slowly outwards, still under compression, so as to broaden the muscle. For smaller muscles, the thumbs can be used. The technique should be repeated several times over each area.

- **Pumping**: a rhythmic focal compression of the tissues, usually best applied into the larger muscle groups and performed with the heel of the hand or a curled fist. The compression may be held into the muscle for a second, released and then repeated.

Tapotement

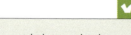

TIP ✔

Tapotement helps to stimulate the body, improve the tone of muscles, increase superficial circulation, and in some instances, reduce pain and induce relaxation.

Tapotement, from the French *tapoter*, meaning to tap, is the selection of percussive techniques generally used in massage to stimulate, tone and energize the body. Rapid, repeated rhythmic striking techniques are applied lightly over the body's fleshy areas. These techniques also help to increase blood and lymph flow, raise skin temperature, superficial tissue metabolism and reduce pain. Tapotement is also an important part of respiratory physical therapy, where it is used to mobilize excess mucous secretions in the upper respiratory tract. There are several techniques, including: hacking; cupping; pounding; beating; pincement. The movement for all techniques, except pounding, comes more from the wrist than from the elbow or shoulder, and the hands should be relaxed enough so as to spring back after striking the skin.

Tapotement is most indicated for pre-event treatments, and can be useful in maintenance and aspects of remedial work.

Tapotement techniques can be classified as follows:

- **Hacking**: wrists are loose but extended, with fingers relaxed, apart and slightly flexed. Rapid alternate chopping-like movements are lightly applied over the fleshy areas of the body.

- **Cupping**: hands are formed into a cup shape with fingers close together. The palmer surface repeatedly strikes the body with a rapid alternating flexion and extension of the wrists. Cupping produces a momentary vacuum-suction type effect.

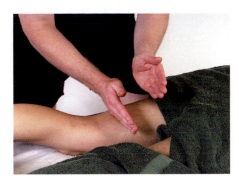

Hacking to the hamstrings

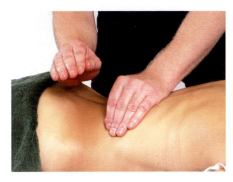

Cupping on the lower back

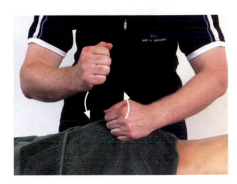

Pounding to the buttocks

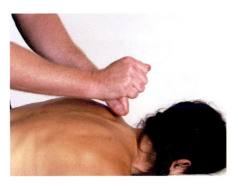

Beating to the upper back

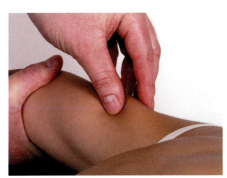

Pincement to the upper arm

- **Pounding**: the hands are formed into clenched fists, and the lateral border of each hand alternately strikes the body. The movement is circular in that the hands move towards the therapist in a rolling or rotating type action, with the movement coming more from the elbow than the wrist. Pounding is the heaviest form of tapotement, most effective on the larger muscle groups.

- **Beating**: the hands are formed into loosely clenched fists. The hands are in a pronated position as the wrists rapidly flex and extend to produce the light beating effect.

- **Pincement**: this is a rapid gentle lifting or plucking of the superficial tissues performed by the rapid alternate grasping of the thumb and fingers. The root of the movement still comes from the repeated flexion and extension of the wrist. It is different from the other percussive techniques in that lightly lifting is the objective rather than lightly compressing.

Stroking

Stroking differs from classical effleurage in that the techniques are more specific and searching, and they also tend to be deeper. Deep stroking, sometimes referred to as muscle stripping, is typically used as part of a

> **TIP**
>
> Stroking is particularly useful in sports massage, and can be either longitudinal or transverse. Longitudinal stroking stretches and decongests specific muscles along their length, while transverse stroking stretches, broadens and decongests specific muscles across the run of fibres.

TIP ✔

One advantage that sports massage has over active stretching is that it can stretch the muscles across their fibres, working to separate them, as well as along with their fibres, drawing them closer together.

TIP ✔

When performing deep pressing, stroking or frictioning techniques, inform the receiver beforehand about the probable effect, benefit and duration. Encourage them to relax and also position the treated regions so as to passively shorten (and relax) the muscles.

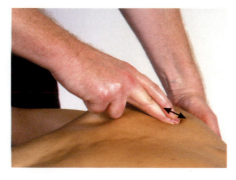

Third finger reinforced with the second

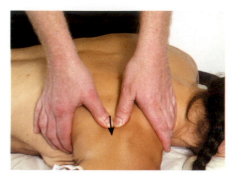

Thumbs supported by each other, side by side

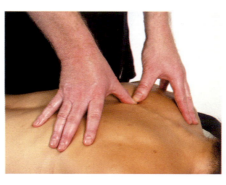

Thumb reinforced by other thumb

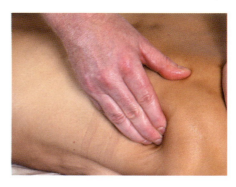

Fingers supported by other fingers

routine maintenance sports massage session because it combines well with other standard techniques and addresses particular muscle tensions. Because deep stroking is applied directly into specific muscles it is also very useful both diagnostically and as a remedial tool. Stroking can be applied with: pads or tips of fingers and thumbs; the ulnar border of the forearm; the olecranon process; the heel of hand; and the knuckles. It is important to protect your own hands, and it is good practice to reinforce your fingers and thumbs, or use alternative methods, whenever there is the slightest possibility of overstressing them.

There are two basic approaches to stroking, both of which require a considerable knowledge of muscular anatomy: longitudinal (along the length of the muscle fibres) and transverse (across the fibres). As with some of the other heavier and more specific techniques, it is often useful, and more comfortable for the client, if the treated muscles are put into a shortened position for the application of stroking. This can be done by simply placing bolsters or thickly rolled towels under certain areas, or by holding or supporting limbs during the techniques. Because deep stroking is direct and intense it should be performed very slowly and carefully. One way of achieving objectives without causing much discomfort is to perform techniques in short stroking steps. Transverse stroking is usually performed systematically throughout the whole length of the muscle.

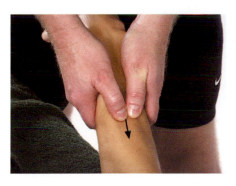

Longitudinal stroking using reinforced thumbs, to wrist extensor muscles

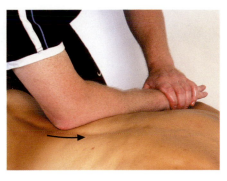

Longitudinal stroking using ulnar border, to paraspinal muscles

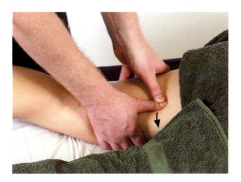

Transverse stroking using reinforced thumbs, across hamstring muscles

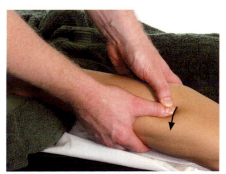

Transverse stroking using reinforced thumbs, across lateral belly of gastrocnemius

Vibrations

Vibrations are rapid oscillatory movements, performed with the pads of the fingers or palms of the hand. The technique may be focused over one region at a time, or performed in conjunction with slow stroking movements. The purpose of vibration is to induce muscle relaxation, stimulate nerve activity and provide pain relief.

Vibration is a subtle, gentle technique and surprisingly difficult to master. The therapist must to be able to rapidly oscillate their contacting hand constantly, for several seconds at a time. Vibration, also referred to as fine vibration or vibratory stimulation, is also often described alongside the technique of shaking, as they are both oscillatory (muscles and tendons can indeed be grasped, vibrated, jostled or shaken), but because shaking is also used in conjunction with joint mobilization techniques, it is described in the next section.

Vibration is begun with initial compression, with either the pads of the fingers, with the palm of the hand, or with a pincer-like grip between the thumb and fingers (the latter is also sometimes described as shaking). Typically, the therapist should then attempt to tense or fixate their upper arm so as to produce most of the vibrational or trembling movements through the rapid alternate contractions of the forearm. The effort required

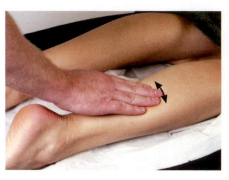

Vibrations using fingertips, to calf muscles

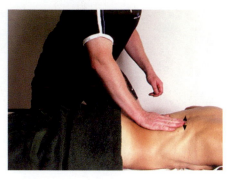

Vibration combined with stroking using palm of hand, to lumbar region

is fatiguing, and therefore is only applied for a few seconds at a time. One variation of the technique is to produce a running vibration through the length of a muscle or limb, where vibration is combined with slow stroking.

Connective tissue manipulation/myofascial release

This selection of techniques has its focus specifically on the superficial tissues (skin; subcutaneous fatty tissues; superficial fascia; deep fascia). The techniques are used to stretch tissues, break adhesions, normalize tensions, reduce fibrous thickening, indirectly reduce joint restrictions and increase local circulations and tissue permeability. They are also particularly indicated for a variety of conditions: the chronic stages of injury to improve the mobility of superficial tissues; fibrosis of the skin and subcutaneous tissues; the later treatment of burns and scarring; post-operative situations.

The terms connective tissue manipulation (CTM) and myofascial release (MFR) generally tend to be regarded as being the same, and the terms are commonly used interchangeably. Both affect superficial tissues and their related muscles, and both usually do not involve a sliding movement over the skin; rather the skin moves with the therapist's hands. There have, though, been subtle differences described between the two: CTM techniques, such as skin rolling, are specifically directed at tightness and restrictions in the accessible connective tissues; MFR techniques are a particular application of CTM which aim to address tightness or adhesions formed within the subcutaneous fascial sheaths and superficial muscles. Both can positively affect limited joint ranges and improve the relative easiness of movement.

The treated tissues are normally stretched to the point of being palpably taut, and held for a second or a few seconds, often until a sense of give or relaxation occurs. Each technique, like all others, should be adapted for each region and for each person individually. In some instances the fingers and thumbs can provide sufficient pressure to cause beneficial changes to the tissues, without having to adapt the client's position. This approach is more likely to be used on very superficial or more delicate tissues, such as on the fascia and muscles of the face and neck. At other times the technique

TIP ✔

Connective tissue manipulation is a technique designed to address restrictions, adhesions and circulatory impairments affecting the skin, subcutaneous tissues, superficial fascia and deep fascia.

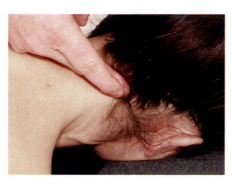

Connective tissue manipulation to the sub-occipital region, with finger tips

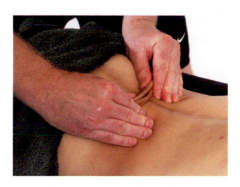

Skin rolling using pads of fingers and thumbs on the lumbar fascia

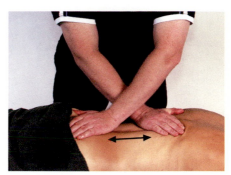

Myofascial release of the lumbar region, with crossed hands

will be enhanced by first putting the affected region into a position of stretch and also by using a stronger contact, such as with the palms or heels of the hands. Often, with this approach, the hands are crossed so as to provide a stronger and easier way of performing the stretching.

Skin rolling, similar to muscle rolling but without the depth and focus to involve muscle tissue, is an excellent way of stretching the skin, subcutaneous fatty tissues and superficial fascia. Once grasped and stretched by the pads of fingers and thumbs, the tissues are further rolled through as the fingers or thumbs press or glide into them, and there may follow a release of tension or restriction in the deeper layers of fascial tissue. This technique is best performed with two hands working closely together, and is often more effective if the technique is performed from a variety of directions over the affected region. Skin rolling should either be avoided, or performed with caution when there is inflammation, instability or fragility due to acute injury, older age, medications or pathology.

CTM or MFR tends to result in either elastic stretching, where the affected tissues return to their normal resting length after the application of the techniques, or plastic stretching, where the length that is gained during the technique remains afterwards, and the tissues are in effect moulded (this is known as plastic deformation).

Excessive contractility in fascial tissue can easily spread to adjacent compartments. Thickening, adhesions, scarring and tightness in the fascia can all affect the smooth movement of muscles and joints. Most instances of excessive fascial tension will be accompanied by hypersensitivity and discomfort. Be aware that normal healthy skin, fascia and muscle tissue have a certain amount of easy elastic mobility and pliability, and where this is not the case, CTM techniques are indicated, in conjunction with other methods.

Joint mobilizations

Joint mobilization techniques are those various methods that aim to maintain or improve the quality of movement at specific joints. Simply, joint mobilizations may be passive, active, resisted or a combination. Passive mobilizations may be performed manually or with the aid of mechanical devices such as continuous passive motion (CPM) exercise machines. In

> **TIP**
>
> There are a variety of joint mobilization techniques. For safe and effective treatment of joint restrictions, the therapist should have good understanding of the acceptable or normal ranges of movement, and then which techniques would be most appropriate for each client.

TIP

Before attempting to mobilize restricted joints, the therapist needs to be able to identify the cause of the restriction, for example: soft tissue shortening; inflammation; arthritic degeneration; mechanical blockage; pain.

TIP ✔

To improve joint mobility, the sports therapist may use: basic massage techniques; passive articulation and stretching; gentle traction and shaking techniques; shearing techniques; deep friction techniques; neuromuscular techniques; muscle energy techniques.

sports or remedial massage therapy the therapist can employ a selection of techniques to improve the movement and health of a joint. Of course, it is always important to encourage active exercise for mobility, strength, endurance, proprioception and well-being, but in the clinic the therapist is able to focus treatment techniques and help make the active components of a rehabilitation programme easier to perform.

By performing mobilizing techniques, the circulation, nutrition and drainage of joints is improved, alongside the more obvious physical benefits of improving or maintaining the amount of movement available.

Joint mobilization techniques can be classified as follows:

- **Articulation**: this is a simple technique which involves the therapist carefully taking the joint through its available ranges of movement. It is good practice to begin gently and within a free and easy range, before taking the movement to the end of the available range. There is usually a slight measurable difference between the comfortable active range and the comfortable passive range. Articulation (the classic form of joint mobilization) is used to assess passive RoM and is a prelude to further techniques, such as passive stretching or muscle energy technique (MET). The therapist should keep in mind the practically relevant concepts of ease-bind and restriction barrier when providing articulatory techniques.

- **Stretching**: passive stretching methods are described in chapter 8.

- **Traction**: this is a technique that gently decompresses or separates structures that are normally very closely associated. It may be performed manually, or in hospital and rehabilitation settings with the aid of weighted pulley systems. The latter is used for such instances as intervertebral disc prolapse, serious fracture or nerve entrapment. Manual traction should always be performed slowly and with great care. It is in itself an assessment technique. When traction brings on pain it may be seen as a positive sign that the stabilizing ligaments are affected, and when it relieves pain it can be a positive sign that compressive forces (disc; fracture; impingement) are involved in the cause of the problem. Sports therapists who perform manual traction should take care to support and hold the body well, and not cause any unnecessary discomfort or aggravation of problems. Manual traction is usually eased into and held for a few seconds at a time, whereas mechanical (medical) traction may be applied for longer time periods. The therapist should take care to work with good posture, often leaning back into the technique and keeping their back upright.

- **Shaking**: this is a rhythmic mobilization technique that employs short-range joint movements. One application of shaking is as a direct technique to the soft-tissues, where muscles or tendons are grasped, lifted up from the underlying bone, and then shaken across their length. Another useful shaking technique is to carefully hold either the hand or foot and simply shake the limb, slowly or briskly, so that the fleshy muscle components are loosened. This is generally performed with the treated limb in a degree of flexion, and encourages relaxation and circulatory drainage. Shaking may also be combined with traction, so that the treated joint(s) can be gently eased apart (decompressed) and then moved side to side or up and down rhythmically. This latter method is similar to the osteopathic harmonic technique, where oscillatory movements (pushing, pulling, shaking, rocking and rolling of limbs) are performed and where there is a natural recoil or rebound response of the tissues to each rhythmic movement. Shaking and harmonic techniques can be performed slowly or rapidly to varying effect. These techniques aim to result in improved circulatory interchange and soft-tissue relaxation, both of which can lead to increases in joint mobility.

- **Shearing**: also called gliding, shearing is a technique that glides one joint surface across its adjacent articulatory surface in a very short range movement. It may involve the stabilization of the adjacent (non-moving) structures. This technique, like most others, is performed slowly with a feel for how the tissues are responding. The areas most conducive to shearing include the neck, shoulder, elbow, wrist, hip and ankle.

- **Neuromuscular and related techniques**: neuromuscular technique (NMT); positional release technique (PRT); strain counter strain (SCS); and MET are described in chapter 9.

TIP ✔

Warning! High-velocity, short-amplitude, thrusting joint manipulation techniques are quite different and separate from the joint mobilization techniques described, and are in the domain of osteopaths, chiropractors, physiotherapists and other specifically trained manipulative therapists. They are potentially very dangerous in untrained hands and should not be attempted by anyone who is not suitably trained.

There are several important safety issues relating to joint mobilization. Firstly, the therapist must take care to not aggravate any inflammatory situations, such as those often seen in cases of arthritis, especially rheumatoid, or any other pathological restriction. If there are any neurological signs and symptoms (such as numbness, tingling, radiating pain or muscle weakness) then such techniques are initially contra-indicated until medically assessed. If there is a subluxation or dislocation of a joint, then this too requires medical attention. Hypomobility of particular joints in a client dictates that the joint would normally be strengthened rather than have its mobility increased. Conditions such as spondylosis or spondylolisthesis are unstable back problems, and therefore should only be mobilized under supervision. Fixed structural conditions and extreme spinal curves require a particularly careful approach. Especially in the elderly and those with known arterial disease (such as arteriosclerosis), there are potential dangers when mobilizing or stretching certain regions, in particular the joints and tissues of the neck. Therefore, neck mobility work should always be performed with great care and with vigilant observation for any unwanted responses to the techniques, such as nystagmus (rapid involuntary eye movements) or dizziness. Be aware that it can take a considerable period of time to improve or re-educate a range of motion at a joint, and in many chronic cases the end result may not be considered ideal, merely improved. Always bear in mind that any undue pain is a warning signal that something is not right.

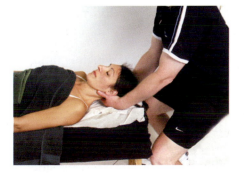 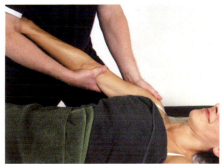 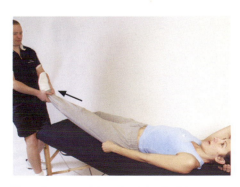

Traction of the neck | Shearing the shoulder joint | Traction combined with shaking to the lower extremity

Lymphatic drainage

Basic lymphatic drainage massage techniques are gentle and useful for a selection of conditions. The actual term lymphatic drainage refers to the normal drainage of tissue fluid and particulate matter into the lymphatic vessels and ducts and onwards back into the general blood circulation. This does occur naturally in good health, but should lymphoedema develop, it may be treated by exercise, specific massage techniques, forms of electrotherapy and other methods.

All forms of massage, to varying degrees, affect the flow of lymph. Indeed, there are a selection of manual techniques which have been developed specifically to influence lymphatic drainage, for a wide range of reasons. Manual lymphatic drainage (MLD) as such is often described as a therapy in its own right. It is beyond the scope of this book to delve deep into the many specific techniques and applications of all MLD systems; however, a short explanation of some simple approaches to improving lymphatic flow, and the rationale behind their use should help to enhance certain sports therapy treatment protocols.

The sports therapist will obviously be aware now of the basic structures that constitute the lymphatic system, and will have knowledge of its fundamental functions. It should be appreciated that the lymphatic system is the body's secondary circulatory system and very much part of its immune system. It is most important that the therapist knows where the main collections of lymph nodes are located, so that when appropriate, they may help to influence the flow of lymph towards them. Of course, there are instances where lymph tissue has been removed or become dysfunctional: such cases may benefit from therapy aimed at helping to divert the flow into other areas. Additionally, it should be understood that lymph, the protein-rich, plasma-like fluid that contains tissue debris and metabolites, and that can accumulate around the tissues in the presence of injury, immobility or pathology, travels from the tissues back towards the general blood circulation by way of the lymphatic vessels. It drains into the larger lymphatic ducts and eventually the subclavian veins. Lymph travels only in one direction, from the tissues towards the heart, and the natural movement of lymph is mainly influenced by the contraction of surrounding skeletal muscles, gravity, body position, negative respiratory pressure, the movement of skin and fascia, and by the presence of valves in the vessel walls, which exist to stop back-flow.

The presence of problems in the soft-tissues (e.g. inflammation; infection; restrictions and tensions; surgical removal of lymph vessels or nodes; post-operative scarring; congenital abnormalities of lymph vessels or nodes; fluid retention) can lead to a condition known as lymphoedema, which is fluid accumulation and swelling resulting from an insufficiency of the lymphatic transportation system. Lymphoedema is often seen whenever there is restricted lymph or venous flow, and for sports therapists it can also be associated with soft-tissue injuries (the swelling from which can cause a sudden overload to the transportation capacity of the lymphatic channels). The pooling of fluids is normally compounded by gravity, hence oedema is usually more pronounced distal to restrictions or abnormalities. Limb girth measurements can help to assess the amount and progress of swelling.

Additional signs associated with lymphoedema, at different stages of severity, include: pitting oedema (where finger pressure into boggy skin leaves a pit or indent in the tissues which remains for a short time); smooth, shiny, hairless skin; dense fibrotic congestion; tissue fragility; ulceration; frequent infections.

Since there is no cure for most forms of chronic lymphoedema, the therapeutic goal is usually to reduce or relieve it. Medically, this would typically involve topical or systemic medications, MLD, compression bandages and remedial exercises. Should the sports therapist be faced with chronic lymphoedema, then they must first encourage the client to obtain medical approval for their treatment: after all, the therapist is not the person to make a decision on the appropriateness of this individual's health-care, especially as there are often underlying problems.

If lymphatic drainage massage therapy is deemed appropriate, then it should be performed correctly for best results. The main basic techniques are: very light effleurage; gentle intermittent pressure stroking; gentle muscle pumping; gentle joint mobilizations. For MLD, the effleurage technique is performed suprafascially (i.e. with a pressure only down to the depth of the muscle fascia) and slowly in the direction of natural flow. The thumbs, fingers or palms can be used to perform this stroke. The intermittent pressure stroking technique is also very light, but generally uses shorter strokes which momentarily, concurrently and repeatedly pump and stretch the tissues, and in particular, those adjacent to main collections of lymph nodes. This technique is perhaps best performed with the fingers or palm of hand. Light, rhythmic muscle pumping, using the palm or heel of the hand, can be used as a general circulatory tonic, and it may be included as part of an MLD strategy, especially over the upper chest area. Performing gentle, rhythmic, passive joint mobilizations helps to create an additional pumping action, which may incorporate a gravitational effect.

> **TIP**
>
> In order for massage techniques to greatly assist lymphatic circulation, knowledge of positions of major lymphatic channels and nodes is essential.

A classic MLD strategy is to begin by first clearing the proximal and any unaffected lymphatic regions, which could typically begin at the neck, contra-lateral limbs and torso. It follows that the axillary (armpit) region should be cleared before the supra-trochlear (elbow) region, and the inguinal (groin) region should be cleared before the popliteal (knee) region. By clearing all proximal lymphatic channels (contra-lateral and ipsilateral) first, the fluid congesting the affected region(s) has somewhere to go when manually drained. In the case of sports injury, the drainage techniques will be applied to the most proximal regions, gradually working down towards the affected area. The therapist should take care to avoid aggravating the injury site in the early stages of healing, and must remember that MLD is a very subtle, gentle treatment. This systematic approach may be repeated several times during a treatment. Elevation of limbs during and between treatments can enhance the effects. It is recommended, also, to use minimal lubricant for the effleurage technique, and no lubricant for the intermittent compression technique. Lymphoedema should benefit from daily or twice daily treatments, over a period of a few weeks, or for as long as symptoms pervade. It is usual to perform MLD first, if combining it with other therapeutic techniques.

As mentioned earlier, there are several well-documented approaches to MLD. Because MLD for chronic problems is more complex than simply

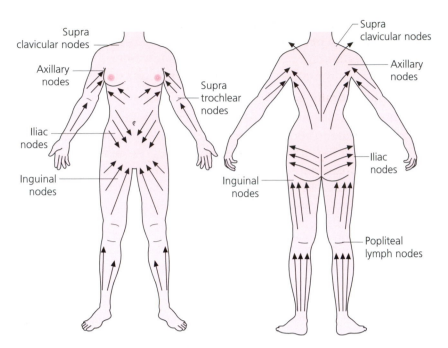

Lymphatic drainage approaches

stroking, pumping and mobilizing, it is recommended that interested therapists undertake specialized training in this area.

REGIONAL CONSIDERATIONS

Although all regions of the body are unique, with each requiring an individualized approach in treatment, it is pertinent to highlight one or two important issues that have relevance to the safe and effective practice of sports and remedial massage.

Abdomen

The abdominal region is a vulnerable area because it houses many vital organs and is poorly protected by musculo-skeletal structures. Of course, the rectus abdominus, external and internal obliques and transversus abdominus are important muscles, and they normally benefit greatly from sports massage therapy. Be careful to avoid deep pressure into the abdomen and underlying organs, and also be aware of the possibility of a full bladder or bowel. Any aching or pain of dubious nature should be medically assessed. Pregnancy is an obvious contra-indication to abdominal massage. For some, menstruation also can be a reason to avoid treatment. Abdominal massage, however, can be very useful for digestive and respiratory problems, and is often provided as part of a relaxation session. There are several approaches to attending to the abdomen:

- For general (non-specific) abdominal massage, the client is typically positioned so as to relax the abdominal muscles (knees supported and flexed), and gentle effleurage, petrissage and stroking techniques are performed in line with the direction of digestive flow (clockwise).

- Superficial lymphatic drainage techniques can be directed towards the inguinal nodes.

- For specific abdominal muscle treatment, have the client slightly tense the muscles (ask them to lift their upper body up a little, keeping knees bent), be aware of muscle fatigue and the fact that deep work into tensed muscles can be quite uncomfortable.

- Work from a side-lying position, and apply lateral pressure or stroking into the abdominal muscles.

- Use light effleurage, and lifting and picking-up petrissage techniques where possible.

Neck

When the client is lying prone, if there is no face hole or cradle, it is good client care to encourage them to alter their neck position from time to time, so as to prevent unnecessary stiffness. The side-lying position can be a very useful position (neck is supported on one side) for attending to neck problems. Avoid heavy pressure into the anterior and lateral neck regions. Clients with kyphosis and forward head will require a pillow for support when lying supine. Work with intent to promote muscle and postural balance. Avoid heavy pressure on spinous processes. As mentioned earlier, be particularly careful when working on older client's necks, and on those with known arthritic or arterial disorders, and of course remember that the presence of neurological signs and symptoms (numbness, tingling, weakness, radiating pain) around the neck, across the shoulder or down into the arm or hand, means that massage treatment is contra-indicated, until approved.

Back

Be aware that not all clients can remain comfortable lying prone, supine or side-lying for any length of time. Bolsters and pillows come in very handy, for support in any position. Back pain can result for a variety of reasons, and is not always related to the tissues of the back – problems in the hip, hip flexors, gluteals, sacro-iliac joint, abdominal muscles, hamstrings or chest muscles, for example, are all common causes of back pain. Work with intent to promote muscle and postural balance. Avoid heavy pressure on spinous processes. Be aware of the contra-indications associated with back (and sciatic) pain.

Shoulder

This region specifically involves the humerus, scapula and clavicle, and all associated joints and muscles. The shoulder is also in close relationship with the neck, arm, upper back and chest. As always try to encourage muscle and postural balance, focusing on the release of tight muscles and fascia, and ideal postural positioning of upper arm and scapula. Try to keep in mind the position and action of all main muscles acting on the shoulder.

Arm

Most athletes will appreciate thorough treatment of the arm muscles. Massage of the arm can be a very relaxing and freeing experience. Remember that we all use our hands all the time, and also the fact that the arms hang downwards, making lymph and venous return an uphill task. The therapist will need to develop skill in supporting the arm while working on it, working in different positions, and also working both single-handedly and with both hands.

Hip

This region is strongly weight-bearing and specifically involves the femur, ilium, ischium, pubis, and all associated joints and muscles. It is also closely related to the lumbar region, pelvic girdle and lower extremity. Inequality of leg length, on either side, can easily lead to hip problems. Osteoarthritis is a common problem for older age groups. The area is treated well with massage, particularly in prone and side-lying positions (stretching and other techniques can be approached with additional positionings). Be aware of the professional boundaries associated with this region. Always keep the client well draped, only exposing the area being treated, and avoid any movements that cause embarrassment to the client, such as any technique that causes the gluteal cleft to open (which must remain covered in any case). In this regard it is often best to stroke towards the cleft rather than away from it, and also it is considered less intimate if the forearm, rather than the hand, is used to treat the gluteal region.

Leg

The legs get a lot of attention in sports massage, and rightly so. They can be effectively treated in all positions, and the best strategy often incorporates prone, side-lying and supine positioning. The knee, ankle and foot are common sites for problems, and the therapist should, as always, take care to assess the problem before treating it. Muscle strains are prevalent in the hamstrings, calves and quadriceps. The ilio-tibial band is also a common problematic tissue, and when tight can be slowly manually stripped to release its tension. Remember that radiating (sciatic) pain down the leg is more likely to arise from the lower back or posterior pelvic region, and in these cases treatment to the pain in the leg will do nothing to improve the problem. Attention to leg biomechanics is particularly important for sports involving running. Always be careful to avoid direct treatment of varicose veins, and be observant for such conditions as phlebitis, thrombosis and ulceration.

Chest

The ribs and sternum are the main protectors of the chest. The other skeletal structures directly related are the shoulder girdles and the thoracic spine. The pectorals, intercostals, sternocliedomastoids, diaphragm, obliques and abdominals are the predominant muscles having an effect on the thoracic cage. The effort for respiration comes from the chest and specifically the main and accessory muscles of respiration. Respiratory disorders (e.g. asthma, bronchitis) often gain great benefit from massage therapy, but medical approval should be sought. Respiratory decongestive and postural drainage therapy, including percussion and vibration, is performed routinely by physiotherapists for patients with excess mucus. Relaxation breathing, abdominal breathing and other remedial exercises can greatly assist respiratory function. Postural problems of this region include kyphosis, scoliosis, forward head, rounded shoulders and barrel chest. Heavy breasted women sometimes suffer with rounding of the shoulders, and very often they will have sensitive upper chest muscles. Here, the therapist must work with very careful positioning, draping and application of techniques, so as not to cause any distress to the client.

PRE-EVENT MASSAGE AND PREPARATION

The pre-event massage plays a very useful and additional part in the athlete's preparation for competition. It normally takes place between 20 minutes and an hour before the event, and lasts 5 to 15 minutes. It certainly must not be considered as the warm-up – merely a part of it. Although this type of massage has useful physical effects (increasing circulation; warming muscles and joints; improving the neuromuscular response; muscle toning), there is also a great deal of psychological benefit to the player.

As previously mentioned, some players have a preference for using superficially warming preparations (liniments) on the skin before the game, and this is fine. However, other athletes may prefer to remain clothed during pre-event work, and the therapist should develop massage skills that do not require oils, creams, powders or lotions.

Be aware that over-vigorous, heavy or deep massage will more likely cause a decrease in performance. The techniques used pre-event tend to be a little more brisk and invigorating than post-event or remedial work, though not to the point of causing the athlete to tense up or suffer discomfort.

Typical techniques used in pre-event massage include: effleurage; petrissage; vibrations; shaking; tapotement; mobilizing; stretching. The emphasis must be on preparing the major muscles and joints that will be used most in the activities that follow. In team situations and where many treatments are required, the therapist may utilize **electro-massage** equipment to provide stimulation.

When presented with an athlete for the pre-event session it is very much a case of responding to their needs. If they are already well warmed-up, then

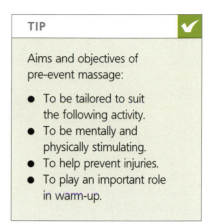

TIP

Aims and objectives of pre-event massage:

- To be tailored to suit the following activity.
- To be mentally and physically stimulating.
- To help prevent injuries.
- To play an important role in warm-up.

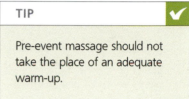

TIP

Pre-event massage should not take the place of an adequate warm-up.

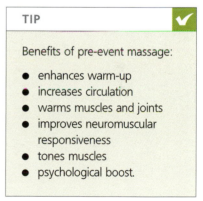

TIP

Benefits of pre-event massage:

- enhances warm-up
- increases circulation
- warms muscles and joints
- improves neuromuscular responsiveness
- tones muscles
- psychological boost.

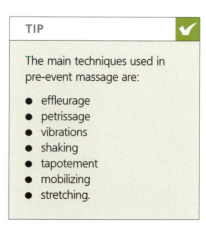

TIP

The main techniques used in pre-event massage are:

- effleurage
- petrissage
- vibrations
- shaking
- tapotement
- mobilizing
- stretching.

TIP

The techniques used in pre-event massage tend to be performed less deeply, more briskly and for a shorter duration than other massage applications.

TIP

The beneficial effects of pre-event massage are greatly increased when the therapist knows the sport, its physical requirements, the player, his mind-set, preferences and injury problems very well.

it might be best to focus on flexibility. If they are cold, then warming is a priority, and if they are nervous a little calming and relaxation may be in order.

Some athletes, and coaches, may prefer to use pre-event massage on the day before. This strategy can allow for greater recovery from training and offer relaxation the night before. It will also reduce the mild anxiety of worrying about preparation on the day and being able to access their pre-event treatment in a time schedule that really has its main emphasis on an active warm-up. In this instance, the pre-event treatment is more akin to the traditional post-event or maintenance massage, as the strenuous activity is not about to follow immediately.

All athletes have their own particular way of preparing for a good or, hopefully, excellent performance. Obviously, in the full scheme of things, with the instigation of cyclical and periodized training schedules, the well-prepared and coached athlete will probably have a whole season's activity planned out and each event or game they are involved in is part of that schedule. Therefore, it is considered ideal when the athlete is fit, focused and fully primed for each major event. Anything that assists their preparation, whether week to week as part of their normal training schedule or on the day is certainly going to be appreciated, and sports massage provides great assistance.

Athletes should avoid over-long or over-vigorous warm-ups, especially in hot conditions, because of the possibility of causing unnecessary fatigue, depleted energy stores or dehydration.

It is well known that, particularly in team sports such as football, rugby and hockey, where competitive seasons are long and arduous, players are not always 100 per cent fit. In such cases, where the player is deemed fit enough to play by the club's medical staff, coach, manager, sports therapist or him- or herself, then the sports masseur must work to improve injury problems, reducing excess muscle tension and soreness.

Other preparative considerations for the day of the competition include: ascertaining the location of organizer's office or desk; clarification of start times; ascertaining the location of treatment area, changing rooms and toilets; making sure all appropriate clothing and equipment is ready and perfectly functional; taping or strapping materials, if used, are available; adequate and appropriate foods and drinks are prepared; first aid kit is well stocked.

It is difficult to recommend one standard pre-event routine which would comprehensively prepare any athlete for their sport. As their skills and experiences grow, with particular sports and individual athletes, the sports therapist will be able to develop their own routines with specific techniques and approaches. In many instances, passive stretching, joint mobilizing and other methods such as electro-massage or heat will be incorporated into these treatments.

DURING-EVENT MASSAGE

Also referred to as inter-event massage, this is very much along the same lines as pre-event massage, but is possibly complicated by the occurrence of new injuries, aggravation of old injuries, muscle or mental fatigue or muscle cramp. Of course, care must be taken not to aggravate injuries with massage – cooling is the normal approach. By kneading, squeezing and pumping muscle groups, circulation is enhanced and fatigue reduced. Cramp is usually best attended to by gently stretching the affected muscle, possibly with a little massage as it settles down (direct compression techniques work well), and sometimes with ice treatment. There are instances when cramp will respond by moving the origin and insertion of the affected muscle closer together, or by use of the reciprocal inhibition technique (discussed in chapter 9). The athlete should also be offered water or appropriate sports drinks.

During-event massage may take place in the intervals at competitions, for example, at half-time or before extra-time in a football match, or between heats at an athletic meeting. It is about keeping the player in a prepared state, and reducing any discomfort or fatigue. There is also the opportunity of being able to offer psychological encouragement and fresh tactical ideas (obviously in conjunction with the manager or coach).

POST-EVENT MASSAGE

Post-event massage normally takes place half an hour to two hours after the activity, and it marks the end of a competition or heavy training session. It should not take the place of an adequate cool-down. Post-event massage is generally a relaxing treatment, somewhat deeper and more searching than pre-event, and therefore a useful hands-on diagnosis and identification for minor injuries, muscle spasm and pain. Certainly, it must be performed with care so as not to aggravate any acute problems, and the depth of techniques can be progressively increased as the superficial muscles relax. The intensity of delayed onset muscle soreness (DOMS), a particularly common problem affecting athletes, should be reduced when adequate massage therapy is applied soon after exertion. Players and athletes attending for post-event treatment may also require injury attention, which usually means either RICES or referral for medical assessment. The therapist should be alert to the signs and symptoms of hyperthermia (headache, nausea, chills, unsteadiness, pallor, sweating, thirst), heat stroke (confusion, incoherent speech, aggressiveness, weakness, reduced sweating) and hypothermia (shivering, euphoria, lethargy, disorientation), all of which could possibly be seen after an extreme event, especially in hot or cold conditions. These conditions are potentially serious and will require appropriate first aid, monitoring and possibly medical attention.

Typical techniques used in post-event treatments include: effleurage; petrissage; longitudinal and transverse stroking; shaking; vibration; and stretching. These are preferably performed with a slower frequency, as the emphasis is on relaxation and recovery, although if there are many people requiring attention, then techniques will need to be applied with more haste. Again, techniques are focused on the main working muscles and joints of the preceding activities. Of course, the whole body is used in any sport, but for most sports, there will usually be a particular emphasis on

TIP

Aims and objectives of post-event massage:

- to be tailored to suit the preceding activity
- to be mentally and physically relaxing
- to help return the body to normal pre-exercising state
- to help removal of metabolic waste products.

TIP

Post-event massage should not take the place of an adequate cool-down.

TIP

Benefits of post-event massage:

- enhances cool-down
- helps the athlete to recover from exertion
- helps the athlete to return to pre-exercising state
- helps to remove the accumulation of metabolic waste products
- helps to relax the athlete
- helps to identify and treat minor injury problems
- helps to reduce pain and DOMS
- maintains and develops the working relationship of the therapist and athlete
- psychological boost.

TIP

The main techniques used in post-event massage are:

- effleurage
- petrissage
- longitudinal and transverse stroking
- vibrations
- shaking
- stretching
- ice for areas of inflammation.

either lower body predominance (running, cycling, football), or upper body predominance (throwing, tennis, swimming). In the ideal situation all major muscles are attended to.

At the sports event, for various obvious reasons, the therapist will prefer the athlete to be clean and showered. However, this is not always possible and, as ever, the therapist must work around the situation and make the best of it. At least, the athlete should be asked to remove dirty, wet or muddy clothing, and also to wipe dirt from their body. Oils, creams and lotions are generally preferred for post-event massage, but because sometimes this is not appropriate, the therapist must be able to work through clothes or towels.

Remember, if the athlete is not known to you, to perform at least a verbal consultation with them prior to treatment, and during the session, encourage feedback from them. It may be wise to ask athletes attending for event-massage to fill in a basic information and consent form while they wait for treatment.

Basic post-event massage routines

Obviously, as previously discussed, each sports massage is different, and the objectives vary each time, especially for different sports and whether there are injuries to contend with. A massage routine is really only a guide, or basic structure, upon which specific adaptations can be applied. In the case of post-event massage, always keep the fundamental principles in mind, work with the athlete and state of body that is being presented to you, and try not to do harm. The following routines are merely suggestions, and as skills and experiences grow the therapist will develop their own routines and add additional techniques and approaches. In many instances passive stretching and other methods will be incorporated into these treatments.

BASIC POST-EVENT SPORTS MASSAGE ROUTINE

Legs (prone lying)

1 Superficial effleurage to whole of one leg
2 Deep effleurage to thigh
3 Palmer kneading to thigh
4 Broadening to thigh
5 Wringing/picking-up to thigh
6 Rolling to thigh
7 Transverse stroking to thigh
8 Longitudinal stroking to thigh
9 Effleurage to thigh
10 Vibrations to thigh
11 Effleurage to lower leg

12 Palmer kneading to lower leg
13 Broadening to calf muscles
14 Wringing/picking-up to calf muscles
15 Rolling to calf muscles
16 Transverse stroking to calf muscles
17 Longitudinal stroking to calf muscles
18 Thumb kneading around Achilles tendon and ankle
19 Effleurage to lower leg
20 Vibrations to lower leg
21 Effleurage to whole leg
22 Shaking to whole leg
Repeat all techniques for other leg

Back, shoulder and arms (prone lying)

1 Superficial effleurage (from lower back, up between scapulae and out over shoulders)
2 Deeper effleurage (as above, or reinforced hands one side at a time)
3 Palmer kneading (up the back)
4 Picking-up and rolling to trapezius (at top of one shoulder)
5 Wringing and rolling (down and up one side of torso)
6 Thumb kneading (up and down erector spinae group)
7 Effleurage to whole of back
8 Thumb and finger stroking and kneading over and around scapula
9 Thumb and finger stroking to mid-trapezius and rhomboids
10 Picking-up to deltoids
11 Reinforced small and large circle kneading over and around scapula
12 Repeat 4, 5, 8, 9, 10 and 11 on other side of back
13 Figure of eight reinforced kneading of both shoulders
14 Effleurage to whole of back
15 Stroking vibrations to back
16 Effleurage (single-handed) to upper arm
17 Picking-up (single-handed) to triceps
18 Broadening to triceps
19 Longitudinal and transverse stroking to triceps
20 Picking-up (single-handed) to biceps
21 Effleurage (single-handed) to forearm
22 Picking-up (single-handed) to wrist extensors
23 Longitudinal stroking to wrist extensors
24 Effleurage (single-handed) to whole arm

Legs (supine lying)

1 Superficial effleurage to whole of one leg
2 Deeper effleurage to thigh
3 Palmer kneading to thigh
4 Broadening to thigh
5 Wringing/picking-up to thigh
6 Rolling to thigh
7 Thumb and finger kneading around knee joint
8 Transverse stroking to thigh
9 Longitudinal stroking to thigh
10 Deeper effleurage to top, sides and undersides of thigh (knee flexed)
11 Deep reinforced stroking to hamstrings (knee flexed)
12 Kneading to calf (knee flexed)
13 Vibrations to thigh
14 Kneading to dorsiflexors
15 Longitudinal stroking to dorsiflexors
16 Thumb and finger kneading around ankle
17 Kneading of dorsal and plantar aspect of foot
18 Effleurage to dorsal and plantar aspect of foot
19 Effleurage to whole leg
20 Shaking to whole leg

Repeat techniques for other leg

Neck, chest, shoulders, arms and hands (supine lying)

1 Effleurage across upper chest, out to each shoulder simultaneously, and up to occiput (standing at head of couch)
2 Picking-up to left and right pectoral regions
3 Thumb and finger kneading to left and right upper pectoral regions
4 Effleurage (as in 1)
5 Finger kneading (single-handed) to left and right paraspinal muscles of neck
6 Thumb and finger kneading to left and right upper trapezius
7 Longitudinal thumb stroking to both left and right upper trapezius
8 Effleurage (single-handed) from occiput down towards both left and right shoulders
9 Effleurage (single-handed) to whole arm
10 Picking-up (single-handed) to biceps
11 Broadening to biceps
12 Longitudinal and transverse stroking to biceps
13 Deep effleurage to upper arm
14 Kneading (single-handed) to wrist extensors
15 Kneading (single-handed) to wrist flexors
16 Longitudinal stroking to wrist flexors
17 Thumb kneading to palmer and dorsal surfaces of wrist, hand and fingers
18 Deep effleurage to forearm
19 Shaking to whole arm
20 Effleurage to whole arm
21 Repeat 9–20 for contra-lateral arm and hand

MAINTENANCE SPORTS MASSAGE

TIP

Aims and objectives of maintenance massage:

- to help in the prevention and detection of injuries
- to aid recovery from intensive training
- to improve flexibility, mobility, tone and responsiveness of the body
- to help improve individual body awareness.

Maintenance massage is what the athletes often like the best. It is usually something to look forward to, is performed generally in a one to one, relaxed environment, and attends to the athletes' current concerns, needs, and aches and pains. Typically, it is a time to get to know your client better and to offer them good treatment and advice. The treatment session may take the form of a fairly standard routine, covering all major muscle groups, or it may focus on particular body regions such as the legs or back.

The techniques used in maintenance massage include: effleurage, petrissage, tapotement; frictions; vibrations; longitudinal and transverse stroking; passive mobilizing and stretching; soft tissue release; muscle energy techniques; thermal therapy; electro-massage.

Clearly, sports massage, or sports therapy, whether dubbed pre- or post-, maintenance or remedial, is all about helping the athlete. The variations of approach are blurred by what is actually presented to the therapist each time, and as such, a maintenance session can easily become a remedial session.

REMEDIAL APPROACHES TO TREATMENT

TIP

Aims and objectives of remedial massage:

- to help treat and rehabilitate soft-tissue injuries
- to promote the body's own healing mechanisms
- to help prevent injury recurrence
- to help improve muscle and postural imbalance and biomechanical problems.

The practice of remedial massage therapy, to benefit, normalize or improve musculo-skeletal and other problems involves the diligent use of all the techniques previously discussed, plus, when applicable, those covered in the next three chapters (deep frictions; passive stretching; soft-tissue release; neuromuscular techniques; positional release techniques; muscle energy techniques; electro-massage). For sports injuries in particular, the sports therapist has a fine collection of massage and related techniques to add to their other main skill in providing remedial exercises.

An effective process for treating a new injury, over as short a period of time as is possible, demands:

- A good initial consultation and assessment, which identifies the key problems, forms the early objectives and provides the athlete with reassurance.
- A sensible first treatment that does not aggravate the injury, but does offer useful advice.
- A responsible follow-up session, where the progress is assessed, objectives reviewed, and the treatment and recommendations modified to suit.
- A treatment, management and home-care strategy that is understood, monitored and progressively developed by all concerned.

When treating injury or other physical problems, the therapist has to develop a strategy to achieve initial objectives, which are based on the consultation and assessment findings. First of all the therapist must decide on which muscles, joints or other tissues are in need of remedial attention. The next step is to select the best techniques and equipment, and to provide the appropriate intensity of treatment, being very aware that inappropriate techniques and intensities can easily worsen any condition.

As a general guide, acute injuries require careful anti-inflammatory, non-aggravating approaches, which encourage pain relief and control swelling. At this stage, it is often indicated to apply cold therapy and support strapping. It can also be useful to gently massage above the site of injury to encourage lymphatic drainage. Particularly in the acute stage, the client will benefit from confident treatment and reassurance.

In sub-acute situations the treatment protocol is dictated by the severity of the injury, and whether inflammation (redness, swelling, warmth, pain, impaired function) has subsided. If signs of inflammation are still present, it is usually best to continue cooling, avoid aggravating the affected region and apply safe, passive, pain-free mobility exercise, combined with light lymphatic drainage massage around and above the injury site, remembering that, with moderate and severe injuries, the cellular proliferation phase of healing can sometimes last for as long as a few weeks. Electrical modalities, such as ultrasound, may be tentatively employed during this phase. As signs and symptoms subside, the treatments intensify.

The later stages of injury treatment, during the remodelling and maturation phase of healing, become more aggressive, with heat, deep localized frictions, stretching techniques, electrical modalities and remedial exercises commonly used in conjunction. These methods are discussed further in the following chapters.

AFTER-CARE

It is an important part of the sports therapist's work to provide useful advice and recommendations for their customers. The after-care that a client receives directly relates to the presenting circumstances. Factors influencing the after-care and advice offered, include: whether the client is new; whether it is the first time they have received sports therapy; whether they are being treated for an injury, postural, biomechanical or other problem; whether they are experienced with treatment and exercise.

Initial basic advice immediately following a therapy session might be to drink some water, take further rest, eat light and avoid alcohol. It is important to explain to your client, especially if they have received remedial massage techniques, that there can sometimes be a minor degree of muscle soreness or stiffness in the tissues for 24–36 hours after the treatment.

If there are any particular objectives to work towards, which there usually are, such as the rehabilitation of an injury or general improvements in flexibility, then it is usual to make further recommendations. Whatever is advised, the therapist should make sure it is the right advice, and explain everything clearly, and then clarify the client's understanding. Clients always appreciate written (or word processed) notes detailing the particular recommendations.

After-care recommendations may include:

- further treatment or referral
- in the case of injury, avoiding all aggravating activities (requires discussion)
- support, taping or orthotics (requires explanation)
- self-massage (requires demonstration)
- cold or heat applications (requires explanation)
- specific mobility, flexibility, strength, endurance, stability and proprioceptive exercises (requires demonstration and coaching)
- in the case of the inexperienced exerciser, the importance of adequate hydration, warm-up, cool-down and appropriate intensity, duration and frequency of exercise (requires explanation)
- adaptations to training routines (requires discussion)
- alternative exercise programmes (requires discussion)
- adaptations to existing exercise equipment or purchase of new (requires explanation and suggestions)
- relaxation techniques (requires explanation, demonstration and coaching)
- dietary adaptations (requires discussion and explanation).

CHAPTER SUMMARY

Massage is a traditional, relatively low-risk, holistic therapy that works to support the body's own healing processes. Sports massage is the systematic manual manipulation of the soft-tissues, designed to produce specific responses in the athlete, and ultimately improve performance. Remedial massage incorporates a selection of well-documented manual techniques, which have been developed to improve certain conditions. There are very many applications and benefits of sports and remedial massage.

It is very important for the sports therapist to create the right environment for practice. Knowledge of what constitutes a safe and effective working posture is important. Being a skilled sports or remedial masseur or masseuse demands an ability to provide techniques with specific degrees of force, intensity, control, direction, leverage, frequency and duration, relative to the individual's condition and the objectives of the treatment. It is important to understand the classifications, effects, benefits, indications and contra-indications of each technique. Providing appropriate after-care is also an important part of the sports therapist's service.

Knowledge Review

1 What is the difference between sports massage and remedial massage?

2 List ten potential benefits of sports massage.

3 Describe the main safety issues relating to the client, the therapist and the environment in the practice of sports massage.

4 What are the advantages and disadvantages of using: (i) no lubricant; (ii) massage oil; (iii) massage lotion; (iv) talcum powder?

5 Describe the following techniques: (i) wringing, (ii) muscle rolling, (iii) hacking, (iv) longitudinal stroking, (v) connective tissue manipulation, (vi) traction, (vii) manual lymphatic drainage.

6 In what ways can sports or remedial massage treatments be made more individualized?

7 Explain how pre-event massage differs from post-event massage.

8 Why is after-care important?

WEBSITE

Visit the companion website at www.thomsonlearning.co.uk/ healthandfitness/ward where you will find the answers to these questions for you to check your progress through the book.

chapter 8

PASSIVE STRETCH AND FRICTION TECHNIQUES

Learning Objectives

After reading this chapter you should be able to:

- understand basic principles of stretching and flexibility
- provide safe and effective passive stretching for clients
- recognize the purpose, objectives and implications of providing deep soft-tissue techniques
- incorporate deep friction massage and soft-tissue release techniques into remedial treatments

Once the sports therapist has grasped the basic theoretical principles of sports massage and gained some practical hands-on experience in providing it for clients, the next logical step is to be able to introduce passive stretching and remedial friction massage techniques into their treatments.

Stretching has always been a part of any well-rounded fitness or athletic training programme. It has also always been a major component in any musculo-skeletal rehabilitation programme. However, not everyone, whether athlete or not, stretches regularly, properly, comprehensively or remedially. It is a natural instinct to have a little stretch when feeling tired, having just awoken or when feeling a bit stiff, but for many people stretching does not go beyond that. We know that massage, especially sports massage, helps to stretch the soft-tissues, and this is one of the main reasons for recipients finding benefit in such treatments. Therefore, it makes sense to enhance the potential benefits of massage, in treatment, with the application of additional specific stretching techniques.

Deep friction techniques are basically very localized stretching techniques that are applied, when indicated, to break up adhesions and help strengthen the scar tissue that forms after injury. Deep friction techniques are sometimes described as being the most remedial of massage techniques, but this is really to underestimate the potential effectiveness of any of the other advanced massage-related techniques. The soft-tissue release (STR) method of treatment, also discussed in this chapter, is simply a combination of passive (or active) stretching with a deep frictional component.

As the sports therapist begins to confidently incorporate passive stretching, joint mobilizations (see previous chapter) and deep specific remedial work into their treatments, then their practice really starts to open up. Classic hands-on massage, effleurage, kneading and tapotement will always be fundamental and useful, but if the therapist is able to move, position and support the client specifically for a range of indications and objectives, and from there is able to provide further advanced dynamic treatment techniques, then the client receives more effective therapy and gains increased confidence in the therapist, and the therapist gains greater satisfaction from working with a wider variety of techniques and from being able to offer the client a better treatment. In essence, as the therapist gathers experience and confidence, and increases their therapeutic repertoire, then their work basically becomes more exacting, more exciting and more interesting.

PRINCIPLES OF STRETCHING AND FLEXIBILITY

To understand stretching is to understand mobility, flexibility, muscle positions, indications for stretching, types of stretching, safety issues relating to stretching, and methods of making stretching specific for each application.

Mobility and flexibility

Mobility and flexibility may be defined in several ways. They may be taken to mean the same thing, and used interchangeably, or they may be used in subtly different contexts. The measurable amount of movement available at a joint, or range of joints, can be described as the individual's mobility. Mobility may also be seen as the individual's functional ability to move, either specific joints or generally. Mobility is affected by the posture and biomechanics of the person, by their injuries, body type, pathologies, fitness regimes, age, occupation and lifestyle in general. Therefore, mobility tends to be associated with the relative quality of movement at a joint or series of joints. Flexibility, too, may be defined by the range of motion an individual demonstrates at a joint or joints, but it may also be used to describe the ease of adaptation into the altered (stretched) position, and therefore it is often more associated with the amount or quality of extensibility in the soft-tissues (muscles, tendons, fascia, skin), which obviously also relates to the overall range of movement. When describing aspects and concepts in mobility and flexibility, it can be useful to apply other related terms such as suppleness, pliability, extensibility, elasticity, malleability or plasticity. Correspondingly, terms such as stiffness, rigidity, immobility, restriction, tightness or tension relate to situations where mobility or flexibility is impaired.

The degree of flexibility an individual has is gauged against generally accepted norms and against what could be realistically expected for the individual concerned, given their age, state of health or fitness. Ranges of movement, as discussed in chapter 4, may be measured with the aid of a goniometer or tape measure, or by observation. Prior to any treatment, it is important to assess all appropriate active-functional and passive movements. Similarly, the restriction barrier and quality of end-feel apparent in the tissues, during observed and palpated movements, should also be ascertained before any particular therapeutic plans are formulated.

Muscle, postural and biomechanical balance is always something to work towards. Being flexible in one region of the body, does not mean that an individual will be flexible in all other areas. A strong indication for remedial massage and flexibility work is the improvement of muscle balance.

Without regular stretching, muscles and joints tend to experience restricted flexibility. Restricted flexibility and muscle elasticity leaves the individual vulnerable to injury. When a muscle is called upon to stretch suddenly (dynamic functional stretch) in a game or any other incident, if it is unable to reach the necessary length, then something has to give, and it will be the structure of the muscle that will tear. Although well recommended by most experts, stretching is still often neglected or paid insufficient attention by exercisers.

Factors affecting flexibility:

- type of joint (the specificity of flexibility)
- elasticity of muscle, tendon, fascia, skin and ligament
- muscle mass
- body fat
- body type
- ability to relax
- body temperature
- age
- sex
- injuries and pathologies
- postural and biomechanical deviations
- environmental temperature
- time of day
- fitness level
- normal fitness training routine undertaken
- occupation.

Just as having poor flexibility has potential consequences for restricting functional abilities and increasing the individual's vulnerability to soft-tissue injuries, the situation of increased flexibility, or hyperflexibility (hypermobility), presents its own set of potential problems. A hypermobile joint is one that demonstrates an excessive range of motion or laxity. This situation can arise due to injury, classically to the major supporting

TIP

For ideal health and fitness, the muscles of the body are strong, supple, responsive, resistant to fatigue and in balance with one another.

ligaments of a joint. Hypermobility can also be a congenital or pathological problem, or arise as a result of inappropriate training and activities. It may affect just one region, or be prevalent throughout the musculo-skeletal system. Either way, hypermobility is usually attended to with strength rather than flexibility training, and perhaps support to affected joints during potentially aggravating activities.

Indications for stretching:

- to loosen tight muscles
- to help mobilize restricted joints
- to improve postural imbalance
- to help improve biomechanical efficiency
- to improve relaxation of the muscles
- to improve circulation
- to improve neuromuscular responsiveness
- to help prevent injuries as part of a warm-up
- to help improve performance
- to help improve recovery from training and competition
- to help reduce exercise-related muscle soreness
- to help treat soft-tissue injuries, adhesions and scar tissue
- to improve flexibility
- to develop body awareness
- to feel good.

> **TIP**
>
> Do not be tempted to apply or recommend stretching in the case of an acute strain or sprain. The injury requires a short period of rest with no aggravating activities, and possibly RICES and other measures.

Yoga and the martial arts

Stretching has long been a component of health-improving regimes. One of the oldest and still most popular exercise systems is yoga (meaning union). Yoga is an ancient Asian discipline which, alongside spiritual purification, meditation and union with the divine, teaches breathing (*pranayama*), stretching and postures (*asanas*) for their health-giving benefits. Hatha yoga, astanga (power) yoga and other variants are now taught daily at many fitness centres in the Western world. Similarly, the various **martial arts**, which originally developed because of the importance the Eastern cultures placed upon the need to live long, and attack or defend, are now deeply integrated into all cultures, and for a variety of benefits. The physical crux of both yoga and the martial arts has always been strength, flexibility, agility, co-ordination, balance and endurance, and not that much has changed since these systems were originally developed.

Stretching is a big subject. The fitness, physiotherapy and sports medicine fraternities have for a long time fiercely recommended stretching as a vital ingredient of exercise regimes, especially for injury prevention and rehabilitation. As the business of fitness has grown, so too have the debates that follow. Refining the specific applications of exercise is how the scientific research must help the industry. We must continue to welcome new findings, challenge older ideas, perceptions and practices, thoroughly investigate newer procedures and successfully integrate those strategies that are conclusively proven to be useful. There are many ways in which the different approaches, techniques and indications of stretching, for example, lend themselves to the research process. Individuals and groups can usefully add to the existing knowledge base by focusing their attentions into such areas as the effectiveness of stretching in the prevention of sports injuries or by examining the advantages of one stretching approach, say passive developmental, over a combined muscle energy technique (MET) and massage approach, for example. Well-organized clinical trials help to improve what the sports therapist can offer in terms of best treatment approaches and best advice for clients.

Stretching, therefore, has a selection of practical approaches. It will always either be active or passive, or, in the case of muscle energy techniques, involve a resistance component. Stretching may also be classified as being dynamic, ballistic or static. There are preparatory stretches, developmental stretches, maintenance stretches and remedial stretches. The therapist also needs to have a working understanding of the body's stretch reflexes.

Active stretching

Active stretching is performed solely by the athlete. A more specific explanation would make the distinction that active stretching involves the contraction of agonist and synergist muscles in order to cause a stretching of their antagonistic muscles. The contraction of the agonist muscles, in this instance, helps to automatically relax the stretching antagonistic muscles by way of reciprocal inhibition, which is discussed later in the text.

Passive stretching

Passive stretching, also referred to as relaxed stretching, is typically taken to describe techniques performed for the athlete by the therapist or partner, and where there is little or no effort on the part of the athlete, and they relax. Instances where the athlete uses certain apparatus, such as a stretch station in a gym, or where they assume a position of stretch by holding the body part themselves, are also considered as passive stretching. Passive stretching can often reach beyond the range achievable actively.

Dynamic flexibility

Dynamic flexibility is that range of movement available during normal active movements. In an exercise context, dynamic stretching, also referred to as mobility training, is about rhythmically moving muscles and joints through their easy ranges, and gradually increasing their available ranges, without force. Dynamic stretching is used as part of warm-up and preparation for sports, and tends to be repetitive in its performance, for example, shoulder shrugs and circles, and elbow and knee bends.

Static stretching

Static stretching is simply stretching and then holding the position, whether actively or passively performed. Different, therefore, from dynamic stretching.

Ballistic stretching

Ballistic stretching is also dynamic and rhythmic, but tends to be more aggressive, involving a bouncing or rebounding momentum into stretch positions. Because muscles are exposed to a rather sudden stretching during ballistic work, they tend to tighten at the end of the range because the stretch reflex is activated. The stretch (or myotatic) reflex is an automatic and basic protective mechanism that causes a muscle to tighten (contract) when it is placed rapidly into a position of stretch. During a sudden stretch, muscle spindles, specialized sensory receptors within the muscle fibres, are also stretched. These then instantly transmit signals to the spinal cord, where a motor impulse is conveyed back to the affected muscle group, initiating a contraction. The same events occur during deep tendon reflex testing, such as the patellar tap, where the quadriceps contract immediately following the sudden stretch produced by the brisk tapping of the patella tendon. This mechanism helps to reduce the possibility of injury during sudden overstretching, but in terms of trying to develop flexibility, the ballistic approach is not good, and actually has injury implications in itself, often leading to microtrauma in the affected muscles. Ballistic stretching is still often used in preparation for such activities as martial arts classes, dance classes and football or rugby matches, and may well help prepare for the dynamic nature of those types of activities, but ballistic methods are generally considered outmoded for the majority of purposes. Certainly, it is now rare to see anyone bouncing up and down to try to touch their toes.

Preparatory stretching

Preparatory stretching is the type of stretching that is performed before full activity is undertaken. It is customary to warm-up (raise heart rate, body and working muscle temperature and breathing rate) and gently mobilize before preparatory stretches are employed. There has been research published in recent years suggesting that preparatory stretching is not necessarily the great injury preventer that the fitness industry once claimed. That said, most research evidence is relative to the circumstances in which it is contextually placed, and therefore such findings should be further investigated and challenged. Most coaches and athletes would probably choose not to discard preparatory stretching. It is still always seen at training sessions and major sporting events, and is a big part of the overall preparation process. Preparatory stretching typically attends to the main muscles used in the sport. The stretches are commonly held for around 10–15 seconds at a time, and often not to the extreme ranges of motion or to the point of pain. Because competitive athletes are often not absolutely 100 per cent fit (minor injuries, muscle soreness, etc.), preparatory stretching can help to reduce discomfort and tightness before strenuous activity is performed. For the therapist, the pre-event massage treatment will normally incorporate passive preparatory stretching. An active pre-event warm-up is the best practice for injury prevention, and muscles will be more amenable to stretching after this.

Developmental stretching

Developmental or relaxation stretching is used to relax muscles, decrease tightness and increase the normal extensibility. This type of stretching is performed slowly: the stretch is eased into and developed as relaxation occurs, and typically lasts for around 15–30 seconds at a time, often repeated a few times during one session for any problematic regions. It is normal to expect gradual improvements over a period of weeks for tightened muscles.

Maintenance stretching

Maintenance stretching is more of a routine approach to helping keep muscles and joints in good working order and helping recovery from hard training. It is common to stretch all major muscle groups during a maintenance session, but with extra emphasis on the main muscles used in particular sports. Maintenance stretches are typically held for 15–30 seconds.

Remedial stretching

Remedial stretching is a particularly important skill area for the sports therapist. Re-educating muscle fibres and joints, treating injuries, addressing muscle tightness and imbalance are common clinical objectives. Remedial stretching is typically combined with many of the massage techniques, soft-tissue release, neuromuscular and muscle energy techniques and thermal therapies. There are some practitioners who will employ pre-heat, massage, an active warming-up of the tissues, or even ice prior to providing stretching techniques. Heat increases circulation and can help to relieve discomfort and relax muscles. Massage has many potential benefits, and can prepare the muscles well for stretching. Ice helps to reduce pain (and therefore the mild discomfort of a developmental stretch), so can be a useful application both immediately before and during passive stretching. The remedial approach may demand that more concentrated treatments are needed, which can mean techniques being repeated and returned to during a session, stretches possibly held for longer periods, and an increased frequency of treatments, until the problems have resolved or improved.

During a stretch the particular angle of the involved joint is altered, typically either reduced (flexed) or increased (extended). Then deep down, as the muscles stretch, the bundles (fascicles) of myofibrils (muscle fibres) are elongated, and the degree of overlap at the myofilaments (contractile proteins, actin and myosin) in the sarcomeres (segments containing the myofilaments) decreases. Typically, as all sarcomeres inside the affected bundles reach their maximal length, further stretching causes the connective tissues around and within the area also to be lengthened, including areas of **fibrosis** or scar tissue – therefore this can help to reorganize and improve the functional capacity of such tissues. Remember that, during stretching, because of the leverage required, it is more likely that muscles are lengthened (stretched longitudinally) than broadened.

The therapist should try to develop practical skill in being able to offer a selection of passive stretching positions for their clients, some of whom will not be able to assume all positions comfortably, and therefore variations and alternatives will be required. This will improve their ability to be able to respond to most presenting problems. Also, the therapist must think about how they will support the client during the flexibility work, especially if they are expecting to hold the position of stretch for more than a few seconds. The way in which the stretch is to be localized to the affected tissues also needs consideration. There is little point in offering generalized stretching when specific adaptation is required.

To localize passive stretches involves several factors:

- identifying the problematic tissues
- positioning the client appropriately
- stabilizing the closely associated regions to restrict or control unwanted movements
- stretching slowly and carefully
- observing client response
- gaining feedback from the client during the movements.

Fine-tuning a stretch (incorporating minor adjustments into the movement), such as adding a touch of rotation or abduction into a flexion movement can also help to localize the stretch into the tissues requiring it.

Perhaps the best way of avoiding causing problems with passive stretching is to have a good **awareness**, based on the assessment of the expected range of motion, keeping an awareness of what structures are involved and related to the movement, and providing all stretches slowly, carefully with feedback.

To provide safe passive stretching:

- assess the region first
- discuss the objectives with the client
- explain the procedures to the client
- encourage relaxation and smooth breathing
- do not stretch acute injury or inflammation
- do not routinely stretch hypermobile joints
- localize and if appropriate stabilize the region to be stretched
- be aware of the normal range of movement expected for each individual client
- begin within safe and easy ranges of movement
- keep mind on job and observe client response
- gain feedback from client during stretch

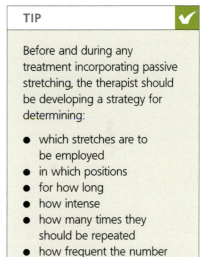

TIP ✔

Before and during any treatment incorporating passive stretching, the therapist should be developing a strategy for determining:

- which stretches are to be employed
- in which positions
- for how long
- how intense
- how many times they should be repeated
- how frequent the number of sessions.

- take care to use correct positioning, leverage and force
- take care not to place inappropriate stresses on joints, ligaments, tendons, intervertebral discs or meniscal cartilages
- remember that cold muscles respond less well to stretching
- work with the basic principles of intensity, duration and frequency in mind
- do not cause undue pain during stretching (mild discomfort can be acceptable for more athletic clients)
- do not overstretch.

Always bear in mind that flexibility is an individual thing. Some people are more flexible than others for no apparent reason. Stretching is not a competition either. Flexibility is important, and some regular stretching helps to maintain it, and remedial stretching is important when it is needed.

Common Passive Stretching Techniques

The following collection of stretches are all viable for inclusion into general and remedial massage treatments. The list is far from comprehensive, as there are many other subtle variations to be discovered and practised.

Cervical region

- Neck flexor stretch, supine. Clavicle and ribs should be stabilized. Main affected muscles are sternocleidomastoid and scalenes. It can help to have the client's head off the end of the couch, supported by the therapist's hand. Slight rotation and/or lateral flexion can be employed.
- Neck extensor stretch, supine. Shoulders should be stabilized. Main affected muscles are trapezius, splenius, levator scapulae and upper erector spinae.
- Neck rotator stretch, supine. Main affected muscles are trapezius, sternocleidomastoid, scalenes and deep rotators.

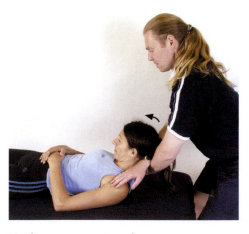

Neck extensor stretch

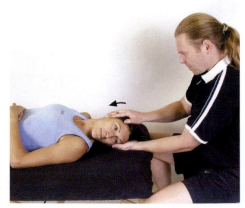

Neck rotator stretch

- Neck lateral flexor stretch, supine. Shoulder should be stabilized. Main affected muscles are trapezius and scalenes.

Thoracic and lumbar region

- Trunk extensor stretch, supine. Put feet together, and flex knees, hips and trunk (taking knees towards chest). Main affected muscles are the lower erector spinae group, quadratus lumborum and latissimus dorsi.
- Trunk extensor stretch, side-lying.
- Trunk rotator stretch, supine. Upper torso stabilized. Main affected muscles are lower erector spinae, obliques, and deep rotators.
- Trunk lateral flexor stretch, side-lying. Client stabilizes themselves with arm overhead. Main affected muscles are quadratus lumborum, obliques, ipsilateral erector spinae and latissimus dorsi.

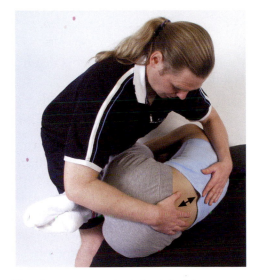

Trunk extensor stretch, side-lying

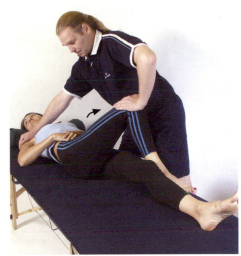

Trunk rotator stretch

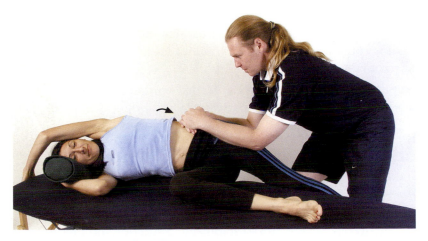

Trunk lateral flexor stretch

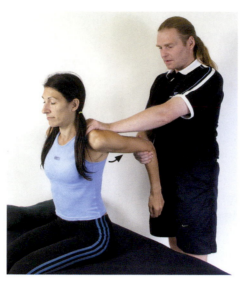 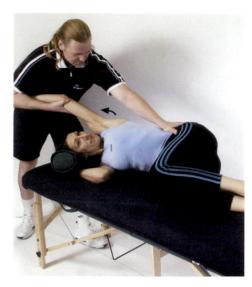
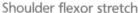

Shoulder flexor stretch   Shoulder adductor stretch

Shoulder region

- Shoulder flexor stretch, seated. Upper torso stabilized. Shoulder is taken into extension. Main affected muscle is anterior deltoid.
- Shoulder extensor stretch, supine. Abduct arm to 90°, and horizontally adduct across the chest. Main affected muscle is posterior deltoid.
- Shoulder abductor/lateral rotator stretch, seated or prone. The arm is taken into medial rotation, elbow flexed, and eased into a stretch behind the lower back. Main affected muscles are anterior and medial deltoids, supraspinatus, infraspinatus and teres minor.
- Shoulder adductor stretch, side lying. Pelvis stabilized. Arm abducted over head. Main affected muscles are latissimus dorsi and teres major.
- Shoulder medial rotator stretch, supine. Shoulder stabilized. Arm is abducted to 90°, elbow flexed, and taken into lateral rotation. Main affected muscles are subscapularis and teres major.
- Shoulder lateral rotator stretch, supine. Shoulder stabilized. Arm is abducted to 90°, elbow flexed, and taken into medial rotation. Main affected muscles are infraspinatus and teres minor.
- Shoulder horizontal adductor stretch, supine. Main affected muscles are pectoralis major and anterior deltoids. Shoulder is abducted to 90–150°, and then horizontally abducted.
- Shoulder scapula retractor stretch, prone. Medial border of scapula is gently lifted and abducted. Main affected muscles are rhomboids and trapezius.

Elbow region

- Elbow flexor stretch, seated. Upper torso stabilized. Shoulder and elbow are taken into extension. Main affected muscles are biceps and brachialis.
- Elbow extensor stretch, seated. Torso stabilized. Shoulder and elbow are taken into flexion. Main affected muscle is triceps.

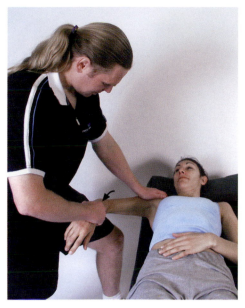

Shoulder lateral rotator stretch

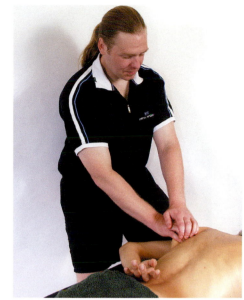

Scapula retractor stretch

Forearm and wrist region

- Wrist flexor stretch, seated. Forearm supinated and taken into extension. Main affected muscles are the common wrist and hand flexor group.

- Wrist extensor stretch, seated. Forearm pronated and taken into flexion (loosely clenching the fist can increase the intensity). Main affected muscles are the common wrist and hand extensor group.

Hip region

- Hip flexor stretch, supine. Contra-lateral limb taken into hip and knee flexion, and stabilized. Hip taken into extension. Main affected muscles are psoas and iliacus.

- Hip flexor stretch, prone. Sacral region stabilized. Hip lifted up into extension. Main affected muscles are psoas and iliacus.

- Hip flexor and knee extensor stretch, supine. Contra-lateral limb stabilized. Similar to hip flexor stretch, but knee is additionally taken into flexion. Main affected muscles are psoas, iliacus and rectus femoris.

- Hip extensor stretch, supine. Hip and knee taken into flexion. Main affected muscle is gluteus maximus.

- Hip abductor stretch, side-lying 1. Contra-lateral limb is uppermost and fully flexed. Stabilize hip at iliac crest. Lift limb from underneath the knee (flexed) into adduction. Main affected muscles are gluteals and tensor fascia lata.

- Hip abductor stretch, side-lying 2. Contra-lateral limb is lowest and fully flexed. Compression over iliac crest stabilizes hip, and limb is taken into adduction. Main affected muscles are gluteus medius and minimus, and tensor fascia lata.

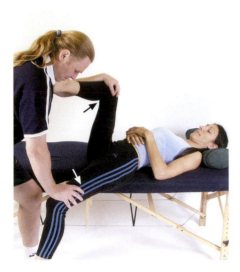

Hip flexor stretch

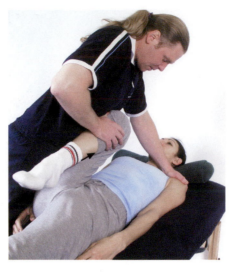

Hip extensor stretch

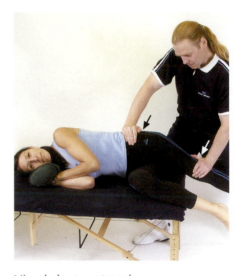

Hip abductor stretch

- Adductor stretch, supine. Knee flexed. Stabilize contra-lateral hip at anterior superior iliac spine (ASIS). Knee is flexed, and hip is taken into abduction. Main affected muscles are pectineus, adductor brevis, magnus and longus.

- Hip adductor stretch, supine. Knee is extended, and hip is taken into abduction. Main affected muscles are gracilis, adductor magnus and longus.

- Hip lateral rotator stretch, supine. Contra-lateral leg crossed over. Stabilize ipsilateral hip at ASIS. Take hip into adduction and medial rotation. Main affected muscles are piriformis, quadratus femoris and gluteus maximus.

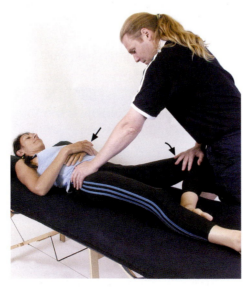

Hip adductor stretch

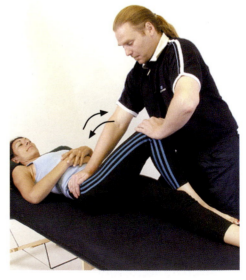

Hip lateral rotator stretch

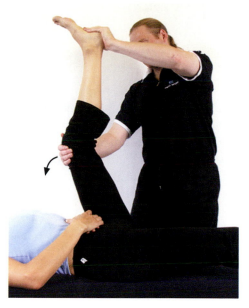

Knee flexor stretch

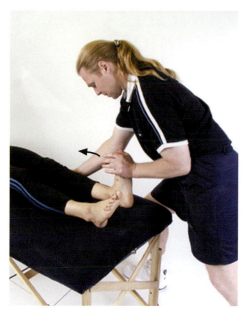

Ankle plantarflexor stretch

Knee region

- Knee flexor stretch 1, supine. Knee partially flexed and supported, and hip taken to 100–120° of flexion. Main affected muscles are proximal hamstrings.
- Knee flexor stretch 2, supine. Knee extended and supported, and hip taken to around 90° of flexion. Main affected muscles are distal hamstrings and proximal gastrocnemius.
- Knee extensor stretch, prone. Sacral region stabilized. Knee taken into flexion. Main affected muscles are quadriceps. The ankle dorsiflexors can also be treated at the same time.

Ankle and foot region

- Ankle dorsiflexor stretch, supine. Knee extended, and ankle taken into plantarflexion. Main affected muscles are tibialis anterior and extensor digitorum longus.
- Ankle plantarflexor stretch, supine. Knee extended, and ankle taken into dorsiflexion. Main affected muscle is gastrocnemius.
- Ankle plantarflexor stretch, supine. Knee partially flexed and supported. Ankle taken into dorsiflexion. Main affected muscles are soleus and flexor digitorum longus.

The way in which stretching can be combined with deep friction techniques is described later in this chapter, and other active approaches to flexibility improvement are discussed in chapter 12.

TIP

Golden rules for passive stretching:

- discuss objectives
- explain procedure to client
- take care to position the client
- be aware of alternative positions for specific circumstances
- be aware of normal and expected ranges of movement
- take care to support and stabilize client
- encourage relaxation
- obtain feedback
- work within the limits of discomfort
- remember that improvements and gains are achieved by gradual and regular treatment and training.

PRINCIPLES OF DEEP FRICTION TECHNIQUES

Many of the techniques available to the sports and remedial massage therapist are closely related and often share similar explanations and categorizations, theoretical benefits and practical approaches. Thumb and finger *frictions*, for example, are sometimes categorized as being a sort of deeper type of petrissage, while *deep friction*, although sharing similarities with deep transverse stroking and connective tissue manipulation (CTM) techniques, are usually described in a class on their own. Frictions, therefore, as opposed to deep friction, are relatively deep, circular, transverse or longitudinal, short sweeping type movements normally applied with thumbs or fingers which are used to help loosen tight tissues and increase the circulation. This approach is often used on the paraspinal muscles and anywhere else where particular muscle or fascial tension is evident.

Deep friction is a classic manual therapy technique championed by sports therapists, bodyworkers, physiotherapists and even orthopaedists. The most common application of deep friction is where very localized, sufficiently deep, short, repeated transverse thumb strokes are performed across the specific site of a soft-tissue lesion. Because the typical approach is to work across the run of fibres, the method is also known as transverse friction and cross-fibre friction, or simply deep tissue massage.

Deep friction differs from deep transverse stroking in that the latter is less specifically applied to a lesion; rather it is used to release tension and to decongest areas more generally, but still through specific regions at a time. The similarities between the two are that they both travel slowly across fibres, they both typically employ the use of reinforced thumbs or fingers, they both help to break apart adhesions in the tissues, and they both may affect the body reflexively.

The crucial objective for the therapist is to pinpoint the exact location of the lesion. There is every chance that deep transverse friction applied to normal healthy tissue will result in a fresh additional (though minor) lesion. Next, the nature and severity of the problem must be assessed. Client questioning, close observation, careful palpation and physical testing should be

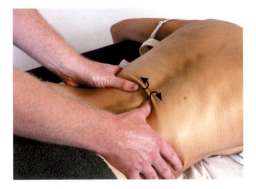

Circular frictions applied with thumbs to the paraspinal muscles

conducted before any remedial work is performed. If still acute and inflamed, like any other massage technique, deep friction should not be applied. The '10 second test' can be a useful way of helping to ascertain whether inflammation is still present. If pressure into the affected tissue causes pain to ease, or at least not to exacerbate, then it is often okay to continue. If, on the other hand, pain increases, the problem is possibly still inflamed – but this is a very rough guide.

Once the problem area has been identified and declared fit to receive deep friction, then the client should be positioned appropriately. One key to effective application is the amount of stretch that is placed on the affected tissue during treatment. As a very general rule, the more superficial the lesion, the more likely it is that a slight stretch is used. The variable tension–pressure factor appears to have quite a strong influence over the precise accessing and localization of the affected tissues, and therefore the effectiveness of the technique. If the region is too relaxed, shortened and softened, then there is the possibility that the depth of friction applied may penetrate to deeper, undamaged tissues. Similarly, if the tissues are too stretched, the technique may not be able to penetrate deeply enough. Typically, though, muscles are often put into a position of relaxation (shortened) so that the therapist can access fibres more easily, and tendons are often placed into a slight stretched position, remembering that tendons by nature are less bulky than muscles. This particular aspect of frictioning is variable, especially allowing for the different body types and muscle tone and tension that are seen in clients, and the amount of pressure and intensity that the therapist is able to comfortably apply themselves.

Deep friction techniques do not usually require lubrication. The control and localization are often better if there is no lubricant on the skin. Normally, with deep frictions, there is very little movement over the skin (or over other tissues superficial to the lesion) by the therapist's hand or arm, and the skin moves with the hand or arm as the affected tissues underneath receive their attention. The range of frictional movement is normally less than 2 cm, which keeps it focused on the problem. The speed of movement is not rapid, it merely needs to be sufficiently rhythmic to perform the desired action in as short a time as possible. The recommended time-scales for treatment vary among practitioners. Applying deep, specific, repeated frictions, within the realms of client tolerance, for one to three minutes should provide sufficient manipulation of the affected fibres, and if repeated two or three times per week this should encourage optimal recovery, especially when combined with all other relevant sports therapy methods. Some experts recommend longer treatments, of, say 5–15 minutes, but any clinical decision is always more easily made when years of experience back it up. Longer applications of friction may be more appropriate for more chronic situations. The therapist may also choose to recommend and demonstrate self-friction massage techniques to their clients.

The most common approach to deep friction is with reinforced thumbs (the treating thumb is strengthened and guided by the therapist's other thumb). Reinforced fingers, knuckles, the ulna border of the forearm, and when greater depth is required the olecranon process of the elbow can be used.

TIP

Effects of deep friction:

- can help to relieve pain
- reduces and prevents adhesions in post-acute injuries
- increases local blood flow (hyperaemia)
- helps to remodel and optimize the newly forming scar (collagen) tissue of injury
- treats lesions in muscle, tendon, ligament and other connective tissues
- helps to improve joint mobility and muscle extensibility.

TIP

Main indications for deep friction:

- post-acute strains and sprains
- adhesions and developing scar tissue
- repetitive strain (overuse) injuries, such as tendinosis, tenosynovitis and plantar fascitis.

TIP

Remember that older, younger, frail and unwell people tend to tolerate less well heavier, deeper, intense and prolonged techniques, and also be aware that RoM is likely to be less for older than younger people.

There are instances where a pincer-like grip technique can be employed, and this approach uses the fingers and thumb of one hand. Some therapists choose to use a plastic or wooden massage tool, but for friction these offer less in the way of palpatory information and overall control. Remember that the therapist's whole body is involved in any treating movement, and that any heavy pressure should come more from the core than from the periphery.

Ice applications are sometimes used immediately prior to deep friction techniques. This approach helps to numb the tissues so that the deep work can be performed more comfortably. Using ice after treatment can help control the degree of any new inflammatory reactions occurring in the region as a result of the treatment, remembering that deep friction does actually cause a fresh (controlled and therapeutic) injury, which the body then responds to with its reparative reactions.

A selection of potential benefits may follow from the application of deep friction techniques onto soft-tissue injuries. The main aims of such techniques are to encourage optimal repair and normalization of injured tissues, breaking apart disorganized scar tissue and fibrosis and properly aligning fibres longitudinally. It is often thought that these deep methods will, or are meant to, cause pain. However, the technique, when performed correctly, may actually have the opposite effect, in that although sometimes initially painful, it can gradually lead to a state of localized analgesia or numbing. There are several possible explanations for the reduction in pain. Analgesia (relief from pain) may result from: activation of the pain-gate; dispersal and reduction of localized pain-provoking metabolites; central release of endorphins.

Contra-indications to deep friction techniques include all those normally associated with other massage techniques. Extra care should be taken to avoid deep friction where there may be a possibility of haematoma or calcification (myositis ossificans) resulting from the injury. Caution must also be applied when confronted with fragile skin, neighbouring infections, unstable or hypermobile joints, systemic connective tissue disorders, rheumatoid arthritis or osteoporosis, among others.

Safety issues with deep friction:

- Treatment must be localized to the lesion.
- Be aware of all contra-indications.
- Do not use on acute injuries.
- Do not use when unsure of the nature of the problem.
- Do not be overly heavy.
- Work within the client's tolerance.
- Where the affected lesion is close to bone, try to avoid compression.
- Avoid deep pressure into possible endangerment sites.
- Do not overtreat.
- Take care to perform with good technique, not unduly stressing your own hands.

Common deep friction techniques

Deep friction techniques are only of use if applied directly to the affected tissue. The following examples simply illustrate ways in which deep friction techniques can be applied.

- Supraspinatus insertion. Seated position, with arm, extended and internally rotated so as to gently stretch and expose affected tendon. Therapist uses reinforced fingers.
- Supraspinatus belly. Seated position. Therapist uses thumb or reinforced fingers.
- Biceps belly. Seated position, with elbow partially flexed to relax muscle. Therapist uses pincer-like grip.
- Pectoralis major belly. Supine position, with elbow flexed and arm partially abducted to relax muscle. Therapist uses pincer-like grip.
- Quadriceps tendon (supra-patella tendonitis). Supine position. Therapist simultaneously presses down and pushes up the distal border of the patella so as to expose the tendon's insertion for reinforced finger friction.
- Lateral collateral knee ligament. Supine position. Ligaments are often treated in both shortened and lengthened positions. Therapist uses reinforced fingers or thumbs.
- Gastrocnemius lateral belly. Prone position, with knee partially flexed to relax muscle. Therapist uses reinforced fingers or thumbs.
- Achilles tendon. Prone position, with knee extended and foot in dorsiflexion, to gently stretch tendon. Therapist uses pincer-like grip.
- Lateral ankle (calcaneofibular) ligament. Side-lying position, with ankle in slight inversion, to gently stretch ligament. Therapist uses reinforced fingers or thumb.

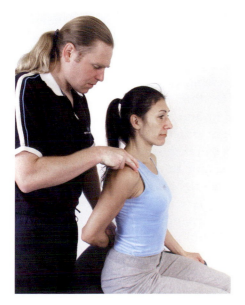

Deep friction to supraspinatus tendon

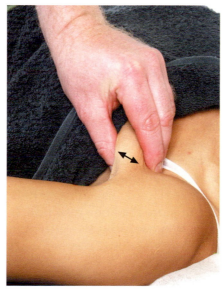

Deep friction to pectoralis major

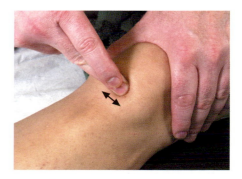

Deep friction to patellar tendon

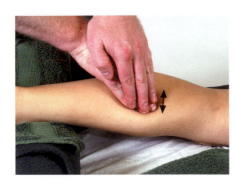
Deep friction to gastrocnemius

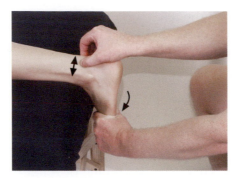
Deep friction to Achilles tendon

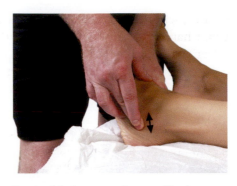
Deep friction to calcaneofibular ligament

PRINCIPLES OF SOFT-TISSUE RELEASE TECHNIQUES

Soft-tissue release (STR) is basically a combination of stretching and deep friction. Also referred to as a muscle release technique, STR can be used to locally stretch lesions both transversely and longitudinally, and offers the therapist a little more flexibility in approach. The stretching is usually passive, but active stretches can also be usefully employed.

As with standard deep friction techniques, the indications must be right, the affected tissues properly identified and no contra-indications presented. The main advantage of STR is that by employing the leverage of a stretch, the therapist's deep contact point onto the problem site does not move – this remains static – and as the joint is mobilized, the affected muscle, tendon, fascia and skin below the contact point should receive a very short, repeated localized stretching (frictioning). If the movement is rotational, then the resultant frictioning is transverse (cross-fibre). If the movement is lengthening, then the effect is one of a localized longitudinal stretching.

Obviously still requiring explanation to the client, careful positioning, appropriate range of movement and client feedback and involvement, STR is a technique on its own, and can be brought into any remedial treatment to offer additional benefit, and release of tight structures. Typically, the client is positioned so that the affected area can be effectively stretched to some degree. It is not always necessary to be able to take a limb through a full range of motion, because as the tissues get tighter, the contact point loses its positioning. The movement is usually repeated several times, and possibly in more than one direction, but this depends on the range offered by the joint in question. The treated muscle is normally put into a shortened position prior to applying the strong contact. Deep pressure should always be applied gradually. Remember to angle pressure away from any bony prominences.

Passive STR requires that the therapist develops a certain dexterity in being able to both apply a specific pressure into the affected tissue with one hand or arm, while at the same time stretching the related region with the other hand. Getting the client to actively move the region has particular advantages: the therapist can focus on applying the specific pressure; it is less tiring for the therapist; the client can control the amount of movement involved; there is a degree of reciprocal inhibition (discussed in the next chapter).

If the depth and intensity of the technique are reduced, usually with a broader contact area (e.g. palm of hand or forearm), and possibly a greater range of motion employed, then STR can also be used as an advanced form of passive (or passive–active) stretching, rather than as a direct deep frictional technique. In this case, the technique is very similar to the stabilization approach used in some passive stretching approaches. Similarly, it may also be used as an advanced CTM technique when the contact pressure is reduced to a depth above the muscles. In these applications, the end point of the stretch may be held for a few seconds.

Common soft tissue release techniques

The following examples are far from comprehensive, as many variations and applications can be developed.

- Trapezius belly. Supine or seated position. Active stretch into slight rotation and lateral flexion. Therapist applies local pressure into muscle with reinforced thumbs.

- Wrist extensor tendon. Seated position. Therapist articulates the forearm through short-range pronation and supination with one hand, whilst applying deep pressure with thumb of other hand.

- Quadriceps belly. Supine position, with client close to foot of couch. Beginning with knee in extension, the client actively flexes the knee as the therapist applies deep pressure into affected region with reinforced thumbs.

- Hamstring origin. Prone position with knee flexed. Therapist articulates the hip through short-range internal (medial) and external (lateral) rotation with one hand, while applying deep pressure into the affected tendon with olecranon process of elbow.

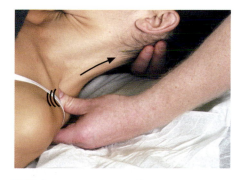

STR for upper trapezius

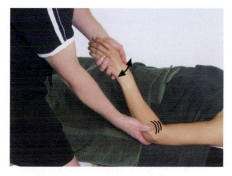

STR for wrist extensor tendon

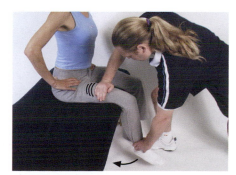

STR for quadriceps

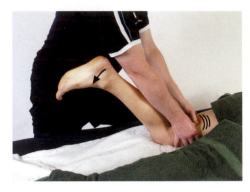

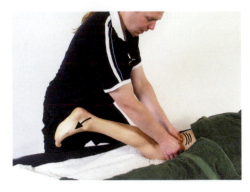

STR for hamstrings, start position STR for hamstrings, end position

- Hamstring belly. Prone position with knee flexed. The client actively extends the knee, while the therapist applies deep pressure into the affected region with reinforced thumbs.

- Hamstring belly. Prone position with knee flexed. The therapist articulates the knee, whilst applying broad based contact with palm of the other hand to perform more generalized releasing.

CHAPTER SUMMARY

This chapter has looked at flexibility, stretching, frictioning and soft-tissue releasing. Regular stretching helps to maintain or improve an individual's flexibility, and restricted flexibility can leave the individual vulnerable to injury. Various factors affect flexibility: everything from the type of joint involved to the age of the individual. There are various practical approaches to developing flexibility, and the therapist must develop strategies for determining which stretches are to be employed, in which positions, for how long, how intense, how many times and how often. Safe passive stretching requires a very careful approach from the therapist.

Deep friction is another classic **manual therapy** technique, where very localized, sufficiently deep, transverse strokes are directed at the specific site of a soft-tissue lesion. Soft-tissue release (STR) is a combination of (passive or active) stretching and deep friction, and can be used to locally stretch lesions, both transversely and longitudinally.

Knowledge Review

1 What is flexibility?

2 What factors can affect an individual's flexibility?

3 Briefly describe the various forms of flexibility training.

4 What are the advantages of performing passive stretching for clients?

5 Describe the important safety issues relating to passive stretching.

6 What are deep friction techniques, and how should they be performed?

7 What are the main indications for friction techniques?

8 What are the main safety issues relating to the use of friction techniques?

9 Describe the soft-tissue release technique.

10 Describe how you would provide: (i) passive stretching to the hip flexors; (ii) deep friction technique for a calf strain; (iii) STR for the pectoralis major muscle.

WEBSITE

Visit the companion website at www.thomsonlearning.co.uk/healthandfitness/ward where you will find the answers to these questions for you to check your progress through the book.

chapter 9

NEUROMUSCULAR, POSITIONAL RELEASE AND MUSCLE ENERGY TECHNIQUES

Learning Objectives

After reading this chapter you should be able to:

- understand the basic principles of neuromuscular techniques
- identify and treat soft-tissue trigger points
- understand the basic principles of positional release techniques
- understand basic principles of muscle energy techniques
- incorporate neuromuscular, positional release and muscle energy techniques into remedial massage treatments

The sports therapist has at their disposal an extensive collection of advanced massage-related techniques, any of which may be selected for use, and in combination, whenever the indications arise. The best treatments are always geared towards helping the client achieve a better level of fitness and health or a speedy recovery from injury. Neuromuscular, positional release and muscle energy techniques are particularly useful advanced manual methods, and they can fit easily into any sports therapy treatment. Once the sports therapist has developed a basic understanding of the potential effects and practical approaches of such techniques, they will soon find themselves incorporating them competently, fluently and regularly into their practice.

The reason that this collection of treatment techniques has been put together in one chapter is because they each share certain similarities, in terms of how they work, and what they are indicated for. Although all massage techniques have a varying degree of both mechanical (direct) and reflexive (indirect) effects, these particular techniques are all used to positively influence the state of tissues via the activation of specific neurological responses. In effect, the sports therapist attempts to engage and affect the nerve pathways relating to a problematic tissue, segment or region by way of specific pressure, stroking, positioning, active contractions, and passive or active stretching.

Neuromuscular technique (NMT), positional release technique (PRT) and muscle energy technique (MET) have all become well-regarded and established manual therapy techniques. The development process that has lead modern practitioners towards standardized applications and also to newer related and refined approaches has evolved from work performed in the 1940s and 1950s by pioneering physiotherapists and osteopaths. These days, these particular manual treatment techniques are routinely employed by massage therapists, sports therapists, osteopaths, chiropractors and physiotherapists. The underpinning theories to all of these methods strongly relate to the functional relationship of the nervous system to the musculo-skeletal system and then how these particular relationships can be influenced, by the techniques, to effect improvements or normalization in problematic tissue.

The three broad categories each of NMT, PRT and MET are further broken down into distinctly separate but closely related applications. Although each individual clinical treatment must always be approached carefully, the practitioner should be aware, and work with the knowledge, that there may be a small degree of trial and error when utilizing these techniques, in some instances. NMT requires that the therapist both palpates (assesses) and treats with the same technique at the same time, and it is the tissue's response to the technique that guides the treatment. Similarly, PRT involves carefully searching for a position of ease, which often involves a series of fine adjustments until that position is discovered. MET involves a sequence of controlled muscular contractions performed by the client against the resistance of the therapist, with a selection of objectives in mind. There is no guarantee that any of these techniques will satisfactorily achieve their objectives, and whether they do depends upon a variety of factors. The ability of the client to work with the therapist is a factor. These methods require that the client can feedback and sufficiently inform the therapist of their (subjective) experience of pain and tightness (and reducing pain and tightness), and also, in the case of MET, be able to actively contract (and relax) in the required manner. There are many clients who will struggle to take such an effectively active role in their treatments, and the therapist must accept this situation and be able to offer alternative approaches, at the same time not making the client feel awkward or uncomfortable. The very nature and severity of the presenting problem also always has an influence on its ability to be effectively resolved by such conservative measures, and this also affects the time-scales of improvement.

If a particular problem is considered amenable to massage treatment, and not in need of non-conservative approaches (surgery) or other more medically conventional methods, then it will also be amenable to NMT, PRT or MET, each of which can be adapted in terms of intensity, duration and frequency to suit both the person and the nature of the problem. These techniques are also normally used in combination with each other and with other massage methods, and obviously also with exercise and lifestyle recommendations.

TIP

The types of problems typically responding well to NMT, PRT and MET:

- excessively tense musculature
- restricted joint mobility
- muscle, postural and biomechanical imbalances
- superficial circulatory impairments
- trigger point pain referral
- soft-tissue adhesions (fibrosis)
- superficial hypersensitivity
- muscle flaccidity (reduced tone and weakness)
- organ malfunction.

PRINCIPLES OF NEUROMUSCULAR TECHNIQUES

This basic premise for NMT is that the careful, slow, localized searching palpation, performed with either thumb or fingertips, also forms the treatment, i.e. as the tissues are being palpated (with sustained or intermittent pressure or with short stroking movements), they are also being treated. The benefit therefore is that NMT is both diagnostic and therapeutic.

NMT is typically performed in three ways:

1 Short, slow, searching and precise strokes, normally performed with thumb or fingertips, although sometimes the ulnar border of the forearm can be used. These are applied both longitudinally and transversely over the problematic tissues. The depth of the strokes can be increased as the sensitivity reduces or if deeper muscles and tissues are to be targeted, and the actual speed of the stroke is not quick. It is usual to use a very small amount of lubrication. These techniques should not cause discomfort. The amount of time spent treating a particular region may vary from one to several minutes, depending upon the response of the tissues. **Origins**, **insertions** and the bellies of affected muscles should all be targeted. Be aware that there are mechanical and reflex effects with this approach. The area may also be treated, left for a period, and then returned to later in the session.

2 Direct continuous or intermittent pressure, usually applied with thumb or fingertips, but also the olecranon process of the ulna, or sometimes a wooden or plastic pressure bar, is used (a 'knobber'). This technique is also sometimes referred to as ischaemic compression. Once tissue sensitivity or tension has been identified, a direct pressure gradually applied into the associated muscle can be an effective method of reducing the symptoms. Pressure that increases pain should be abandoned. The direct, continuous approach may be applied for between 5 and 60 seconds at a time, and may be repeated several times during a session. The intermittent approach is simply an alternating on–off pressure technique, with pressure held on for a second or two, and off for a second or two. Direct NMT is typically used as a main approach to addressing trigger points.

3 Integrated neuromuscular inhibition technique (INIT) combines direct NMT with PRT and MET, and is discussed later in the chapter.

There have been a selection of differing approaches described by the experts in this field, but for effective results with NMT, the strategy must involve identification of problematic tissue. Problematic tissues may be hypersensitive, tightened, hardened, restricted, oedematous, congested, fibrosed or nodular, or contain trigger points. These tissue abnormalities may be the result of a recent injury, training overload, period of illness or emotional problem, or they may be associated with a more chronic situation, having developed over a longer period of time.

Acute injuries are often accompanied by a protective muscle spasm, which is the body's natural response to help restrict any further damage. Chronic problems, such as postural imbalance, repetitive stress injury, organ dysfunction and conditions such as arthritis or fibromyalgia, can all lead to what has been described as a 'facilitated' situation, where neurologically related tissues become hypersensitive or hyperirritable due to constant dysfunctioning. The facilitation may be local and/or segmental to the main problem area(s). A common consequence of local facilitation is the development of trigger points, which are so named because, when active, they refer discomfort to other regions. Segmental facilitation is where the sensory and motor nerve circuits serving the affected tissues become hypersensitive, often leading to excessive muscular tension and tenderness in the paraspinal muscles relating to the spinal segment from which the problematic tissues receive their innervation. This situation is often observed where there is organ malfunction, and the spinal segment serving the organ becomes facilitated. Whenever a region has become facilitated, it is likely that any further physical, environmental, emotional or other stress to the area will easily intensify the situation.

Observation of postural deviations, imbalanced musculature and restricted movements, combined with questioning relating to the associated functional experience for the client, and their feedback during treatment helps guide the palpatory process. The techniques of palpation are also the techniques of treatment, and these are continued and adapted as the tissues begin to respond. Light pressure or stroking detects sensitivity, tightness and fibrosis, and as the pressure or stroking is further applied, the sensitivity and tissue tension can be expected to reduce if the technique is being successful. Of course, any increase in pain or sensitivity during assessment suggests an acute problem and inflammation, and the approach should be abandoned in the short term. The same contra-indications as for other massage and remedial treatments apply to NMT.

Reductions in sensitivity, restriction, contracture and trigger point activity, and increases in circulation and drainage following NMT mainly occur due to the resulting inhibition of both the sensory receptors and the motor nerves within the soft-tissues, and in particular, within the muscles. In effect, NMT helps to calm and 're-set' neural circuitry, which then leads to a normalization in the resting level of muscular tension, and is often a preferable initial approach to the more reputedly aggressive methods (such as other massage techniques, mobilizations, stretching or electro-therapy).

Clients should be allowed to anticipate the treatment techniques and be encouraged to try to breathe and relax into the light but specific pressure or stroking of NMT. Obviously, pressure is increased only gradually as the discomfort begins to dissipate. Often, any initial discomfort reduces as the technique is applied and as the client relaxes and allows the effect to occur.

Common NMT approaches

The following examples simply illustrate ways in which NMT can be employed.

- NMT: thumb-tip stroking with fingers positioned to create a supportive bridge. The thumb moves slowly towards the fingers. The movement is repeated several times, and in a variety of directions, over the affected region.

> **TIP**
>
> Common signs and symptoms of a facilitated region:
>
> - skin and muscle hypersensitivity
> - muscle spasm
> - reduced tissue elasticity
> - increased local sudoriferous gland activity (sweating)
> - trigger points
> - reciprocally inhibited antagonist muscles.

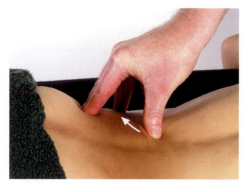

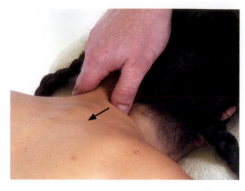

NMT to lumbar paraspinal muscles   NMT to cervical paraspinal muscles

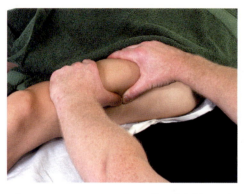

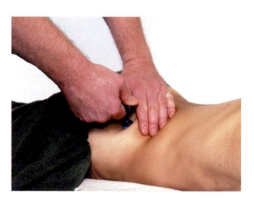

Direct pressure NMT to iliotibial band   Direct pressure NMT to gluteal region
                                          using pressure bar

- NMT: reinforced thumb-tip stroking to thoracic region.
- NMT: thumb-tip stroking to the cervical paraspinal muscles.
- NMT: direct pressure approach using reinforced thumb-tip to iliotibial band.
- NMT: direct pressure approach using plastic pressure bar to gluteus medius.

TRIGGER POINTS

When postural imbalance, overuse of muscles or compensated body movements develop and continue unchecked for periods of time, very specific areas of hypersensitivity, tenderness and tightness can develop in the related tissues. A trigger point, which can easily result from such a situation, is a specific point in a muscle which can cause a referral of pain and aching to other areas. Trigger points are typically housed in postural muscles and specifically within tightened bands of muscle, often near the origin or insertion, and when palpated feel nodular or lumpy. The reason for the typically nodular formation is because the affected muscle has become hypersensitive and irritable, and can be locally contracted. There may also be associated adhesions and thickening of the affected fibres.

TIP

Trigger points often correspond with motor points in the muscles and also with commonly used acupuncture points.

Common causative factors of trigger points include:

- postural and biomechanical imbalances
- trauma (injuries)
- overload in exercise training or physical work
- excessive exposure to cold or damp
- psychological or emotional distress
- soft-tissue disorders
- organ dysfunction
- illness
- toxicity (strong medications; environmental exposure)
- insufficient rest or sleep
- poor diet
- other trigger points.

It is not uncommon for clients to attend for treatment complaining of a nagging, aching pain in the arm, neck or head, or down the leg, but with no evidence of actual injury in the affected area itself. In such cases, the cause is often trigger point pain referral. Trigger points can be identified by the therapist, firstly by listening to the client's explanation of symptoms, and then by carefully palpating the suspected tissues. It is not unusual to reproduce the pattern of pain referral simply by pressing into the trigger point. The point will also often be sensitive to touch, and the associated muscle fibres may 'twitch' (reactively tighten) when pressed.

The common diagnostic factors relating to trigger points are as follows:

- Trigger points have typical pain referral patterns.
- Often the trigger point is outside the area of pain.
- Often the area of referred pain is cooler than surrounding tissues.
- When pressed, there is often a localized twitch response.
- There is often local tenderness.
- The trigger point is often housed in a taut band of muscle.
- There is often weakness in the affected muscle.
- There is often a restricted RoM in the associated joints.

Trigger points are often described as being 'active', when they are the client's main cause of discomfort (or are easily activated to do so), or 'latent', where they do exist in the tissues, and are usually tender themselves, but do not normally cause too much trouble. Latent trigger points may become active if postural, biomechanical, nutritional or environmental factors or poor health are manifest. Distally located 'satellite' trigger points can sometimes develop over a period of time, and these are characteristically activated by the primary trigger points.

Having a working awareness of how trigger points tend to refer their pain helps the therapist to identify their exact location. For example, trigger points in the supraspinatus rotator cuff muscle can typically refer pain to the top of the shoulder and also down the lateral aspect of the upper arm. Therefore, a client with pain in these regions, without other obvious causes,

> **TIP**
>
> Trigger points are hypersensitive areas located usually in muscle tissue. They are typically housed within a taut band of postural muscle, are tender to the touch, produce a 'twitch' response, feel nodular and characteristically refer an aching type of pain, or other sensation, to related body areas. The patterns of pain referral associated with each specific trigger point are typically similar between individuals.

TIP	

Muscles that can commonly contain trigger points:

- mastication muscles
- sternocleidomastoid
- splenius
- scalenes
- trapezius
- levator scapulae
- rhomboids
- erector spinae group
- quadratus lumborum
- supraspinatus
- infraspinatus
- pectorals
- abdominal muscles
- wrist extensors
- gluteals
- tensor fascia lata
- quadriceps
- hamstrings
- calves.

TRIGGER POINTS: MUSCLES AND COMMON PAIN REFERRAL PATTERNS

Temporalis: temporal region; around the jaw; above the eye.

Masseter: ear; around the jaw.

Sternocleidomastoid: back of head; around the ear; forehead; chin; anterior neck.

Splenius: top of head.

Anterior scalene: upper chest; upper arm.

Upper (cervical) erector spinae: occipital region; posterior neck; medial scapula region.

Upper trapezius: posterior neck; around the jaw; temporal region; back of head.

Levator scapulae: lateral neck; medial scapula; posterior shoulder.

Lower trapezius: posterior neck; shoulder region.

Rhomboids: medial and superior aspects of scapula.

Supraspinatus: top of shoulder; lateral upper arm.

Infraspinatus: anterior shoulder; lateral upper arm; lateral forearm.

Pectoralis major: chest region; medial arm.

Rectus abdominus: abdominal region; lumbar region; pelvic region; groin.

Wrist extensors: above elbow; dorsal aspect of forearm and wrist.

Lower (lumbar) erector spinae: lumbar region; abdomen; posterior pelvic region.

Quadratus lumborum: lumbar region; hip region; groin.

Gluteals: around iliac crest; lower lumbar region; posterior and lateral hip region; posterior and lateral upper and lower leg.

Tensor fascia lata; anterior and lateral thigh.

Quadriceps: anterior thigh; around patella.

Hamstrings: posterior thigh, knee and upper calf.

Tibialis anterior: shin region; dorsal region of foot.

Gastrocnemius: calf region; heel region; medial foot.

Soleus: heel region.

Peroneals: lateral lower leg; around the lateral malleolus.

may well have trigger points in that particular muscle, and pressure into the point (in the muscle) will usually reproduce the symptoms.

Trigger points are treated in a variety of ways and the sports therapist will be able to combine treatment techniques. Direct or intermittent compression NMT can be particularly effective, especially when followed with cooling of the affected area, gentle stretching and/or PRT and MET approaches. Clearly, the therapist should also attempt to help the client identify and reduce causative factors.

Common treatment strategies for trigger points are as follows:

- general massage techniques
- NMT
- PRT
- MET/INIT
- ice and stretching

- heat
- ultrasound
- TENS
- remedial exercise programme
- correction of causative factors.

PRINCIPLES OF POSITIONAL RELEASE TECHNIQUES

Positional release techniques are relatively gentle, indirect treatment techniques, and in simple terms, aim to position the client in such a way that their localized pain or tissue tension is dissipated or greatly reduced. As the affected body area is carefully positioned, neurological and circulatory changes gradually occur, which then lead to positive functional changes in the tissues and a reduction in pain. Both students and clients are often quite amazed at the effectiveness of these relatively easy and gentle techniques.

For the clinical sports therapist, positional release techniques are particularly useful where there is: muscle spasm associated with sub-acute injury; localized muscle tension, tender points or imbalance; soft-tissue restriction to RoM (including contractures associated with arthritis); trigger points; facilitated tissues. PRT, like NMT, is a very useful approach when faced with conditions where a more direct approach could be considered inappropriate (e.g. acute spasm; sensitive, frail individuals).

> Most of the positional release methods involve motion into ease, away from bind, utilising a slackening, crowding or 'folding' of dysfunctional tissues, in order to facilitate muscle spindle resetting and improved function.
>
> LEON CHAITOW (2002)

Although muscle spasm is an important physiological reaction, providing a warning signal that something is not quite right and a splinting protection for injured structures, it is also often the main cause of pain and restriction in acute and sub-acute problems. To reduce the spasm it is necessary to reset the affected neural circuits, encourage freer movement and reduce pain. It is crucial, however, to bear in mind that an acute episode of neck or back pain, especially with neurological symptoms, or any other more serious injury requires a far more tentative approach, and probably medical attention. Intervertebral disc protrusions and soft-tissue ruptures are all too easily aggravated in the early stage of healing. In such instances, the acute RICES approach (emphasizing rest) is probably the wisest initial strategy. Therapists should never treat conditions that they do not have confidence (or sufficient training) in correctly assessing. When in doubt, referral is the safest policy, simply because sports therapists are not front-line (primary) health-care practitioners.

Although there are several well-documented approaches to PRT, probably the two most well-known methods are strain counter strain (SCS) and functional (positional release) technique (FT).

Strain counter strain

The application of SCS is a very interactive process, involving four basic components: palpation to identify the tender points associated with a dysfunctional region; passively positioning the affected body part so that a particular tender point is eased (no longer tender or painful, or at least reduced); holding the position of ease for a sufficient time so as to allow the nervous system and the local tissues to functionally adapt, thereby reducing sensitivity, pain and spasm, and increasing the ease of active movement; and reassessing the tender point in the original position and also the client's ability to move the affected region. Typically, the time required for these effects to occur is between 60 and 90 seconds. The client should be encouraged to relax as much as is possible during each component. Additionally, during SCS, the client must be able to report to the therapist on the degree of pain experienced at the identified tender point during the repositioning.

A useful way of helping the client to gauge their altering pain experience during these movements is to ask them to rate their pain on a scale of 0 to 10 (10 being extremely painful, 0 being no pain at all). The therapist needs to be able to explain the technique well and to comfortably support the client during each component. A confident holding approach greatly improves the effectiveness of this technique. It is very important not to cause any form of additional pain during these movements, and also to be aware of the safe normal ranges of movement for each joint.

Each SCS technique requires, firstly, the client's starting position (prone, supine, sitting or side-lying) and, secondly, the initially performed main passive movement (e.g. flexion, extension and rotation) of the body parts. There then follows a subtle fine-tuning approach, whereby the therapist employs a selection of very small passive movements, one 'built' on to the other (e.g. slight amounts of further flexion, extension, rotation, lateral flexion, compression, elevation, protraction).

The most effective approach to SCS usually involves the affected tissues being taken carefully into relaxed and shortened positions, possibly reproducing the initial strain position, (strain, counter strain) and also often exaggerating the deviated position associated with excessive muscle tension. For example, a tender point in the upper back may reduce if extension combined with slight lateral flexion, rotation and compression towards the point is employed. It can also be useful, when treating the neck, torso or pelvis, to bring in subtle limb movements on top of the movements of the affected region. Remember that, because the position of ease is to be held for a minute or more, the therapist needs also to be correctly positioned so as to avoid straining themselves.

Often, it is the starting position for the SCS technique that provides a large part of the search for the position of ease. The client should be positioned so that the movements to follow can be easily performed. Limb positions and pillows or bolsters can also be used to refine the starting position, remembering that the affected tissue may require a passive, relaxed shortening, from all angles.

SCS: typical method

1 From consultation and assessment decide where treatment is to be focused.

2 With slow, careful, methodical palpation, search the soft-tissues for tenderness, sensitivity, trigger points or pain referral.

3 Explain the technique to client.

4 Help the client assume the most appropriate position for effective performance of SCS.

5 Encourage the client to relax, and to report back on their experience of pain at the tender point (use a scale of 0–10).

6 Using finger palpation as a guide, provide very careful, subtle passive movements in such a way as to reduce the tenderness at the point.

7 When close to finding the position of ease, very 'fine-tuning' movements are employed.

8 Hold the position of maximal ease for up to 90 seconds (the depth of palpating pressure should be reduced during the holding component, but light contact should remain).

9 Carefully (slowly) return the body part back to its resting position, and reassess.

Functional technique

Functional positional release technique (FT) is quite similar to SCS, the main difference being that, as well as the client's perception of pain being a modifier of the passive positioning into ease, the therapist uses, through palpation and assessment of the ease of movement during each subtle component, their own sense of awareness of the reducing tension in the tissues. Therefore, the skill in applying effective FT is being able to carefully manoeuvre the body part while feeling for a sense of release and freedom from restriction, but very locally. Like SCS, the end position of maximal ease is held for up to 90 seconds, and then the body part is gradually returned to its resting position for reassessment.

There is often room for slight experimentation when using PRT. The therapist, while simultaneously locally palpating and working with feedback from the client, applies a selection of subtle movements (e.g. flexion, extension, rotation, compression) to the affected body region and attempts to evaluate the effect that each slight movement has on the tissues, until a position of maximum ease is attained. Commonly, strains and tender points affecting the anterior aspect of the body are positioned into variants of flexion, while those affecting the posterior of the body are placed into variants of extension.

Obviously, as with most methods in sports therapy, PRT strategies are usually best combined with other therapeutic techniques. However, PRT is often a very useful first-line approach and can often be followed with NMT, MET, thermal therapy, general massage, remedial exercises and after-care advice.

> **TIP**
>
> During the functional positional release technique, the therapist, during passive movement, palpates locally for reducing tension and also feels for an easing of motion in all directions. The pain from a tender point, although relevant, is less of a guide to the modification of this technique. Certainly, though, this technique must not cause or increase any pain. The therapist attempts to discover and hold a position of maximal ease.

Common PRT (SCS and FT) approaches

The following examples simply illustrate ways in which PRT can be employed.

- PRT: start position (side-lying on least painful side) for painful, restricted neck extensor muscles.
- PRT: end position for painful, restricted neck extensor muscles (employing variations in extension, lateral flexion, rotation, and compression).
- PRT: start position (prone) for painful, restricted lumbar extensor muscles.
- PRT: end position for painful, restricted lumbar extensor muscles (employing variations in hip extension, abduction, lateral rotation and compression).
- PRT: start position (sitting upright) for painful, restricted shoulder muscles.
- PRT: end position for painful, restricted shoulder muscles (employing variations in shoulder elevation, flexion, abduction and rotation).

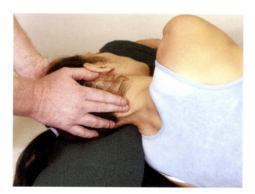

PRT for painful, restricted neck extensor muscles (start position)

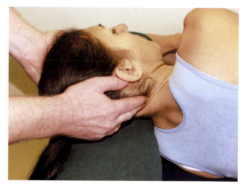

PRT for painful, restricted neck extensor muscles (end position)

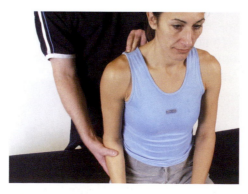

PRT for painful, restricted shoulder muscles (start position)

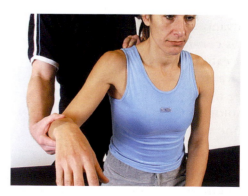

PRT for painful, restricted shoulder muscles (end position)

PRINCIPLES OF MUSCLE ENERGY TECHNIQUES

The various muscle energy techniques used in sports therapy can be incredibly useful for a selection of objectives, depending upon how they are applied: reducing muscle tension or spasm; increasing RoM; increasing body awareness; improving proprioception; breaking apart adhesions; increasing muscle tone; improving functional strength. Therefore, there are a variety of applications and achievable objectives with MET, and many clients like the advanced interactive approach that MET offers. As with NMT and PRT, MET builds upon the basic massage therapy techniques and foundations to offer additional methods of achieving therapeutic objectives, and similarly combines well with all other related techniques. Once the therapist has gained skill and confidence in guiding, positioning, supporting, mobilizing and passively stretching their clients, then the next obvious progression is to develop their practice with these valuable and very flexible procedures.

Early MET theories and applications were originally described as indirect osteopathic methods in the late 1950s, and have been in continual development and adaptation ever since. However, the roots of MET lie in the proprioceptive neuromuscular facilitation (PNF) techniques used in physiotherapy.

> PNF is best defined by first defining the individual terms. *Proprioceptive* refers to stimuli aroused within an organism through the movement of its tissues. *Neuromuscular* pertains to the nerves and muscles. *Facilitation* is the hastening of any natural process.
>
> CHUCK HANSON (IN HALL AND BRODY 1999)

The PNF approach to treatment, which mainly incorporates therapist-instigated functional patterns of movement, was originally used as part of rehabilitation programmes in the treatment of neurologically related pathologies, such as spinal cord injury and stroke. Although the potential for achieving effective improvements with PNF depends to an extent upon the seriousness of the presenting condition (and the skill of the therapist), impairments in muscle fibre recruitment and the associated functional movement patterns, may respond, over time, to a selection of manually resisted movements. Similarly, shortened, restricted muscles can be more effectively encouraged to relax and lengthen with such an approach.

The co-ordinated movements commonly described for the purpose of advanced PNF strategies are typically of a diagonal pattern, whereby it is considered that combined movements (e.g. flexion with rotation or extension with abduction), whether for the head, trunk, upper or lower extremities, are functional. Additionally, the therapist works with the understanding that to develop smooth controlled movement (basic motor skill) involves initiating (or re-educating) a specific series of muscle contractions (and associated relaxations or inhibitions) in all the involved agonists, synergists, fixators and antagonists in the particular movements.

By loading specific muscle groups during a particular movement, a variety of neurological components responsive to such a process are affected, in particular, the afferent (sensory) and efferent (motor) impulses. The result of this can be an improved recruitment of fibres in the contracting (agonist) muscles and an improved relaxation in the antagonistic groups. Proprioception, which is about balance and co-ordination, can usually be trained and developed very well, especially in the absence of underlying neurological pathology, and where such problems exist it is often an important functional objective to improve upon.

PNF, therefore, is used in a variety of rehabilitation settings, and its advanced use requires a deeper understanding of neurologically related pathologies. It is probably generally considered more the domain of physiotherapy.

> Muscle energy techniques involve a voluntary contraction of a muscle in a specifically controlled direction at varied levels of intensity against a distinctly executed counterforce applied by the sports therapist.
>
> WILLIAM E. PRENTICE (1999)

There is the possibility of confusion when discussing PNF or MET – the terms are sometimes used interchangeably and taken to mean the same thing. The PNF (or partner assisted) stretching, often described in textbooks, is a simplified application of PNF that is used to effect improvements in flexibility, and the basic protocol is the same as one particular method of MET (post-isometric relaxation). The similarities do not end there. Both PNF and MET can employ various types of manoeuvres, angles, holds and contractions to achieve their objectives and, like many of the widely used manual techniques, there can be a blurring of principles and applications, especially where different, but related, professional bodies adopt similar methods.

MET means involving some degree of muscular effort (energy) from the client. The degree or intensity of effort can always be altered to suit the objectives, and it may be that the effort is produced either in the muscles requiring the attention (agonists) or in their paired opposites (antagonists).

As always, the techniques work best following correct identification of problematic tissues. MET is most commonly used to help bring about improvements in flexibility, but can also be used to improve muscle relaxation, tone and strength, and ultimately functional improvements. The main variations of MET are described as follows.

Post-isometric relaxation (PIR)

The PIR approach is probably the most common and least confusing application of MET. Basically, the muscle or group to be treated is assessed for structural integrity and for its RoM (the restriction barrier is identified). The therapist then positions the treated muscle short of its restriction barrier (often a mid-range position is easiest) and asks the client to (isometrically) contract the muscle against their equal (unyielding) resistance. The intensity of the contraction can be altered to suit the ability of the client, but is typically between 25 and 30 per cent of maximal. The contraction is normally held for about 7–10 seconds, and the client should be encouraged to breathe smoothly during the exercise. The client should then be asked to relax, and following the contraction (and a slight relaxation phase of 1–3 seconds), the muscle is passively lengthened (stretched) and taken to, and hopefully just past, the previously identified restriction barrier. This sequence is usually repeated several times until no further improvements are observed. It can be useful to hold the final position in a longer (developmental) stretch for 20 seconds or so.

The reason for using this particular strategy is because a muscle will normally relax following a contraction. The physiological response, which involves the Golgi tendon organs and the muscle spindles, results in a (short-term) inhibition of motor impulses to the affected muscle, which means that the muscle is in a relaxed state and more amenable to being lengthened. PIR also causes, during the contraction phase, a degree of fatigue in the affected fast-twitch muscle fibres, which means that they will offer less resistance to the stretching that follows.

Both the client and the therapist need to be positioned carefully for the safe and effective application of these techniques. The client may be prone, supine, side-lying or sitting upright, depending on their condition, ease of movement, body type and the muscle groups being targeted. Fine-tuning of the various positions can be made by the use of pillows and bolsters, and by the positioning of the client's limbs. The therapist should consider these factors before beginning any treatment techniques. For relatively fit and mobile clients the positionings required will be similar to those detailed in chapter 8 (passive stretching). Those clients who are older, less mobile, arthritic or injured may well require adapted positions and assistance. Therapists should also be careful to position themselves carefully because they will need to be able to support their client, as well as resist their muscular efforts.

The following examples simply illustrate ways in which PIR can be employed:

- PIR: start position (prone) for shortened quadriceps. The restriction barrier is identified, and then the limb is brought back just short of the barrier. The therapist provides equal resistance to the client's contraction of the quadriceps.
- PIR: end position for shortened quadriceps. Following contraction, the limb is passively taken to its new restriction barrier.
- PIR: start position (supine) for shortened lateral shoulder rotators. The restriction barrier is identified, and then the limb is brought back just short of the barrier. The therapist provides equal resistance to the client's contraction of the infraspinatus and teres minor.
- PIR: end position for shortened lateral shoulder rotators. Following contraction, the limb is passively taken to its new restriction barrier.

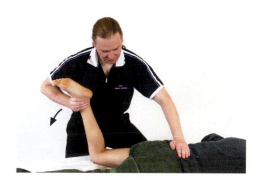

PIR for shortened quadriceps (start position)

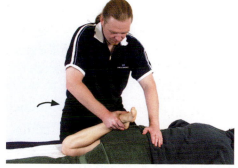

PIR for shortened quadriceps (end position)

TIP

RI is the relaxation of an affected (agonist) muscle following isometric contraction of its opposing (antagonist) muscle.

TIP

For both PIR and RI, increasing the duration of contraction may be an effective alternative to increasing the intensity of effort to obtain better results.

Reciprocal inhibition (RI)

The RI MET approach works with the fact in mind that many muscle groups function as antagonistic pairs. That is, as one (agonist) muscle contracts to produce its force, its opposite (antagonist) muscle must relax. For example, as the biceps and brachialis muscles work to flex the elbow, the triceps (the opposite, antagonistic elbow extensor muscle) must relax, otherwise no movement will take place. This is a functional, automatic, physiological reciprocal inhibition response to normal activity. The same principle can be applied in treatment, by contracting one muscle to create relaxation in another (its opposite).

RI can be used in conjunction with PIR, and other methods, but it is probably most useful where contraction of the agonist is not appropriate, such as when there is acute injury, inflammation, spasm or cramp. Therefore, to cause a relaxation in the affected muscle, its antagonist is contracted (isometrically), which should cause no discomfort or further aggravation to the affected muscle. After contraction of the antagonist, relaxation of the agonist may be the only initial objective (reducing muscle spasm, for example), and it may not yet be appropriate to apply any developmental stretching. RI therefore, is often a useful early treatment technique, which should cause no irritation to an acute problem.

The basic components of the technique are similar to PIR. It is usual to identify the restriction barrier in the agonist muscle first of all. It is probably easiest to use a mid-range position to contract the antagonist, at a mild to moderate intensity (20–30 per cent of maximum). The contraction should be held for between seven and ten seconds, and afterwards the previously identified restriction barrier may be reassessed and possibly held (without discomfort) for a few seconds. Again, the whole sequence can be repeated several times. A careful progressive treatment strategy would not involve strong stretching in the acute stages of healing, so other useful techniques might include: ice; supportive strapping; light massage above and around the injured area; ultrasound.

The following examples simply illustrate ways in which RI can be employed.

- RI: start position (supine) for restricted (long) hip adductor muscles. The restriction barrier in the adductors is identified. Short of this point, the therapist provides equal resistance to the client's contraction of the hip abductors.

- RI: end position for restricted hip adductor muscles. Following contraction (of the antagonists: mainly gluteals and tensor fascia lata, the limb is passively taken to its new restriction barrier.

- RI: start position (sitting) for restricted neck rotation to the right. The restriction barrier in neck rotation is identified. The therapist provides equal resistance to the client's contraction to the left.

- RI: end position for restricted neck rotation to the right. Following contraction (of the antagonists), the neck is passively taken to a new restriction barrier.

Of course, in addition to offering benefit in more acute situations, RI can also be used as part of a whole treatment strategy to improve specific

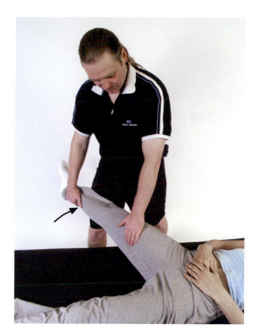
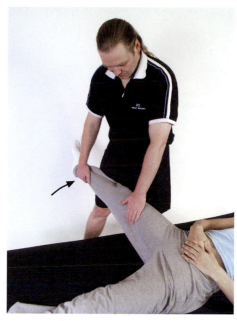

RI for restricted hip adductors
(start position) (contracting abductors)

RI for restricted hip adductors
(end position)

restrictions in flexibility, and when combined with PIR, it has been referred
to, more specifically, as the contract relax antagonist contract technique.

> Deciding whether to use the PIR or the RI method can be very simple. When the barrier
> position is fixed, the patient is asked to try the technique in both directions. If one feels
> uncomfortable, then only the other should be used. If neither causes any discomfort,
> then the two methods can be used alternately.
>
> MEL CASH (1996)

Contract relax antagonist contract (CRAC)

The CRAC technique simply combines the PIR and RI techniques to
produce increases in flexibility. The technique begins, as the others,
with identification of the restriction barrier. The affected muscles are
then isometrically contracted against the equal resistance of the therapist.
Following a brief relaxation phase (one to three seconds) the client is then
asked to isotonically contract the antagonists. In other words, the client
firstly contracts the shortened muscle, and then contracts its opposite
muscle so as to cause an active stretching of the agonist. This may or may
not be in combination with the additional passive stretching applied by the
therapist. The whole sequence, therefore, incorporates the principles of PIR,
where a muscle will relax following a contraction, and RI, where contraction
of an antagonist muscle causes an automatic relaxation in its (opposite)
agonist.

The following example simply illustrates how CRAC can be employed:

- CRAC: start position (supine) for shortened hamstrings. The restriction
  barrier is identified, the limb is brought back just short of the barrier, and
  the therapist provides equal resistance to the client's contraction of the
  hamstrings.

 TIP

CRAC combines the principles
of PIR and RI to facilitate
improved specific flexibility.

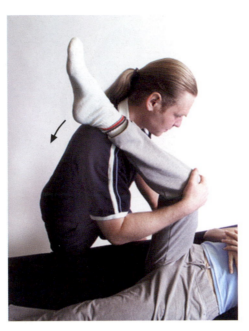
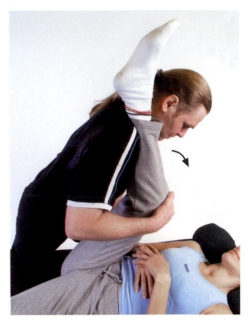

CRAC for shortened hamstrings
(start position)

CRAC for shortened hamstrings
(end position)

● CRAC: end position for shortened hamstrings. Following isometric contraction of hamstrings, and a brief relaxation phase (PIR), the client is asked to isotonically contract their quadriceps (RI) as the therapist simultaneously assists in taking the limb to its new restriction barrier.

Integrated neuromuscular inhibition technique (INIT)

INIT is an advanced application that combines PRT, NMT and MET. It may at first appear complicated, but once the basic principles of these three techniques have been grasped they can be mixed and matched for a variety of applications.

INIT is probably most useful where trigger points or muscle spasm is evident, and it offers a very localized and thorough manual approach to such specific problems in the soft-tissues.

A typical INIT approach might be, first of all, having identified the localized problematic tissue, to perform an intermittent inhibitory pressure (NMT) for between 10 and 30 seconds. Then, while maintaining thumb or finger contact on the point, attempt to passively locate a position of ease (PRT), and hold this for about 30–60 seconds (with no effort at this point from the client). Following this second technique, the client is then asked to contract (isometrically) the muscle in which the problem is manifest, against the equal resistance of the therapist, for between 7 and 10 seconds (at around 30 per cent of maximum intensity). This contraction is then followed by a brief relaxation phase (PIR) and a careful passive stretching of the same muscle, which may be held for 20–30 seconds. This sequence of techniques may be repeated two to three times.

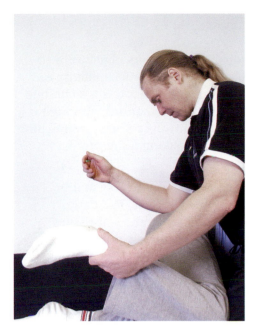

INIT for shortened piriformis
(NMT component)

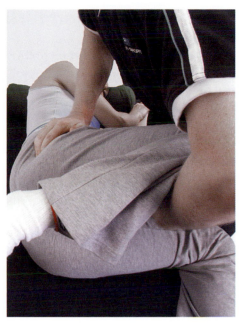

INIT for shortened piriformis
(PRT component)

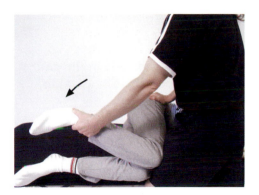

INIT for shortened piriformis
(isometric contraction component)

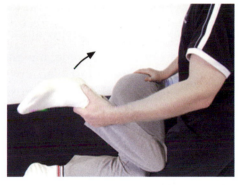

INIT for shortened piriformis
(end position)

The following treatment sequence simply illustrates how INIT could be employed:

- INIT: start position (side-lying, hips and knees flexed) for piriformis tender point. Intermittent inhibitory pressure (NMT) is applied into the tender point, typically using elbow pressure.
- INIT: the client is placed into a position of maximum ease (PRT) for 30–60 seconds.
- INIT: the client is asked to contract the affected (piriformis) muscle for seven to ten seconds, at about 30 per cent of maximum intensity.
- INIT: end position. Following isometric contraction (PIR), the muscle is passively stretched, taking the hip into medial rotation.

Isolytic contraction technique (ICT)

> **TIP**
>
> ICT involves, very carefully and specifically, stretching, through a controlled range of movement, a contracting muscle.

ICT is not a regularly used technique, probably because its objective is to cause micro-trauma to fibrotic tissue. It has, therefore, some similarity to the deep friction and soft-tissue release techniques, in that it is a technique to use on areas exhibiting adhesion and scar tissue formations, although it does not actually apply a direct friction; rather it involves a strong stretching of a contracting muscle (lengthening the fibres), making it therefore a muscle energy technique.

This is not a technique to use on the frail or elderly, on acutely injured clients, or, because of its vulnerability, on the neck region. The basic protocol involves identifying the existence of fibrosis in the soft-tissues (muscle or fascia). The client should then be appropriately positioned so that, while they are performing a contraction with the involved muscles, the therapist can effectively overcome that contraction to stretch out the affected (contracting) area. The contraction, therefore, is eccentric (lengthening) and the therapist's resistance is greater than the effort of the client. The start position is usually best in the mid-range, and the actual degree of movement is usually not large, as the therapist attempts to target localized problematic tissue and stabilize related body areas. The speed of the technique may be varied (from a slow stretch to quite a quick stretch), and, if indicated and comfortable, can be repeated several times in one session. ICT is not recommended for most clients or treatment sessions, as other more controlled methods are usually more preferable.

The following example simply illustrates how ICT could be employed:

- ICT: start position (supine, hip and knee flexed) for fibrosis in the gluteal and lateral rotator muscle groups. ASIS is stabilized. Client is asked to push out against the therapist's resisting hand.

- ICT: end position for fibrosis in the gluteal and lateral rotator muscle groups. The therapist overcomes the effort offered by the client to produce a stretching of the contracting muscles.

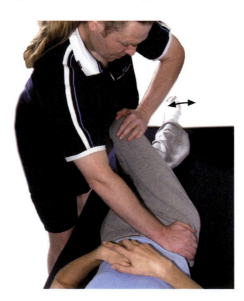

ICT for fibrosis in gluteal and lateral rotator muscles (client provides some muscular effort against that of the therapist)

Isotonic concentric contraction technique (ICCT)

ICCT is an MET used to tone and strengthen, improve proprioception and rehabilitate muscles and joints. Not only is ICCT an MET, but it is also a form of manual muscle training, useful for both rehabilitation and close-up personal training. It is worth remembering that, because of the reciprocal innervation related to the antagonistic pairing of major muscles, in some instances the excessive tone, or hypertonicity, manifested in one muscle or group can lead to an inhibition situation, and resultant reduction in tone, or hypotonicity, and weakness in its opposite muscle or group. Typically, isotonic exercises are incorporated into the rehabilitation programme after isometric work has been performed for a period of time.

Once the particular muscular weakness has been identified, whether related to injury or not, the client is positioned so that they can perform an isotonic (concentric) contraction against the lesser effort (resistance) of the therapist. The concentric (shortening) contraction is performed over about two to four seconds, through a comfortable range of movement, using a maximal effort that is achieved gradually, not suddenly. This exercise can be repeated in terms of repetitions (five to ten) and sets (one to three, with rest periods in between). This form of rehabilitation exercise can be adapted to include isometric holds at various positions, with different angles, and also isotonic eccentric (lengthening) contractions.

The following example simply illustrates how ICCT can be employed:

- ICCT for weakened quadriceps: start position (sitting upright, with legs hanging down). Client contracts quadriceps muscle against therapist's manual (lesser) resistance.
- ICCT for weakened quadriceps: end position. Client's efforts overcome the resistance of the therapist during the concentric (shortening) contraction. The whole sequence can be repeated several times, possibly including an isometric component, and the intensity of force can be adapted to suit the client's ability.

> **TIP**
>
> ICCT incorporates manual resistance to the muscular efforts of the client. It is used to improve muscle tone and strength, improve proprioception and can form a useful part of the functional rehabilitation process.

CHAPTER SUMMARY

This chapter has looked at a selection of advanced massage-related techniques. The theoretical principles behind neuromuscular, positional release and muscle energy techniques may be difficult to grasp at first, but all can be relatively easily be incorporated into remedial treatments and used positively to influence the state of tissues via the activation of specific neuromusculo-skeletal responses. In effect, the sports therapist attempts to engage and affect the nerve pathways relating to a problematic tissue, segment or region by way of specific pressure, stroking, positioning, active contractions, and passive or active stretching. Such techniques combine other methods well, and offer the client a more practically varied treatment, with the associated increases in benefit.

WEBSITE

Visit the companion website at www.thomsonlearning.co.uk/healthandfitness/ward where you will find the answers to these questions for you to check your progress through the book.

Knowledge Review

1 From the following list of acronyms, write down the full title of each treatment technique: NMT; PRT; SCS; FT; MET; PNF; PIR; RI; CRAC; INIT; ICT; ICCT.

2 List the main indications for using the above techniques.

3 Describe the three ways in which NMT can be applied.

4 Describe the difference between SCS and FT.

5 How does PIR differ from RI?

6 Describe how you might approach treating a tight quadriceps muscle group using a PIR strategy.

7 Describe how you might approach treating a painful neck rotation situation using an RI strategy.

8 Which MET strategy can be used to improve the tone, strength and proprioception of muscles? Describe the basic protocol for this technique.

chapter 10

ELECTRO-THERAPY, CRYOTHERAPY AND THERMAL THERAPY

Just as the sports therapist has at their disposal an extensive collection of hands-on advanced massage and exercise therapy techniques, they may also call upon a selection of electrical and thermal equipment, which enhance their treatments, improve healing times, increase therapeutic benefits and offer even more variety for clients.

Today, the modern high-tech sports therapy clinic may well be equipped with all manner of electrical therapeutic devices, some being clearly more useful and versatile than others. It certainly is far from essential to spend a fortune buying a lot of expensive equipment – indeed the only really essential equipment is the couch, towels, clinical disposables and your hands! That said, if the client is offered a pre-heat treatment prior to massage, then, because thermal therapy can help to make muscles and joints more supple, the physical side of the sports therapist's work can be made a little easier and the overall client experience can be more pleasant. Thermal therapy does not need to involve expensive equipment (hot water can be easily used to prepare hot towels or a moist heat pack). Similarly, it is not difficult to have ice available for the treatment of acute injuries or trigger points. If the therapist has a good quality electro-massage machine, the task of loosening and relaxing tight muscles can be made a little less demanding, and many clients enjoy and appreciate the variety offered by such devices. Certain items of equipment such as electronic muscle stimulators or ultrasound machines can be very useful for specific indications: the former mainly for passive muscle toning exercises; the latter mainly for the treatment of strains, sprains and other soft-tissue injuries.

Having a selection of well-maintained and functional therapy equipment can help make the job more interesting for the therapist and even more beneficial for the client. It is, however, important that the therapist does firstly develop their hands-on skills before expecting any piece of high-tech equipment to do the job for them. Also, therapists should not incorporate any piece of equipment into their practice for which they have not received sufficient training or obtained insurance.

ELECTRICAL THERAPY EQUIPMENT: GENERAL SAFETY FACTORS

Treatment should never be provided without first performing appropriate consultation and physical assessment, and this is especially important where electrical equipment is to be used, because the potential for harm can be great. There are many safety issues regarding the use of such equipment, and the sports therapist must always work with these in mind. It is particularly important to ascertain whether the client is suitable to receive the proposed treatment and, if so, whether there are any areas of their body requiring special care. Once the therapist is satisfied that the client is fit to receive treatment, they will need to discuss and agree on the objectives and then explain what the treatment entails.

ELECTRO-MASSAGE

Electro-massage may also be referred to as mechanical massage. Massage machines can provide either very vigorous and deep treatment, or alternatively very gentle treatment, depending upon which machine is being used and what adjustments it has. Electro-massage machines replicate to some degree many of the standard manual massage techniques, but they also offer a selection of their own specific and very useful benefits. There is a wide range of massage machines on the market, for both home and professional use, and there are three main types: gyratory vibrators; percussors; audiosonic vibrators.

The effects and benefits of electro-massage therapy are very similar to those of manual massage: general and local circulations are improved; lymphatic drainage increases; local tissue temperature is raised; tense muscles become more relaxed; weaker muscles can become more toned; aches and pains may be relieved; general relaxation increased. Most of the heavy-duty massage machines are best suited to areas of bulkier muscle or excess

SAFETY WITH ELECTRICAL EQUIPMENT

- Always read manufacturer's instructions prior to using electrical equipment.
- Ensure that the equipment has been checked and labelled safe for use by an authorized electrician.
- Check that all switches, leads and plugs on the equipment are secure and functional.
- Do not use equipment that is faulty.
- If the equipment is mounted on a stand, ensure that the base is secure, that leads can safely reach the mains socket and that the equipment will not cause any obstruction.
- Be aware of how the lead trails, making sure that it cannot cause anyone to trip over it.
- Do not overload mains sockets or extension leads.
- Do not work electrical equipment anywhere near water.
- Make sure equipment is cleaned and applicator heads sterilized before use.
- Check that all attachments are clean and functional, and when used, securely attached.
- Prior to application, the treatment must be explained to the client.
- Make sure the client has removed all jewelry prior to electrical treatments.
- Never surprise the client with modalities or expect them to know what is coming next.
- Make sure all controls are set to zero before switching the equipment on.
- Intensity controls should be turned on last, increased gradually, and switched off first.
- Where appropriate, test the equipment on yourself before using on client.
- Commence treatment and encourage client feedback.
- Work with awareness of recommended treatment times.
- Try to gauge client's response to the treatment.
- Adjust the treatment time and intensity to suit the client.
- Never leave machines unattended when plugged in.
- Clean equipment and store away safely after use.

TABLE 10.1 Advantages and disadvantages of electro-massage therapy

Advantages	Disadvantages
Less tiring for the therapist	Can be expensive to buy
Produces quicker effects	Requires regular servicing
Reduces treatment time	Requires storage space
Useful in team situations	Requires specific skills to operate safely
Useful in pre- and post-event situations	Less personal treatment
Adjustable intensities	Requires more careful monitoring of client's response to treatment
Interchangeable attachments	Less palpation during application
Can provide deep and vigorous treatment	Can be heavy and cumbersome for some therapists
Can target specific tissues	Can cause problems if used incorrectly
Enhances manual massage treatments	Some clients do not like electro-massage therapy
Adds variety to treatment sessions	
Some clients prefer electro-massage therapy	

adipose tissue. The audiosonic machine is a much lighter machine, having a different set of applications. Particularly positive and more specific effects may be gained when the machine has a selection of attachment heads for different applications and intensity adjustment controls.

Gyratory vibrators

Gyratory massage machines may be either the floor-standing type (commonly known as the G5 machine) or the hand-held portable type. The movements generated by these machines are rapid and repetitive (25–60 cycles per second), combining back and forth movements, in the horizontal plane, with up and down movements, in the vertical plane. The G5 is a particularly robust machine, designed for more continuous use, and it is very adaptable, having a selection of attachments (made from either sponge, rubber or polyurethane) each for a different effect. The machine must always be switched off when changing attachment heads.

G5 treatments require that a light application of talcum powder be applied to the skin so as to reduce surface friction during movement of the applicator heads (oil may damage the equipment). There are specific heads available that can be used with hot water, providing additional benefit. After use, the heads should be washed in soapy water, dried and then sanitized in an ultraviolet cabinet. Disposable plastic covers can be used with some of the heads.

The hand-held gyratory machines can be very useful, particularly when the therapist is working away from the clinic. They have their motor built onto the applicator head (rather than mounted separately on a pedestal), which means that they can be quite heavy, but no additional pressure needs to be added by the therapist during treatment.

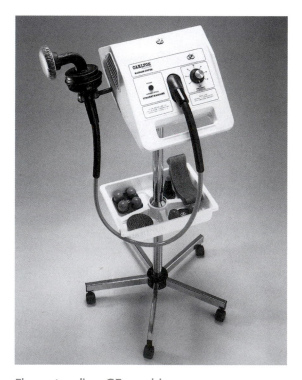

Floor-standing G5 machine

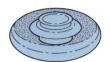

1. Round, smooth applicator

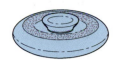

2. Round, smooth water applicator

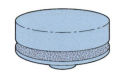

3. Round sponge applicator

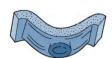

4. Curved sponge applicator

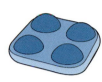

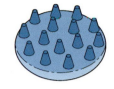

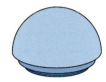

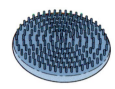

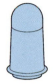

5. 'Eggbox' applicator

6. 'Pronged' applicator

7. 'Football' applicator

8. 'Spiky' applicator

9. Lighthouse

Common applicator attachments for G5 machine

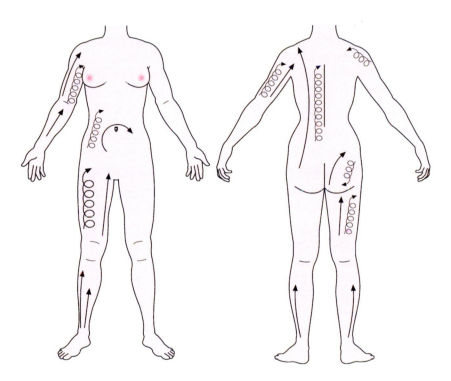

Gliding strokes towards the venous return lymphatic nodes

Round smooth sponge applicator

Round smooth massage head

Curved sponge applicator

Spiky rubber applicator

Rotary movements along muscle length or localized area

Round smooth applicator

Eggbox rubber applicator

Pronged rubber applicator

Football rubber applicator

Lighthouse rubber applicator (used on upper fibres of trapezius muscle)

G5 treatment techniques

Be aware of the following specific safety issues of electro-massage:

- All potential contra-indications relating to manual massage also relate to electro-massage.
- Do not overtreat the client (as erythema, or itching, develops, stop treatment or move on to the next area).
- Do not treat anywhere near pins and plates.
- Choose the correct attachment head for each treatment area.
- Avoid heavy application over bony areas, or areas with little muscle or fatty tissue.
- Avoid neck, kidney and breast regions.
- Avoid excessively hairy areas.
- Avoid uneven pressure of application.
- If performing general massage, work in a centripetal direction or towards the nearest lymph nodes.
- If treating the abdomen, do so gently, with great care, and in the direction of the flow of the large intestine.
- Treatment too soon after injury can increase tissue damage.
- Smaller machines, such as the audiosonic may overheat if used for longer than 20 minutes at any one time.

Percussors

Modern technology has brought about a selection of hand-held percussor machines which are capable of working continuously for longer periods, and with a range of intensities. These machines replicate the tapotement technique, moving up and down very rapidly (typically up to 25 times per second). Obviously, this quick-fire action is much faster than that performed manually, and so these machines offer their own therapeutic benefits, in particular being able to quickly relax tense muscles, increase local circulation and reduce musculo-skeletal pain. Percussors are often better used through clothing or a towel, and perhaps the best approach is to 'park' the machine over a particular region for a short period of around 10–20 seconds before moving on to the next area.

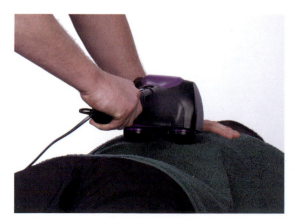

Hand-held percussor machine

Audiosonic

The audiosonic machine is another hand-held appliance. Its motor is much smaller than those of larger massage machines, and it produces a distinctive 'humming' noise. Not to be confused with ultrasound machines, which are completely different, the audiosonic (or 'sound wave vibrator') works through the action of an electromagnet, which when activated by the alternating electrical current, causes a rapid up and down movement of the applicator head (up to 50 cycles per second), but through a very short range of motion. Although quite similar to percussor vibrators, the audiosonic does not 'beat' the skin; rather, it remains in constant contact with the skin. The resulting action creates an alternating compression and decompression of the tissues. The effect is very light on the skin's surface, but may penetrate up to 5 cm deep into the tissues. This means that there is little or no irritation to the skin or over-dilation of surface capillaries, and the subcutaneous tissues can be selectively targeted. The vibrations emitted from the audiosonic machine spread out through the tissues from the applicator head rather like the ripples on a pond. In sports therapy, audiosonic therapy can be used effectively to gently relax tense muscles and increase the reparative circulation through injured muscles, tendons and ligaments.

Most machines feature a master intensity control, a choice of frequencies, and two attachment heads: a flat disc for general massage, and a ball head for accessing the nooks and crannies of joints, or for focusing treatment into fibrositic nodules. Audiosonic therapy can also be used to help reduce tissue sensitivity, in a manner similar in effect to the manual neuromuscular massage techniques. It is usual to use a very light application of oil to allow easy movement of the applicator head (but manufacturers' recommendations should be checked). In application, the head should be moved very slowly back and forth or in a circular manner, over a small treatment area, for up to a few minutes at a time, depending upon the objectives.

TIP	

The audiosonic machine provides a very gentle, but therapeutically useful, treatment. It can be used on tense or sensitive muscles, post-acute injuries such as strains, sprains and tendinosis, and when the intensities are reduced, it may also be used, in certain instances, on the paraspinal, posterior neck, and facial muscles.

TIP	

Do not use an audiosonic machine for longer than 20 minutes at a time, because it may overheat.

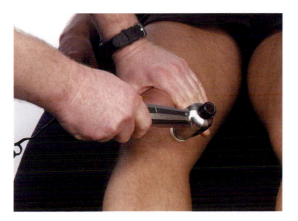

Audiosonic machine

CRYOTHERAPY

Cryotherapy (treatment with cold or ice) and thermal therapy (treatment with heat) are particularly important methods for the sports therapist to be able to confidently apply. One or the other (or both) could easily and appropriately be incorporated into almost any treatment, depending on the therapeutic objectives, simply because they are so therapeutically useful. It is not essential to have expensive cryotherapy and thermal therapy equipment available. It is not difficult to have available basic but effective cooling and heating equipment.

Effects and benefits of cryotherapy

Potentially, cryotherapy can:

- reduce the acute inflammatory response
- cause vasoconstriction, leading to a decrease in local circulation
- decrease local metabolic rate and secondary hypoxic tissue damage
- increase local blood viscosity
- reduce swelling
- cause local anaesthesia and reduce pain
- reduce muscle spasm
- be used as part of the treatment of trigger points
- be used to reduce the discomfort of deep friction massage techniques
- be used to reduce the discomfort of certain remedial exercises
- be used by the client at home to enhance their rehabilitation programme.

The main use of cryotherapy is in the acute stages of injury (as a component of the RICES strategy) to help control bleeding, swelling and pain, but it can also be very useful in the later treatment and rehabilitation stages of healing. Initial tissue swelling (from torn fibres and ruptured capillaries) and secondary hypoxic tissue damage (certainly an undesirable sequelae) are the usual acute inflammatory responses to soft-tissue injury, and the pain that follows (a very sensory and unpleasant experience) is also obviously not wanted. If we have in cryotherapy an effective non-pharmacological method of reducing these responses, then it should always be readily available, both in the clinic and at sporting events. Sports therapists should be able to use cryotherapy safely and effectively, and be able to instruct their clients to use it likewise at home. Like most interventions, it is often the intensity, duration and frequency that dictate the degree of benefit derived, and with cold treatments there are a variety of methods and approaches available. The type of cooling applied should depend on the location, depth and severity of the injury, and the client being treated.

Be aware of the following specific safety issues of cryotherapy:

- Any contra-indications relating to body treatments.
- Do not use cryotherapy where there is decreased or problematic circulation (e.g. arterial disease; cardiac conditions; diabetes).

- Do not use cryotherapy where there is cold hypersensitivity or allergy (e.g. Raynaud's disease, where vaso-spasm and pain can occur, especially in the extremities).

- Do not use cryotherapy where there are areas of reduced or absent skin sensation.

- Avoid cryotherapy over superficial nerves (e.g. peroneal nerve at the lateral popliteal space or radial nerve at the posterior-lateral elbow), because it may cause a nerve conduction block, leading to distal numbness or tingling.

- Reduce the intensity and application time of cryotherapy on areas with little body fat or muscle bulk.

- Do not overtreat with cryotherapy, especially because prolonged treatments do not increase the effectiveness. Tissue death, nerve damage, unwanted vasodilation or frostbite are all possible results of excessive cooling.

- Apply great care (lower intensity and duration) when using cryotherapy for children or the elderly, who are more likely to have a less than efficient temperature regulation system and a reduced ability to communicate their experiences so well.

> **TIP** ✔
>
> The sooner that cryotherapy is applied to an acute injury, the better.

Typically, cryotherapy treatments are applied for between 10 and 30 minutes at a time, even rarely for longer. This should allow for good cold penetration, even with deeper injuries. Where the application is more direct, such as with ice-cup massage, the treatment time may be less, especially if the desired responses appear to have occurred. The usual subjective response to cryotherapy, during application, begins with the cold sensation and a short-duration dull pain, followed by a burning-like sensation, deep aching, and finally a numb sensation. An ice treatment should end as numbness occurs. Regular reapplications can be recommended at a rate of once every hour or two, acutely, and later twice a day, until inflammation has subsided, bearing in mind that the inflammatory response will usually last for 24–72 hours.

Shorter periods of ice application should suffice when preparing to perform deep friction massage, remedial exercise (cryokinetics) or the treatment of trigger points. The cooling, in these instances, may be repeated after the massage or exercise. The benefit of using cold (to relieve pain) in conjunction with remedial exercise is that the amount of muscle atrophy and joint stiffness related to moderate injuries can be reduced. Clients should be instructed to perform their pain-free exercises (mobility or strength work) until the normally experienced mild discomfort returns (usually after about five minutes). The region should be cooled again and the exercise repeated, finishing with a final cold application. This approach to exercise must always be more carefully performed than that without cooling, because there is a danger of worsening the condition by being too aggressive or ambitious in the early and intermediate stages of rehabilitation. When trigger points are being treated, a common approach is to use NMT and/or PRT, followed by cooling the pathway of referred aching, and then stretching the affected muscles (cryostretch).

Cryotherapy equipment

There are a variety of ways of applying cryotherapy:

- ice: crushed ice; ice cube; ice cup; ice lolly; ice bath
- frozen peas
- gel pack
- chemical cold pack
- cold spray
- cooling gel
- cold compression units.

Most forms of cryotherapy are inexpensive and easy to organize. A fridge with a freezer compartment is all that is needed to prepare for ice treatments. Crushed or flaked ice in a plastic bag is a great way of cooling larger areas such as a calf muscle or the knee or shoulder joints. It is safest policy to wrap ice bags with a thin towel to prevent the possibility of tissue death from excessive freezing. If the towel insulating the pack is damp or wet, the cold will penetrate more than if dry, but will still be less than if the pack is applied directly. Any area being cooled should be checked regularly for any warning signs of adverse reactions (e.g. wheals with reddened, raised swollen areas of skin; rash). It is normal to observe pink or reddened skin after cryotherapy. A bag of frozen peas can work just as well as one of crushed ice, and they both mould well to the contours of the body. Gel packs, often produced from a formulated silica gel contained in a sealed vinyl bag, can be a very useful way of keeping cooling equipment handy, and although they are not as aggressively cooling as plain ice packs, they remain flexible when frozen, and can be reused.

Ice bathing is gaining popularity with elite athletes, where after arduous training sessions, a short soak in a cold bath helps to reduce the severity of minor muscle injuries and the inevitable aches and pains. Specific ice baths for clinical injury treatments are most useful when cryotherapy for the hand or foot is required. Because an ice bath could be considered an aggressive method, it is probably best to use a large bowl containing cold water with ice cubes floating in it or crushed ice (slush), and the treatment can be intermittent in application, letting comfort be the guide. Ice baths may be used in combination with thermal baths in a technique known as contrast bathing (discussed later).

Ice cup massage is a particularly efficient method of icing for the sports therapist to use in many clinical situations. By freezing water in a styrofoam cup, the therapist has a ready-made ice applicator complete with insulated sleeve. The top of the cup is peeled back to expose the ice, and the therapist can hold the cup without freezing their own fingers. The client should have towels placed around the treated area because the ice will melt as it is applied. Ice cup massage can be useful for applying cold treatment to very localized areas, such as muscle tears or sites of tendonitis. Some therapists recommend first applying a thin film of massage oil to the affected region to help reduce the potential for adverse effects. The ice massage itself should be performed in a circular manner, without any additional pressure applied.

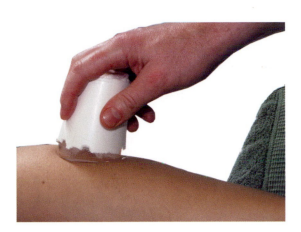

Ice cup massage

Chemical cold packs are specially designed for use when actual ice is not available. They stay at air temperature until activated by squeezing the bag and mixing the chemicals. Although useful in first aid situations, they are not very cold. Cold aerosol (vapocoolant) sprays are also useful when ice is not available. These offer brief but rapid cooling, but are not as effective as actual ice treatment, the cooling only tending to reach superficial tissues. The effect is probably more of mild pain relief than of circulation restriction. The affected area should be sprayed, at a set distance for a few seconds at a time, and care should be taken to avoid possible skin or eye irritation. This technique can be helpful as part of a treatment for trigger points. Cooling gel is another form of superficial chemical cooling, whereby a specially formulated gel can be massaged gently into an injured area, with the effect being similar to that of a cold spray.

Cold compression units are more expensive items of clinical equipment and are most commonly used in post-operative settings and larger sports clubs and rehabilitation centres. The basic idea is that iced water and air are pumped, intermittently, from a base machine into a special sleeve surrounding the client's affected body area. Compression occurs as the sleeve becomes more inflated with air, and it is the combination of controlled cooling and compression that provides a very effective method of reducing inflammation, swelling and pain.

THERMAL THERAPY

Heat therapy can be used clinically to reduce pain, increase local or general circulations, increase soft-tissue extensibility and generally improve the healing in post-acute and chronic injuries. There are a variety of methods of heating the body. Radiation heating is by way of such items as infra-red lamps, and does not involve direct contact with the body. Conduction heating involves direct contact, and examples of this approach are hot packs and baths. The majority of techniques described here are classed as being superficial heating methods.

TIP	

As a very general guide:

- Use cryotherapy for acute and sub-acute injuries and early rehabilitation.
- Use thermal therapy for post-acute and chronic problems, as a pre-heat prior to other treatments, and as a general relaxation method.

Deeper heating methods, where tissues underneath the subcutaneous layers are specifically targeted by specialized equipment, are used by many physiotherapists. Such techniques include shortwave and microwave diathermy, which use high-frequency electromagnetic waves, interferential, an advanced form of TENS that employs dual currents aimed to intersect at the injury site, and ultrasound (discussed later).

Effects and benefits of thermal therapy

Potentially, thermal therapy can:

- cause vasodilation and increased blood flow through a region
- reduce pain (or increase the pain threshold)
- increase local metabolic rate
- help relax muscle tension and spasm
- increase soft-tissue extensibility and pliability
- help reduce joint stiffness and increase range of movement
- increase healing rate of soft-tissue injuries
- improve neuromuscular response (sensory and motor)

THERMAL THERAPY: SPECIFIC SAFETY ISSUES

- Be aware of all contra-indications relating to body treatments.
- Do not use thermal therapy where there is problematic circulation or cardiac insufficiency.
- Do not use thermal therapy where there is acute injury (including strains, sprains, open bleeding and bruising).
- Do not use thermal therapy where there is impaired sensation. Always test for thermal sensation prior to application on local areas.
- Do not use thermal therapy where there are implanted metal pins, plates or pacemaker.
- Do not use thermal therapy on swollen areas.
- Do not overtreat with thermal therapy, because prolonged treatments do not increase the effectiveness. Burning, fainting, dizziness, headache, nerve damage and tissue necrosis are all possible results of excessive or inappropriate heating.
- Apply great care (and lower the intensity) when using thermal therapy for children or the elderly, who are more likely to have a less than efficient temperature regulation system and also a reduced ability to communicate their experiences so well.
- Apply great care (and lower the intensity) when using thermal therapy for pregnant women. Avoid the abdomen and low back.
- Remove all jewelry before applying heat treatments.
- Be careful to avoid eye irritation when using infra-red lamps (use appropriate goggles or shield eyes with dampened cotton wool pads).
- Always adjust the intensity and duration of thermal therapy to suit the client's tolerance.
- The majority of thermal therapy treatments demand that the therapist stay with their client, encourage feedback and monitor their responses.

- help improve recovery from training
- be used in the intermediate and later stages of injury rehabilitation
- be used by the client at home to enhance their rehabilitation programme
- help bring about feelings of increased well-being.

Therapeutic heating in the clinic can normally be provided for the majority of clients, and there are various methods to choose from. There are, of course, many safety issues for therapists to be very aware of.

> **TIP**
>
> Hyperaemia is an increase in the amount of blood circulating through a local area. Erythema is a reddening of the skin due to the dilation of superficial blood vessels.

Testing thermal sensation

It is most important that the client is able to differentiate between hot and cold sensations, especially in the area that is going to receive treatment, otherwise, if the client is not able to report their thermal experience, there is a danger of tissue damage. The usual method for the testing of thermal sensation is to half-fill two test tubes, one with cold water, and one with hot water. Before applying to the client's skin, the tubes should firstly be tested on yourself (so as to make sure that they are not too hot or cold to apply). The client should have a tube lightly placed onto the area to be treated, and be able to report whether it is hot or cold. An alternative method is to simply use a warm spoon and a cold spoon.

Thermal therapy equipment

- General: **sauna**; **steam room**; **steam bath**; jacuzzi; hot bath; hot shower.
- Local: gel pack; wheat bag; moist heat pack; hot towels; paraffin wax; infra-red lamp; heat spray/rub.

Spa treatments

Many sports therapists are trained to set up and organize spa treatments for clients. The most common spa facilities, often available in the larger health clubs and fitness centres, are saunas, steam rooms, steam baths and jacuzzi baths. These are very useful pre-heat treatments prior to massage, as they are great for increasing general circulation and thoroughly relaxing the body. The safe provision of all spa treatments requires that the therapist follows strict health and safety procedures. Another very useful spa treatment, perhaps better classified as a form of hydrotherapy, is hydro-massage, where powerful jets of water are carefully directed at the client by the therapist. Hydrotherapy pool exercise is particularly useful in guided rehabilitation settings, where the warm water can help make mobility exercise easier to perform, especially when hand rails, steps and specially designed aqua resistance equipment is available.

Most clients, particularly those with general stiffness or aches and pains, can easily be recommended to take relaxing hot baths at home, but the temperature should not normally exceed 40 °C. Hot showers can also be very useful home-care measures, especially where neck, shoulder or back pain is an issue.

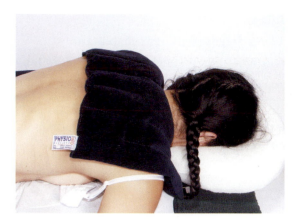

Thermal therapy using wheat bags

Hot packs

In the clinic, heating applications in the form of gel packs, moist heat packs and wheat bags are relatively straightforward to organize. Gel packs (often the same type that can be used for cryotherapy) are easily warmed up by being placed into a pan of boiled water for a few minutes and then wrapped in a thin towel before being applied to the body. Moist heat (hydrocollator) packs require a slightly longer preparation: they are placed into a pan of gently simmering water for about 15 minutes and then taken out using tongs. The excess water is allowed to drip off, the pack is then wrapped in layers of towels and applied to the affected area for between 20 and 30 minutes. The amount of towelling wrapped around the pack can be adjusted to suit the tolerance of the client. Moist heat packs, which can be much more effective than the dry heat packs, penetrate more deeply, open up the skin's pores and encourage a greater localized hyperaemia. They are also a great pre-heat treatment prior to massage. Wheat bags are another readily available form of heat pack. Placed in the microwave for around two to four minutes, these bags provide a similar treatment to that of the moist heat packs (from time to time, add a small amount of water to the bag), and the preparation is minimal. Always be careful not to burn a client with a pack that is too hot, and keep extra towels handy to wrap around them. Most packs come in a selection of shapes and sizes applicable to different body regions, and it is helpful to have a small selection available.

Hot towels

Alternating hot towels are another inexpensive and easy method of performing basic heat treatment. This technique requires that a well wrung-out hot towel is placed onto the affected area, then taken off and immediately replaced by another hot towel (the towels cool off quite quickly). This cycle is repeated several times for 10–15 minutes. Always explain what is about to happen to the client, so that they can remain relaxed and able to describe their experience.

Chemical heat

A heat (aerosol) spray, is similar to a cold spray in that it is very superficial and has a short-lived effect, but they can be useful to some players in pre-event situations, as can topical creams and muscle rubs containing warming properties (a common ingredient being methyl salicylate). Do not combine heat sprays, creams, rubs or balms with other heating methods.

Contrast baths

Contrast baths, combining cold immersion with heat immersion, cause a localized and alternating vasoconstriction and vasodilation. This approach is most often used in the sub-acute stages of healing, where inflammation is subsiding, but where swelling remains. Normally, the treatment begins with a cold immersion of around three to four minutes, followed by a heat immersion of around one minute. This cycle may be repeated several times in one session, typically finishing with a cold application.

Paraffin wax baths

Paraffin wax treatment is a common method for the sports therapist to employ. A specially designed, thermostatically controlled, wax heating bath is required to prepare for this treatment. Specially formulated (pre-mixed) solid white wax (a petroleum derivative) and oil packs are melted in the bath, at a temperature of around 45–50 °C, which turns the wax into a translucent fluid. This is normally a safe temperature to apply the wax directly onto the skin. From cold, it can take the wax about an hour to completely melt, but this depends upon the heating strength of the bath being used. There are two basic approaches to paraffin wax treatment: the repeated immersion method and the painting method.

Because the baths are usually quite portable and not large, only the immersion of hands, elbows and feet is normally possible. The area to be treated should be thoroughly cleaned prior to application so as to reduce contamination, and the temperature of the wax tested by the therapist. All

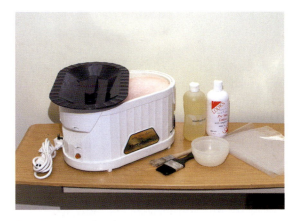

Paraffin wax bath

other safety checks relating to electrical and thermal treatments should be performed, and as always, the client should have the treatment explained to them. The body part being treated should then be dipped into the bath and immediately removed. The wax should be allowed to set (become white) for five to ten seconds before re-immersion. This process may be repeated several times until there is a thick covering of wax on the body part. After the final application, the part should be wrapped in a plastic sheet, wax paper or tin foil, and then covered in a towel to slow down the cooling of the wax. The wax and coverings should be left on for around 10–15 minutes.

If the body part requiring paraffin wax treatment is too large to use the immersion method, such as the back, shoulder or knee regions, then the wax can be applied to the area with a (clean) paint brush (the molten wax is taken from a plastic bowl). The therapist should take care not to spill or drip the wax onto the client (or the floor or couch), and the wax should be brushed on over the area quite quickly (because it does cool quickly) and thoroughly, building up a thick layer of hardening, white wax. As soon as the wax has been applied, the area should be covered with plastic sheeting (or wax paper or tin foil) and a towel. The client should then be encouraged to relax for the duration of the treatment.

Some therapists like to provide an additional infra-red heat treatment in conjunction with paraffin wax treatment (the lamp is directed at the towel covering the wax) so as to maintain the therapeutically beneficial temperature. After sufficient treatment time, the towels and plastic sheeting (wax paper or tin foil) should be removed, and the wax should peel off cleanly. The sheeting should be disposed of hygienically (alternatively, the wax could be sterilized if it is heated in a pan to 80 °C, and then allowed to cool).

Infra-red lamps

The infra-red heat lamp is another useful piece of clinical therapy kit. Infra-red (IR), on the electromagnetic spectrum, lies between visible light and microwaves. IR rays are given off from the sun and any other heating object, such as an electric, gas or coal fire, hot pack or lamp.

IR lamps are described as being true and non-luminous (invisible), or radiant and luminous (visible). These days, most IR lamps are the radiant luminous type, where visible red light is emitted along with the heat. It is clearly much safer in the clinical environment if a heat lamp can be observed to be switched on and be hot (i.e. when the red glow is observed), rather than, as in the case of true IR, not at all obvious. Also, the radiant lamps tend to heat up much more quickly than the true IR lamps. Although the heat can be a little more irritating with radiant IR rather than true IR, it will penetrate through the skin's layers more deeply, it may feel less hot, and the heating effect may be more evenly dispersed.

There are many safety factors to consider when using IR lamps. In addition to all safety issues previously discussed regarding thermal therapy, two specific rules apply. The *inverse square rule* dictates the distance that the lamp should be positioned from the client's body: the intensity of IR radiation decreases as the distance from the lamp increases, and vice versa. Most manufacturers will recommend a specific distance relating to

TIP

Infra-red heat lamps: safety issues:

- Make sure the equipment and the treatment area is safe.
- Be aware of all contra-indications.
- Test the client for thermal sensation.
- Be particularly careful to measure the correct distance (usually at least 50 cm).
- Angle the lamp correctly (so that the incident ray is 90° to the skin's surface).
- Shield eyes if in danger of exposure.
- Record the time of treatment.
- Observe and monitor the client's response to treatment.
- Ask client to report immediately if the heat becomes uncomfortable.

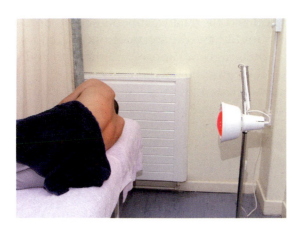

Infra-red heat lamp

the intensity of the lamp, and this should be strictly adhered to (use a tape measure to set the correct distance, which is typically at least 50 cm). Many lamps do have both an on–off switch and an intensity control. IR rays should always be as near to perpendicular as possible to the skin's surface to avoid uneven exposure and possible burning.

Additionally, the lamp and its stand should be fully inspected for stability and function. The bulb should be well fitted, and along with its reflector should be cleaned of any grease, oil or dust. Most lamps are not designed to be used from directly above the client, since a bulb may shatter or fall, or the lamp could be knocked by the client or someone else. Obviously, thermal sensation tests must be performed, and the client should not have any oils or creams on their skin. Whenever in use, the therapist should stay with and monitor the client, and they should be asked not to touch or move any nearer to the lamp. Often the best treatment position for IR is side-lying, facing away from the lamp. If there is any danger of eyes being exposed to the IR lamp, then special goggles or dampened cotton wool pads should be worn. It is not recommended to apply IR to the neck region because it can cause too great an increase in blood flow to the brain.

All that said, infra-red is a useful, and normally safe method of applying heat the body. The typical treatment time is from 10 to a maximum of 30 minutes. It can be quite pleasant for the client if the ray of heat is occasionally broken by the therapist's hand lightly stroking over their skin. If you are at all worried about the intensity of the heat, then do remember that the intensity of the treatment can be adjusted by the intensity control (if the lamp has one) or by moving the lamp further away from the client. Once treatment is concluded, switch off and unplug the lamp, and position it out of harm's way.

> **TIP**
>
> Clients who have received a thorough heat treatment should be encouraged to relax for at least ten minutes afterwards, and to drink a glass of water. This can prevent the possibility of faintness, which, although unlikely, can occur when there is reduced blood flow to the brain and vital organs.

ULTRASOUND

Not all training courses in sports therapy currently offer tuition in ultrasound, the reason being that it is often not part of the main syllabus.

Ultrasound is one particular treatment tool especially associated with the treatment of sports injuries, and specifically with treatment from a physiotherapist. Because sports therapists are now gaining a greater reputation for being able to manage and rehabilitate common sporting injuries, it is only natural that ultrasound should become a part of their own therapeutic repertoire, providing, of course, that the therapist receives sufficient and appropriate training in the method. Ultrasound is a technique to know well and understand before use. It is important to understand not only the main indications, contra-indications, benefits and adversities, but also the way in which the intensity, frequency and timing of the technique, and the size of treatment area can influence the outcome. Importantly, the body's musculo-skeletal anatomy needs to be well known, just as should methods of assessing, identifying and localizing problematic (injured) tissues. Provided here is merely a basic introduction to the subject.

Although ultrasound may be used in medical settings both diagnostically and as a treatment for improving the healing of such conditions as dermal ulcerations, surgical skin incisions and fractures, in sports therapy it is more often used in combination with other modalities and rehabilitation exercises for the treatment of muscle, tendon and ligament injuries. Being regarded as a deep treatment tool, and having both thermal and non-thermal effects, ultrasound may be used for a selection of purposes, and it can be used to treat acute, sub-acute and chronic injuries.

Effects and benefits of ultrasound therapy

Depending upon the intensity and frequency of ultrasound, there are a selection of potential effects and benefits:

- It can be selected to provide thermal or non-thermal effects, according to the stage of healing.
- In acute situations it may enhance early healing and resolution of the inflammatory phase.
- It can be used to perform phonophoresis in the acute inflammatory phase of healing.
- It may help to reduce and control pain.
- It can be used where deep localized heating of tissues is required.
- It can improve local circulation, and therefore the nutrition to a site of injury.
- It can help reduce muscle spasm.
- It may help reduce scar tissue formation.
- It can help prepare shortened tissues for stretching techniques.
- It may improve the healing of chronic tendon injuries.
- It may improve the rate of healing of surgical skin incisions.
- It may improve the rate of healing of fractures.
- It combines well with other modalities and rehabilitation exercises.
- It is comfortable and easy to receive.

In the treatment of acute injuries, non-thermal ultrasound has been shown to cause localized mechanical agitation and increased cellular permeability, which when combined with other beneficial effects such as increased histamine release, phagocyte responsiveness and protein synthesis by fibroblasts, a hastening of the resolution of the early phase of soft-tissue healing occurs. During this early stage of healing, ultrasound can also be used to drive topical anti-inflammatory or analgesic medication directly through the skin's pores into the affected tissues – a technique known as phonophoresis.

Thermal ultrasound is normally employed once inflammation has subsided. Increased localized blood flow and tissue metabolism encourage an improved cellular proliferation and remodelling in injured tissue. Alongside improved supply of nutrients for repair, the heating effects of ultrasound can also help to create an increase in collagen extensibility, making tissue mobilization (and normalization) easier to perform. Additionally, pain thresholds may be increased by ultrasound therapy.

The various effects of ultrasound are caused by the inaudible, high-frequency sound waves that occur as an alternating electrical current is imposed onto a piezo-electric crystal within the transducer (applicator) head. The amount of vibration occurring at the crystal depends upon the size of the crystal and the frequency of the current. When effectively coupled (through the medium of a conduction gel or water), the resulting sound waves pass through the skin and into the body's tissues. The depth of penetration of the waves (and therefore the localization of the technique) is governed by the frequency. The most common wave frequencies used for sports injury treatments are 1 MHz, which penetrates to a depth of 3–5 cm, and 3 MHz, which is for targeting more superficial tissues. The intensity (output) for therapeutic ultrasound, is calculated by dividing the total delivered watts (W) by the effective radiation area (ERA) in cm^2 (W/cm^2), and the usual range of intensities goes from 0.5 to 2 W/cm^2. Additionally, the mode of application may be selected to be continuous, where the effect is constantly applied to the tissues, or pulsed, where it is intermittent (on and off, at pre-set intervals). Continuous ultrasound at higher intensities produces thermal effects, which are most useful in later stage therapy. Pulsed ultrasound at lower frequencies produces the non-thermal effects suitable for more sub-acute and sensitive work.

Ultrasound, when used inappropriately, can potentially aggravate existing conditions or create new problems, and the main contra-indications to treatment are the same as for any other sports therapy modality or treatment.

Be aware of the following specific safety issues of ultrasound:

- Any contra-indications relating to body treatments.
- Do not treat when unsure of the nature of the problem.
- Do not use ultrasound therapy where there is problematic circulation, cardiac insufficiency or a pacemaker.
- Do not use ultrasound therapy where there is impaired sensation. Always test for thermal sensation prior to application on local areas.
- Do not use ultrasound therapy where there are implanted metal pins or plates.

- Do not use ultrasound over bone growth (epiphyseal) plates.
- Apply great care when using ultrasound therapy for pregnant women. Avoid the abdomen and lower back.
- Avoid high-dose ultrasound in areas of inflammation, over fracture sites and breast implants.
- Be careful to avoid central nervous system (CNS) tissue and the eye region.
- Always begin with low intensities.
- Always adjust the intensity and duration of ultrasound therapy to suit the required objectives.
- During treatment, always keep the applicator (sound) head in motion (do not use it in a stationary mode).
- Be aware that burning of tissues can occur with inappropriate or excessive use of high dose ultrasound, particularly in tissues with impaired circulation.
- Reduce intensities of ultrasound over areas with superficial bone.
- Be aware that optimal outcomes are more likely if regular, appropriate dose treatments are employed.
- Encourage feedback from the client, and stop treatment if any discomfort is experienced.
- If during a course of treatment, progress is slow, reconsider your approach and make a decision as to whether referral might be appropriate.

> **TIP** ✔
>
> Sports therapists should undergo a thorough training in ultrasound therapy, and obtain insurance to practise, before offering it to clients.

Ultrasound equipment

The basic equipment required for ultrasound is a calibrated machine (featuring frequency indicator, intensity control and timer), transducer heads (different shapes and sizes are available, but must match the frequencies of the machine) and a coupling gel (or bowl of degassed water).

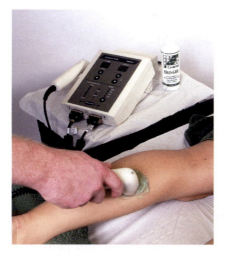

Ultrasound machine, transducer head and coupling gel

Ultrasound techniques

The sports therapist must consider all safety factors prior to any electrical treatment, and this should include identification of contra-indications, thorough checking of equipment, performance of a thermal sensation test, and explanation of the procedure to the client. The client should be appropriately positioned to receive treatment, and the machine should be set up for use, with careful attention to choice of frequency, intensity, transducer head and treatment time. If using direct ultrasound, a generous blob of coupling gel should first be applied to the skin. The transducer should then be placed on the skin and the machine turned on. The transducer head must be kept moving slowly over the skin (at a rate of about 4 cm per second), and the actual area being treated should not be more than two or three times the size of the head, so as to keep the treatment effect localized and of sufficient intensity. Moving the head too quickly can result in lost effect, and not moving the head can result in discomfort for the client and the burning of tissues. The duration of the treatment depends upon the size of the affected area and the stage of healing. For acute injuries, the treatment time will normally be around three minutes (pulsed). For post-acute and chronic problems, five minutes (continuous) is typical. Once the pre-set treatment time has elapsed, the head should be removed, and the both the client's skin and the transducer head cleaned of coupling gel.

An alternative approach is to use indirect (or aqueous) ultrasound (through the coupling medium of degassed, water). In this method, best suited to hands, elbows and feet, the body part and transducer head are placed into a bowl of water, with the head aimed at the affected area. The head does not make contact with the skin's surface (keeping a distance of 1.5–3 cm); this approach allows for a more effective ultrasound application over uneven body contours.

The optimal frequency of ultrasound treatments appears to lie somewhere between one treatment per day or two per week. Client records must be kept with specific regard to the choice of frequency, intensity, timing, method, client response and combined interventions.

ELECTRICAL MUSCLE STIMULATION

Electrical muscle stimulation (EMS), also known as neuromuscular electrical stimulation (NMES), is used to both passively tone and strengthen muscles or to create a gentle, repetitive massaging effect. There are a selection of machines able to provide these effects, some being large and expensive, others being small, inexpensive, battery operated and portable.

EMS involves attaching pads to either the motor points or origins and insertions of specific muscles. These days, there are a selection of currents used in EMS therapy. By employing a low-frequency interrupted direct current (traditionally around 50 Hz or cycles per second), through pads strapped onto specifically targeted muscles, a controlled passive workout

TIP
The motor point, in the muscle belly, is where a motor nerve enters and acts on its muscle fibres to make them contract.

TIP ✓

Some muscles have more than one motor point (e.g. trapezius; gastrocnemius), and some motor nerves are more superficially sited, meaning that they will respond to a lower current. Stronger (regularly exercised) muscles usually require less intense stimulation to achieve strong contractions, whereas weaker muscles can fatigue more easily, tremor and fail to contract appropriately.

can be initiated. There are three main variations to padding technique that have been developed, each providing slightly different benefits.

Paired padding or duplicate padding is where each pad of a pair is placed on the motor points of two separate, but adjacent muscles. If both sides of the body are padded up in this manner, each group can be worked individually, which allows for differences in muscle strength.

Longitudinal or bi-polar padding is where each pair of pads (electrodes) is placed on each end (near to the origin and insertion) of one muscle. This method, which can be ideal for the larger muscles, allows for effective shortening. The pads should be placed parallel to the fibres of the particular muscle, and therefore it is important to be familiar with the shape and run of fibres in the larger muscles.

Split (motor point) padding is where one pad (of a pair) is placed on a particular muscle on one side of the body, and the other pad is placed on the same muscle but on the other side of the body (e.g. left and right gastrocnemius). This method tends to be more commonly used on superficial muscles which require less stimulation, but can contribute towards muscle imbalance, if not carefully monitored. It can be useful, when using larger machines, particularly when there is an uneven number of pads (rather than leaving the free pair of pads lying idle).

Effects and benefits of EMS

Depending upon the chosen frequency, intensity and duration of EMS, there are a selection of potential effects and benefits:

- minimizes muscular atrophy following injury
- improves tone and strength of muscles
- improves endurance of muscles
- improves neuromuscular re-education
- increases local circulation and tissue metabolism
- improves elimination of waste products
- allows early instigation of rehabilitation exercise
- can be combined with active contractions
- can help to improve poor posture or body contours
- promotes an earlier return to active and functional exercise.

Particular care must be taken to identify possible contra-indications prior to EMS. Obviously all equipment should be thoroughly checked, and the procedure fully explained to the client before application. During treatment the client is monitored for comfort and adverse reactions.

There are various reasons for an EMS treatment being problematic: client in inappropriate treatment position; skin not suitably prepared; not starting on zero intensity setting; turning intensity up during relaxation phase; pads incorrectly positioned; pads not securely positioned; pads too wet; pads are frayed or not flat to the muscle; intensity or duration of treatment is too great; large quantity of adipose tissue in area; allergic reaction to the pads.

Working with great care and attention to all details should make EMS a safe and, especially in the case of the early rehabilitation of sports injuries, a very useful modality.

Be aware of the following specific safety issues of EMS:

- Any contra-indications relating to body treatments.
- Carry out a skin sensitivity test to ensure that the client can differentiate between sharp and blunt sensations.
- Do not use EMS where there is problematic circulation, cardiac insufficiency, impaired sensation, implanted metal pins or plates, or a pacemaker.
- Apply great care when using EMS therapy on pregnant women. Avoid the abdomen and lower back.
- Always adjust the intensity of EMS very slowly, and only during the contractile phase of stimulation.
- If the intensity is too high, the treatment time too long, or the relaxation phase too short, muscle fatigue and soreness can occur.
- Encourage feedback from the client, and stop treatment if any discomfort is experienced.

EMS equipment

The larger, modern clinical EMS machines offer a very comprehensive selection of computerized muscle stimulation programmes, a large number of paired pads, and enable more than one body region to be treated in one session.

Small portable units offer a less expensive approach to muscle stimulation. Portable units are designed to be lightweight and easy to use. They typically have only a few controls and facility for two pairs of pads. The range of frequencies may not be as great as a clinical machine, nor such a wide range of programmes built in, but they can nevertheless be used easily by clients at home, and be very effective.

TIP
It is definitely not recommended to use portable EMS or TENS machines while driving or operating other machinery.

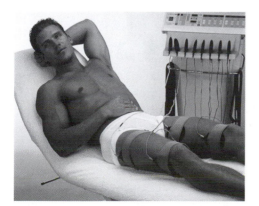

EMS treatment to thigh muscles

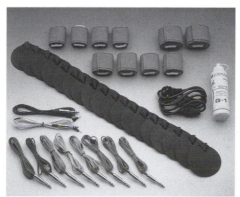

EMS cables, strapping, pads and ionized solution

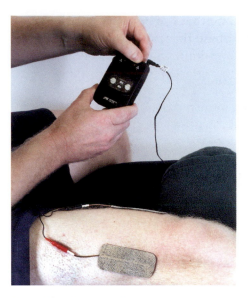

Portable EMS machine

EMS techniques

The therapist must become familiar with the various features of the machine that they are using. Most EMS machines will have: a mains switch; a pulse control (which varies the length of the stimulation and relaxation phases); a frequency control (which controls the number of pulses per second, and therefore the depth of stimulation); an amplitude control (which regulates the intensity at each pad); a mode control (which selects either a monophasic or biphasic mode); a gain control (which increases or decreases all intensity dials at once); a variable control (which causes the stimulation–relaxation phases to become randomized, rather than regular); and a timer (which can be pre-set to allow accurate treatment and automatic cut out).

The client should be positioned comfortably on the couch, and the treated regions supported and placed in a non-end of range position (bolsters or rolled towels can be used). The treated areas of skin should be cleansed to ensure no grease is present. Because the skin has a resistance to electrical current, the electrode pads, usually made of electrically conductive carbon or graphite impregnated plastic, are moistened with an ionized (gel or saline) solution to assist the passage of electricity into the muscle. Each pair of pads should be tested by the therapist on themselves (at low intensity) before being applied to the client (simply place a finger between the moistened pads, and turn the intensity up slightly until a tingling is experienced). The pads are then attached to the body by way of elasticated straps, and fastened (not too tightly) with Velcro. Once the pads are attached, the leads can be inserted into the relevant outlets of the machine, and the appropriate programme selected.

Prior to turning the machine on, the client should be informed of what to expect. Initially, at low intensity, a tingling sensation is experienced followed by relaxation (the stimulation–interval cycle). As the intensity increases, the muscles begin to tighten (isometrically contract). The duration of the

> **TIP**
>
> Never switch the EMS machine on without first checking that all dials are set to zero.

contraction depends on the stimulation time that has been set. Similarly, the duration of the relaxation or interval phase that follows is also predetermined by the therapist. During the stimulation phase, the intensity of each pad can be individually and slowly increased to a comfortably level. The master gain (intensity control) can be used to lift and reduce the overall intensity. Once all pads have been adjusted to suit the objectives of the treatment, the client may have a blanket, or towels, placed over them, to keep them warm. To enhance the effect of the treatment, and especially in the case of injury rehabilitation, the client can be instructed to perform active isometric contractions in conjunction with the stimulation phase of the cycle.

> The stimulation period must be long enough for the muscle fibres to be stimulated and shorten. The interval period must be of a sufficient duration to allow all the muscle fibres to relax and lengthen or muscle fatigue will occur. A client with poor muscle tone or excessive adipose tissue will require longer stimulation and relaxation periods to achieve a full contraction of the muscle fibres being stimulated.
>
> LORRAINE NORDMANN, LORRAINE APPLEYARD AND PAMELA LINFORTH (2001)

Do not overwork the muscles. Providing a relatively short treatment time of 5 minutes (for injuries), 10 minutes (for older or unfit clients) and 20 minutes (for fit clients) at their first session is often the safest policy. If there are no adverse reactions, then consecutive sessions can be gradually intensified, rising to a maximum of 40 minutes per session. For optimal results, treatments are typically provided three to five times per week, for four to six weeks. Some units incorporate an automatic warm-up and cool-down phase into the programme. At the end of the treatment

| TIP | |

Make sure that antagonist muscles (those opposite to the ones requiring stimulation) are not padded up. Muscles cannot perform two opposite movements at the same time.

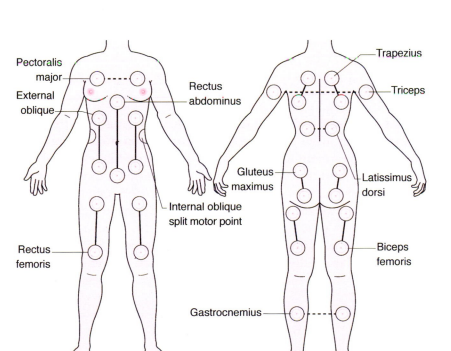

-------- Split motor point   ——— Longitudinal

Sample padding techniques to anterior and posterior body

session, the intensity of stimulation should be reduced only during the relaxation phase to reduce possible discomfort, and the machine should be switched off before the pads are removed. Be careful to avoid tangling the many cables that supply the pads. It is good practice to offer manual massage treatment to help recovery and dispersal of metabolic waste products (post-event style). After use, the pads and straps should be cleaned in antiseptic solution, and sanitized in an ultraviolet sterilizing cabinet.

TENS

Transcutaneous electronic nerve stimulators (TENS) are similar in many ways to portable EMS units. Typically comprising a small hand-held, battery operated (portable) unit, featuring intensity, frequency and mode controls, which send electrical signals to either one or two pairs of strategically positioned pads, TENS is mainly used to help control pain. TENS may be selected to operate with either a high or low frequency, depending upon the therapeutic approach.

High frequency is the conventional TENS approach, where the objective is to inhibit incoming messages of pain via the activation of additional (electronically produced) sensory messages, which are designed to override the individual's pain and 'close the pain gate'. The electrode pads are typically placed over either side of the area of pain, the experience for the client should be a mild to moderate tingling sensation, and no muscle contraction should occur. It is not inconceivable to recommend treatment times of 30–60 minutes at a time, possibly several times per day, in early attention to severe cases.

Low-frequency (higher-intensity) TENS is often described as being acupuncture-like TENS (AL-TENS). This approach can produce a stronger 'pricking-type' sensation, and is typically used to treat acupuncture and trigger points, or along the dermatome in which pain may be referred. The treatment times for the AL-TENS approach tend to be shorter than for conventional TENS. Both high- and low-intensity TENS have been shown to cause the release, within the CNS, of the body's opiate-like pain-reducing chemicals (enkephalins and endorphins), through various pathways of reaction. Often, when pain reduction is a main objective, it can be worthwhile to experiment with both high and low frequencies in an effort to identify which is most effective for the individual concerned.

Sports therapists may like to be able to recommend TENS to clients who are suffering from long-term pain, such as that resulting from a worsening arthritis or a frozen shoulder, but they should remember that its use requires that clients are aware of all safety issues, including knowledge of such contra-indications as pacemakers, nerve and circulatory disorders, epilepsy, superficial skin lesions, and adverse reactions to the treatment. Certainly, a client should never be treated for the pain of something that the therapist does not recognize or understand, and medical approval is strongly recommended in these instances.

CHAPTER SUMMARY

It can be seen from this chapter that the sports therapist is able to select items from a wide range of equipment to offer their clients different treatments, and the best chance of optimal recovery from injury. Obviously, any form of treatment, whether manual or electrical, needs to be tailored specifically to the individual, and this particularly involves selecting the correct intensities, frequencies and durations. The main reason for labouring the health and safety aspects relating to electrical treatments is simply because there is a much greater potential for harm to be caused with these treatments than with manual methods.

Electro-massage can offer great benefits for both the client and therapist. Massage machines can be time and labour-saving, and offer their own specific therapeutic benefits, but they are more impersonal and sometimes cumbersome, and can depreciate the therapist's hands-on skills. The simple use of cold and heat to improve health really is an important aspect of sports therapy. It can be seen that cryotherapy is most useful for acute injuries, while thermal therapy is best in the intermediate and later stages of injury rehabilitation. Ultrasound, which offers both thermal and non-thermal (mechanical) effects, can be used in early and late stages of repair, but only by those trained to do so. EMS is useful for muscle rehabilitation and postural retraining, and TENS is widely used to help control pain.

General over-reliance on equipment is not a good way for the sports therapist to practise, but having the right equipment available (well-maintained and correctly operated so as to supplement your main skills) can be a definite advantage.

Knowledge Review

1 List ten general but crucial safety factors relating to the use of electrical therapy equipment.

2 What are the main advantages and disadvantages of using electro-massage machines?

3 What are the main safety issues regarding the use of cryotherapy?

4 Describe the sensations typically experienced during a cryotherapy treatment.

5 What are the main potential effects and benefits of thermal therapy?

6 Describe how thermal sensation can be tested, and explain why it is an important procedure.

7 List ten methods of applying therapeutic heat treatment.

8 Describe how ultrasound therapy may be used to produce thermal or non-thermal effects, what its main indications for use are, and its main safety issues.

9 What are the main differences between EMS and TENS?

WEBSITE @

Visit the companion website at www.thomsonlearning.co.uk/healthandfitness/ward where you will find the answers to these questions for you to check your progress through the book.

chapter 11

TAPING AND STRAPPING TECHNIQUES

Learning Objectives

After reading this chapter you should be able to:

- develop knowledge of indications, objectives and applications of taping and strapping techniques
- identify important equipment required for safe and effective taping
- develop practical skills of taping for a selection of therapeutic objectives

Athletic taping or bracing used along with a treatment protocol is an excellent tool to assist an injured athlete's return to an activity while not placing him or her at a greater risk for injury. Tape that is applied improperly or for no specific purpose may predispose an athlete to an injury or add to the severity of an existing injury.

THOMAS A. FRETTE AND THOMAS J. REILLY (IN MELLION 1994)

Therapeutic taping, bandaging, strapping and supporting play an important role in sports injury treatment, rehabilitation and prevention. In first aid situations, bandaging can help prevent unwanted movements of injured musculo-skeletal structures, such as suspected joint dislocations, subluxations or bone fractures. Additionally, bandaging is used to compress soft-tissues so as to help reduce the degree of acute swelling, or prevent loss of blood. These are temporary measures used to protect injured tissues from any further aggravation until medical attention is provided.

In rehabilitation settings, taping, strapping or other supportive measures are used to restrict or completely immobilize joint movements. This typically allows the client to perform controlled, progressively remedial exercises without aggravating the injury. Taping is also used to help improve proprioception and soft-tissue-related biomechanical problems. Ultimately, the goal of rehabilitation taping is to assist the athlete with a faster return to activity.

Taping and strapping are also widely used to help prevent re-injury, or help prevent new injury. Some taping rituals are quite normal prior to participation in certain sports, such as rugby, football and boxing.

Whether for acute injury, minor biomechanical malalignment or a chronic problem, taping and strapping can be used whenever there is a need to add support and stability, but there must be a purpose to a tape job, as taping just for the sake of taping can itself be a cause of injuries.

TAPING, STRAPPING AND OTHER SUPPORTIVE EQUIPMENT

In order to minimize confusion, it is necessary to identify just what is meant by the following key terms: bandaging; taping; strapping; bracing; orthotics; supports.

Bandaging

Bandaging is the special piece of material used to cover a dressed wound, or offer acute support to an injured joint, such as a sling.

Taping

The terms taping and strapping are often used interchangeably, but for convenience, we shall take taping to be the use of adhesive rolls of tape, whether elasticated or non-elasticated, permeable to air, water resistant, hypoallergenic or tearable. Tapes come in a variety of different materials and a selection of widths for different jobs. They are usually perforated so that strips can be easily torn off by hand. Some people are adversely reactive to some kinds of tape (or the adhesive); therefore, if taping is still considered important, it will be worth trying a specially formulated zinc oxide or other low-allergy adhesive tape, perhaps combined with an astringent application, which can help reduce the degree of skin irritation.

Strapping

Strapping (or wrapping), therefore, is the application of non-adhesive straps (or wraps), which may also be elasticated or non-elasticated (in strapping for sports or rehabilitation, the straps are usually elasticated). Strapping may be performed with or without the use of adhesive tape, and straps may or may not feature mechanisms for tightening up (e.g. belt buckle type; clip; Velcro). Straps are generally made from a cloth material, and they may be purpose built (specifically designed for particular applications, specific joints, different sized people, etc.), or simply different sized straight rolls for general applications. The special types of protective equipment used in some competitive sports, such as American football or rugby, often incorporate straps into their design. Strapping is also often an integral part of a support device.

Bracing

A brace (or splint) is a specially designed strong support for a joint. They tend to classified as being preventative (prophylactic), functional or rehabilitative. A preventative brace is designed to restrict potentially harmful movement that might be a cause for concern in a particular sport (the collateral knee ligaments are the most commonly protected in this way). Functional braces are designed to allow training to take place, but keep problematic joints to a relatively safe range of motion, and are often used by athletes with some instability (commonly, it is the anterior cruciate ligaments of the knee and the lateral ligaments of the ankle that are offered this kind of support). Rehabilitation braces are usually used following reconstructive joint surgery, and they will offer either complete immobilization (at a predetermined angle) or restriction to a full range of movement, plus they can provide a good deal of protection from unwanted direct forces. Braces are often very technical pieces of equipment, made from a combination of materials, including moulded plastic, metal framework, cloth straps and foam cushioning. The more complex devices may be very finely adjustable, allowing good control of degrees of positioning or movement. Most bracing procedures are usually based on the recommendation of an orthopaedic consultant or physiotherapist. Preventative braces are sometimes used as an alternative to standard protective taping and strapping for sports. They can work out less expensive in the long run, and also may be applied by the player themselves.

Orthotics

Braces are sometimes seen as being orthotic devices, but in sports therapy, orthotics tend be regarded as shoe inserts, designed to help correct, control or support problematic foot motion. These are either semi-rigid or flexible, and are normally custom-made from a mould, although over the counter orthotics are available. Rubber heel pads or cups are also very useful, especially for absorbing heel strike impact (helpful for plantar fascitis, bursitis and heel spurs) or relieving stress on an inflamed Achilles tendon. There are a selection of common athletic problems that can respond to the regular use of orthotics. These include: over-pronation; leg length discrepancy; Achilles tendinosis; heel shear and shock; pes planus; periostitis (shin splints); lower back pain. The measuring for and preparation of custom-made orthotics are specialist skills requiring appropriate training. A biomechanist, podiatrist (chiropodist) or physiotherapist specializing in such procedures should be sought when it is felt that custom-made orthotics will be helpful.

Supports

A support is a specially designed piece of equipment that offers support to a particular body region for a specific purpose. It is typically made from thickly woven slightly elasticated cloth. The support required might be to help restrict certain movements, to help keep a body region warm (heat

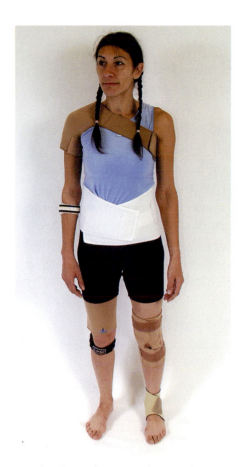

A selection of supportive equipment

retainer) or to help stabilize a body area. They may be specifically recommended by an orthopaedist, physiotherapist, coach or sports therapist, or they may be simply bought over the counter by the player themselves. They are typically worn only during activities that may stress weakened or recovering problems. Over-reliance on supports should be avoided, if possible, as the emphasis should be more on active strengthening and general fitness training for sports, in combination with appropriate treatment. Well-designed support products are now affordably available for most problematic body regions (e.g. lumbar; sacral; shoulder; elbow; wrist; knee; ankle).

There are quite a lot of important items of equipment used in the process of providing effective therapeutic taping and strapping, much of which is one-use only and disposable, which means that it can be quite expensive, and clinical supplies need regular checking and restocking.

Recommended basic taping and strapping equipment

- Bandage scissors (household scissors are too dangerous).
- Tape cutters (specially designed to access tape already applied to the skin).

TIP

Tapes are usually available in different grades. The heavier and more expensive tapes contain a greater number of longitudinal and vertical cloth fibres, making them more able to cope with the demands of physical movement.

TIP

Elastic tape conforms to the contours of the body, and allows for normal tissue expansion. It is used mainly to support and compress muscles, and, when adhesive and applied unstretched, it can be used to provide anchor strips.

TIP

Non-elasticated tape can be used to: support non-contractile structures such as ligaments; restrict joint movements; provide protection against re-injury; reinforce elasticated tape.

- Zinc oxide adhesive, non-elastic tape (several widths, 3.75 cm probably being the most useful).
- Adhesive, non-elastic tape (several widths, from 1.5 to 10 cm).
- Adhesive, elastic tape (several widths, 2.5 and 7 cm being the most useful).
- Cohesive tape (useful because it adheres to itself and not the skin, is quick to apply, and is reusable).
- Underwrap tape (a thin polyurethane foam material, adds padding and protection, and reduces amount of adhesive contact with the skin).
- Heel and lace pads (thin foam squares, positioned over areas vulnerable to friction and blisters, such as the dorsum of the foot).
- Padding made of surgical felt, cotton wool or foam rubber (to fill out uneven regional contours, or to create localized compression to affected tissues, e.g. a cut-out 'horseshoe' for the ankle).
- Astringent skin preparation (can help prevent irritation, ensure that the taping stays in place, and makes its removal easier).
- Lubricating ointment, such as petroleum jelly (for reducing friction over sensitive areas such as: Achilles tendon; dorsum of foot; popliteal space; cubital space).
- Gauze squares (lubricating ointment can be applied to the gauze, by a spatula, and then placed over the sensitive area).
- Adhesive spray (strengthens the tape job, helping underwrap, pads or tape to adhere to the skin more easily, also useful in humid or wet conditions).
- Tweezers (useful for aligning taping components).
- Tape remover, typically a (dehesive) spray (helps make tape removal more comfortable by dissolving adhesive). Specialized wipes are also available to aid in the removal of adhesive residue.

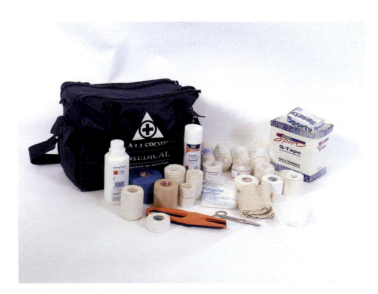

A selection of taping equipment

TAPING AND STRAPPING: SAFETY ISSUES

There are many safety issues relating to the use of therapeutic taping, not least the various contra-indications to the techniques. Common contra-indications include: skin infections (e.g. warts; dermatitis); skin injury (e.g. burns; cut); abnormal skin sensations; active inflammation or joint swelling (gentle, preferably elasticated, compression may be appropriate); allergy to taping materials; conditions where a more aggressive form of stabilization is required; when taping may adversely affect a medical condition (e.g. circulatory disorders).

- Assess the region thoroughly before deciding that taping is the most appropriate intervention.
- Be sure of the therapeutic objectives.
- Be aware of all possible contra-indications.
- Do not use adhesive tape directly on acute injuries.
- Store all taping materials hygienically in a dry, cool place (rolls of tape are best stored standing on their ends).
- Check for allergy to tape, adhesive spray and adhesive remover.
- Do not tape over an area that has been iced (the tissues may increase in size as they warm up) or heated (tissues may diminish as they return to normal).
- Prepare the area of skin to be taped (wash, dry and shave hairy skin, and apply a mild astringent).
- Take care to make sure that the tape job is neat, free of wrinkles, not stretched tightly over skin and comfortably supportive. If it is not right, make it so.
- Never completely encircle a limb with non-elastic tape (keep in mind that muscles must have room to contract and relax).
- Avoid excessive tightness (firm, not tight).
- Be careful to not tape tightly over bony prominences.
- Always check for comfort and circulation following taping application (pinch toes to check for return of colour).
- Do not keep taping on for long periods, and no longer than two or three days (remove tape immediately after training).
- Take great care when removing tape (use tape remover; cut through layers of tape with tape cutters; pull the tape back on itself slowly, rather than 'ripping it off' quickly).
- Clean the area with antiseptic wash after tape removal.
- Do not encourage premature return to activity.
- Discourage over-reliance on taping.
- Always follow conventional approaches.
- Offer after-care advice to the person receiving the taping (e.g. recommend tape removal if abnormal skin reactions or swelling are observed).
- If in doubt about whether to tape, don't!

TIP

The effectiveness of taping reduces over a short period of time, as the chances of skin problems increase (the skin can become macerated – softened and degenerated).

TAPING TECHNIQUES AND APPLICATIONS

There are a variety of taping indications, applications and approaches. In sports therapy, taping is commonly used to: place injured tissues into a pain-relieving position; support torn ligaments (taped into a slightly shortened position); support injured muscles (limiting their full stretch); support injured tendons (usually taped into shortened positions); offer proprioceptive input; prevent injury to vulnerable structures. Most applications of taping attempt to take any possible harmful stress off injured tissues, allowing the body's natural healing activity to occur and continue without too much interruption (obviously this process is stimulated by the use of other therapeutic interventions). With taping, one particular objective can theoretically be approached in a number of different ways, for example there are a variety of ways in which the lateral collateral ligaments of the knee can be taped, as there are a variety of different tapes that can be used. The job of the taper is to provide a taping technique that is comfortable and effective, and their choice of application should depend upon what they have been taught and practised. It has been said that it can take up to 50 practice attempts at one particular tape job before professional competence is achieved.

Proprioceptors (specialized sensory nerve cells) convey messages relating to minute changes in musculo-skeletal position during movement. Proprioceptive exercise is an important part of the rehabilitation of most sporting injuries, as it will encourage optimal muscle response, co-ordination and balance. Taping can provide an additional proprioceptive input (proprioceptive taping). As the body senses the external support (the taping), the individual's conscious awareness of the injured area increases. This increased awareness means that the individual will tend to avoid movements and situations that may further stress the area.

As a general rule of thumb, the larger the body part, the wider the tape that is used (and vice versa). Remember that many non-elastic tapes can be split, by hand or scissors, down the middle to make a thinner strip. Most localized tape jobs do not feature a continuous winding approach (exceptions are when using wide, elasticated, non-adhesive tape), rather, strips of tape are used to create the correct accurate effect. These strips, which are cut (or torn) to appropriate lengths, are overlapped and applied to fit the natural contours of the body part.

When applying several strips of tape over one particular area, there should be a degree of overlap (usually half the tape width) to reduce the possibility of gaps (and the likelihood of skin irritation) and to increase the strength of the support.

Tape anchors are those strips of tape that are firstly applied to the skin, strategically so that the additional strips can be applied more effectively (usually above and below the main focus area). Anchor strips are normally made from elasticated, adhesive tape, and they do not usually completely encircle a limb, unless applied with very little tension. Anchors help to minimize traction on the skin, and they should be applied without any

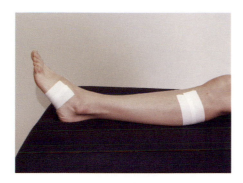

Anchor strips for ankle taping

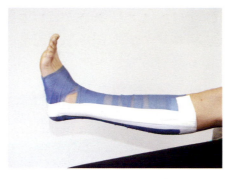

Ankle stirrups, overlying underwrap and anchors

additional tension. Support strips (stirrups) help to restrict lateral movements, and are typically 'U-shaped' loops which are applied more tightly on the affected side of a joint.

Horizontal (transverse) strips provide general stability across the affected joint. Vertical strips, which restrict sideways movements, are applied under tension from the distal anchor to the proximal anchor, typically travelling from the medial to lateral aspect of the joint and vice versa. Check-reins are (typically three) vertical strips applied, over foundational layers, at angles of 10–45° to each other (like a cross, with a vertical line in the middle), and these tend to be used to restrict complete functional extension of joints (such as at the knee or elbow). Reinforcing strips provide extra strength to specific areas, usually when laid onto elastic tape. Compression strips, which are elastic and applied in short stretched pieces, are similar. They are placed over underlying layers of underwrap and low-tension elastic tape and apply focused pressure over a muscular injury site; they should be repeatedly overlapped several times, still working horizontally distal to proximal. The tension of compression strips should be released at the end of the strip.

Heel locks provide support to the subtalar and ankle joints, and usually two overlapping heel locks are applied. A figure of eight pattern can be applied by using a continuous wrap of adhesive, non-elastic tape around a joint to offer extra stability to the job, and to cover any remaining open areas.

Lock (closing) strips, which are applied under little tension, are used to secure the ends of elasticated tape (which can tend to peel away), and neatly finish the tape job.

> **TIP** ✔
>
> Elasticated tape should be allowed to recoil a little before sticking down the last 2–3 cm unstretched.

> **TIP** ✔
>
> A sequence of two alternately angled strips applied over each other, in an overlapping manner, is known as a basket weave pattern.

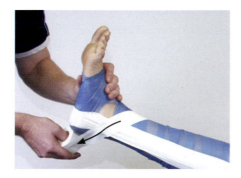

Heel lock 1

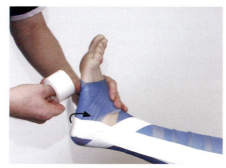

Heel lock 2

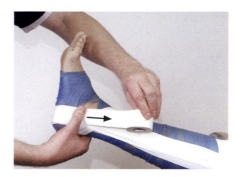

Heel lock 3

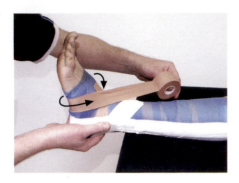

Figure of 8 around the lateral ankle 1

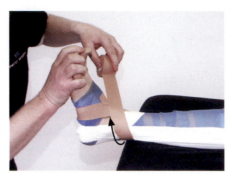

Figure of 8 around the lateral ankle 2

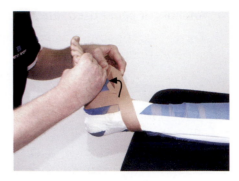

Figure of 8 around the lateral ankle 3

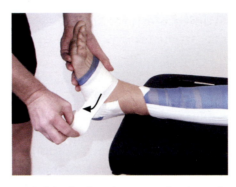

Lock (closing) strips over the lateral ankle 1

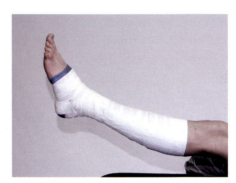

Lock (closing) strips over the lateral ankle 2

Typical adhesive taping process

1 The sports therapist should have all necessary materials prepared and to hand, and, prior to providing any form of taping or treatment, must assess the client and discuss and agree on the objectives. If the client is suitable for a tape job, then the particular application should be thought through and planned. Keep in mind all safety points.

2 Prepare the correct type, width and amount of tape for the job in hand.

3 The therapist and the athlete or client should both be comfortably positioned, so as to minimize unnecessary fatigue or discomfort.

4 The affected region should be washed, shaved of hair and dried.

5 Ensure that the affected structures are in a shortened position (this position may need to exaggerated). It can be awkward for the therapist to apply the tape while at the same time holding the region in a shortened position (the client can assist by holding the region with a belt or length of resistance band).

6 If being used, apply astringent and adhesive spray to the affected region. Lubrication can be applied to gauze squares or special pads over areas of friction or sensitivity. Pressure pads may also be applied to specific sites. Underwrap, when used, goes under adhesive tape, and this can help reduce skin irritations.

7   Anchors, if being used, are the first strips of tape to be applied.

8   Further, overlapping strips are applied so as to neatly cover and support the region.

9   Cohesive tape may be applied if conditions are wet, to help prevent adhesive tape from coming away.

10 Explain how it should feel, ask the client how it feels, and then ask them to try some simple functional movements, similar to what they are intending to do.

11 Check for impaired circulation, and if all seems okay, the job is done.

12 Explain what reactions would necessitate a swift removal of the tape, and explain about how the taping must be removed either immediately after training or competition, or at least after two or three days anyway.

With taping, most joints can be approached in a variety of ways, and the method selected will depend upon the particular nature of the problem, the technical skills of the therapist and the taping materials available. A tape job can in some instances be a very simple, straightforward and effective procedure (e.g. 'buddy' taping of the fingers; one strip patella realignment taping; basic cohesive figure of eight around the ankle). Most applications of taping for rehabilitation purposes, however, can involve a series of intricately patterned layers of different types of tape. Skill in application comes only with repeated practice.

The regions most commonly in need of supportive measures related to sports activities are the foot, ankle, knee, hip, shoulder, lower back, elbow, wrist and hand. The knee joint is a particularly vulnerable joint, and often a tape job is required to support damaged ligaments. A similar joint in basic structure (hinge) to the knee, is the elbow, and several similar taping approaches can be applied to both these joints (e.g. to restrict full movement; to support injured ligaments; to provide gentle compression to muscular strains).

Medial collateral knee ligaments can be taped with the client standing with their knee placed in a slightly varus and flexed position. The taping incorporates: proximal and distal anchors; lubricated pads over hamstring

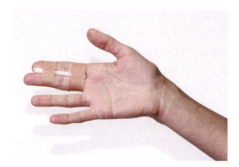

Buddy taping of the fingers. Place a pad between the two fingers, and apply non-elastic adhesive tape above and below the affected joint

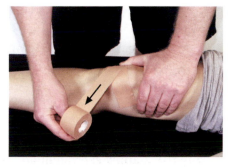

Patella realignment strips. Indicated for patella maltracking and vastus medialis re-education, using non-elastic tape

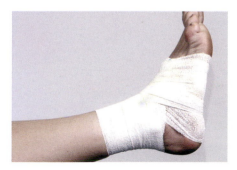

Cohesive figure of eight wrap around the lateral ankle

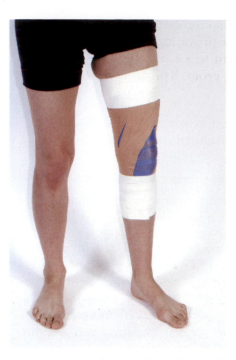

Taped support for medial collateral knee ligaments

tendons; underwrap; several vertical and reinforcing strips to support medial collateral ligament; posterior cross reins to limit full extension; lock strips to finish the job.

Non-adhesive, elasticated wraps are useful for providing support to larger areas, and they are washable and reusable. There are several styles of strapping using this material. In some instances, a wrap can be applied over adhesive tape to offer comprehensive support, but they can as well be very effective when used on their own. Often, once in position, wraps are overlaid with adhesive elastic or non-elastic tape which then provides even greater stability. It is usual to put the affected area into a shortened position with muscular contraction so as not to impede functional contractions or circulation once the tape has been applied.

When using wraps, the techniques tend to incorporate a continuous wrapping of the affected area, and the strapping may be in either a circumferential or spica pattern (see below). When beginning any wrap job, you should start distal to the injury and finish proximal, lifting tissues up a little against the gravitational pull, this helps to reduce the occurrence of swelling. The wrap should be stretched as it is applied to the skin (but not to its full potential length). A wrap may be secured by tucking it in on itself or with elasticated adhesive tape. As with other taping approaches, the wrapping should overlap itself by half a width.

Circumferential (circular) wrapping refers to the basic wrap around method which can be used to simply support a large muscle area such as the quadriceps or hamstrings following a strain, or it may be a component of a more detailed taping approach. A spica wrap is a method that wraps around two adjacent body areas to secure and support a region between the

TIP

Taping should normally reinforce the body's supportive structures, in their shortened, relaxed position.

two. It is characteristically, a continuous looping technique, in a figure of eight pattern, that can be most effective for providing gentle compression and support as well as restricting movement to a safe range. Spica wraps are commonly used to support a shoulder, groin, hamstring or thumb strain or sprain.

TIP

The taping of muscles, to restrict stretching, cannot protect against the possibility of muscular strain from strong contraction.

CHAPTER SUMMARY

Most sports injuries will heal more quickly if they are given the opportunity to do so without being continually aggravated. Because it is virtually impossible to rest an injured structure completely, so as to enable healing to occur, the use of additional support in the form of taping, wraps, braces and other methods allows protected (preferably controlled) activity to be performed. Not only does such support offer protection from an injury worsening, but it will also allow, in many cases, progressive rehabilitation exercise to be undertaken and also general fitness to be maintained. There are also arguments for the preventative benefits that the specific and regular supporting of vulnerable structures, for particular sporting activities, can offer. For various reasons, there are a number of safety issues pertaining to therapeutic taping and strapping, and the sports therapist must be familiar with all of these, not least the various contra-indications, skin reactions and important safety aspects to the techniques themselves.

Sports therapists involved in the delivery of sports injury management should have knowledge and understanding of the different types of support available, and of which particular method is most appropriate for their client. This will include selecting from a choice of manual taping and strapping methods, over the counter elasticated supports, or specialized braces and orthotic devices.

Knowledge Review

1 Why are taping and strapping skills important for the sports therapist to develop?

2 What is meant by the following terms: (i) taping, (ii) strapping, (iii) bracing, (iv) orthotics, (v) supports?

3 What are the basic items of equipment required to provide therapeutic taping?

4 Describe the key safety issues relating to taping and strapping.

5 What is the purpose of the following: (i) anchor strips, (ii) underwrap, (iii) stirrups, (iv) compression strips, (v) cohesive wrap, (vi) spica wrap?

6 Describe when and how adhesive tape should be removed.

WEBSITE

Visit the companion website at www.thomsonlearning.co.uk/healthandfitness/ward where you will find the answers to these questions for you to check your progress through the book.

chapter 12

REMEDIAL EXERCISE TECHNIQUES

Learning Objectives

After reading this chapter you should be able to:

- understand the basic effects and benefits of exercise
- recognize the main safety issues relating to exercise
- prepare for and provide fitness training programmes
- develop knowledge of rehabilitation exercise
- recognize commonly used exercise equipment
- develop knowledge of relaxation exercises

Good or great fitness, ability, performance, looks, energy, health, strength, suppleness, endurance, well-being: these are all things that many of us strive for. Probably what springs to most people's minds when thinking of sports therapy is fitness, exercise and keeping well. It is so well accepted now that exercise is good for us that it can no longer be denied. Exercise can offer an increased activity performance combined with a greatly reduced chance of suffering many kinds of ill-health – you may even enjoy a longer life. The sports therapist is the professional expert to whom exercisers can turn to for professional help and advice.

The subject of remedial exercise is large. Wherever there are targets or objectives to achieve, from reducing body fat, through to improving sporting performance or rehabilitating injuries, and whenever exercise is the key intervention for any of these processes, it can be considered as being remedial. The aim of remedial exercise is to solve or improve upon a wide variety of problems.

Physical fitness may be defined variously as being: the ability to comfortably perform particular physical tasks; the ability to carry out daily tasks without undue fatigue; the ability to function well under exercise conditions; the capability of the cardio-respiratory and muscular systems to function at optimum efficiency.

TIP

Exercise can be defined as the carrying out of considered and considerable physical effort as a means to maintain or improve health and fitness.

Physical fitness in the sporting context is difficult to define since it can refer to psychological, physiological or anatomical states of the body. To most physical education teachers it is seen as a concept obtained by measuring and evaluating a person's state of fitness by using a battery of tests.

R.J. DAVIS, C.R. BULL, J.V. ROSCOE AND D.A. ROSCOE (1991)

Physical fitness, however, is only a part of what has been termed total fitness, which is really the ability of the individual to respond to the many demands of the environment. Total fitness includes physical, nutritional, medical, mental, emotional and social fitness. Being physically fit, therefore, does not necessarily mean being healthy. A typical definition of health is one that describes the situation of being relatively well, and free of illness. It is quite normal to describe an individual's state of health as being either very good, very poor or somewhere in between.

As sports therapists, we need to consider more the individual's health in the present tense (i.e. their current state of health), so that we can help to take it forward. Unfortunately, there are no long-term irrefutable diagnoses for anyone's health. Illnesses or injuries can develop, without warning at any time, for all manner of causes within, or externally from the environment. All we can ever do is consider the presenting facts, and encourage and practise healthy, or healthier, behaviours. As we know, for example, that smoking, excess alcohol, obesity and high stress are bad for our health (and fitness), and to be avoided, we also know that a nutritionally balanced diet, sufficient rest time and regular exercise are good for us, and should be encouraged.

The following factors affect total health and fitness:

- genetics and heredity
- previous and current illness, injury, disability and medications
- education, influences, experiences, knowledge and cognition
- emotional health (confidence; motivation; stability; contentment; personal relationships)
- occupation
- hobbies and interests
- body awareness
- body composition
- exercise history and training methods
- cardio-vascular endurance
- muscular strength, endurance and power
- mobility and flexibility
- co-ordination, balance, speed, timing, reaction, rhythm, agility and skill
- recovery, rest and relaxation time
- diet and nutritional status
- smoking, alcohol and recreational drug use
- utilization of medical care, preventative and remedial treatments and advice
- environment, facilities and resources (domestic; working; sporting; community)

TIP	

In order to attain a high level of physical fitness, the individual must train regularly, appropriately and sufficiently vigorously.

TIP	

The physical fitness achieved through exercising for the main purpose of maintaining and improving aspects of health is correctly termed health-related fitness.

TIP	

Health is typically defined as the state of being well and free from illness.

The health-related components of physical fitness include strength, aerobic endurance, muscular endurance, flexibility and body composition. Skill-related physical fitness includes balance, co-ordination, speed, agility, power and reaction time.

JENNIFER STAFFORD-BROWN, SIMON REA AND JOHN CHANCE (2003)

THE EFFECTS AND BENEFITS OF EXERCISE

The reason that regular exercise training can be so effective for improving health and fitness is because the body has an ability to make adaptive responses. The adaptations that occur are specific to the type of training that is performed regularly. In simple terms, the systems of the body respond specifically and differently to aerobic training, muscular strength, power and endurance training, stability training, flexibility training and specific skill training. This may be further broken down to short-term and long-term adaptations. In the short term, although a newly instigated exercise programme may feel like hard work to some, soon (in just a matter of a few weeks) the exerciser will begin to feel more aware of their body, develop feelings of increased well-being and reduced stress, and their co-ordination, endurance and general ability will begin to improve. Over time, body composition and posture observably improves, as do all components of fitness that are being trained (e.g. strength; power; speed; flexibility; cardio-vascular endurance).

The general benefits of regular well-structured exercise are:

- It promotes good health.
- It helps prevent ill-health.
- It enhances mental health.
- It encourages feelings of well-being.
- It maintains and improves fitness.
- It promotes optimal posture, suppleness, strength, endurance and body composition.
- It helps to reduce the severity of certain health disorders.
- It helps to promote the optimal growth and development of children.
- It helps to minimize the deleterious effects of the ageing process.
- It helps to improve the performance of activities of daily living.
- It improves the athletic performance.
- It helps to offset the negative effects of increasingly sedentary lifestyles.
- It helps to reduce the negative effects of stress.
- It fully enhances an holistic approach to healthy living.

Experienced exercisers and athletes know well the benefits, but are usually keen to find ways to improve their fitness. A training routine can be improved and modified in many ways, for example: subtle adjustments to basic technique; altering weekly routines; varying the exercise environment; instigating new training concepts and ideas; incorporating new items of equipment; psychological and motivational approaches; one to one training;

TIP

A high level of skill-related physical fitness is what is required of competitive sportspeople.

TIP

The body will respond positively to a regular well-planned exercise programme. The SAID principle reminds us of the body's Specific Adaptation to Imposed Demands. This means that the type, intensity, frequency, duration and focus of the exercise regularly undertaken will determine in which ways the individual will respond over a period of time.

TIP

Sports scientists analyse the effect of exercise upon the tissues during a particular activity and at periodic intervals in a programme of regular training. They identify and explore the advantageous responses and the detrimental responses of the body to exercise.

training in groups; longer-term cyclical preparation for competitions; skills focusing; introduction of biomechanical and technique analyses; regular fitness testing; working more closely under the guidance of exercise experts.

EXERCISE: SAFETY ISSUES

Perhaps the most important aspect for the sports therapist to consider, when providing and managing exercise and sporting activities, is the prevention of problems (injury prevention strategies are discussed in chapter 5). Main preventative issues to consider are: minimizing the potential for hazards and making the exercise environment as safe as is possible; making sure first aid facilities are available; screening participants for contra-indications prior to involvement; making sure correct exercise and protective equipment are available and functional; ensuring games and competitions are appropriately officiated; making participants aware of signs and symptoms indicating that they should stop exercising.

When gym or personal training programmes are being designed, it is very important to perform a detailed consultation, taking notes on your client's medical history, occupation, lifestyle, and previous and current involvements with exercise and sports. Preferably, a **physical assessment** and fitness test is also provided early on so that all factors can be considered in the preparation of the exercise plan. With exercise classes (such as aerobics or circuits), a very simple **physical activity readiness questionnaire** (PARQ) can be completed prior to participation. The PARQ is a standardized and basic form which aims to help the instructor decide whether the individual is safe to participate, or whether a doctor's approval is required. Similar, but usually more detailed, screening forms are completed when joining a fitness club, and this is an essential process for various health, safety, ethical and legal reasons.

Even well-trained, relatively fit athletes can be subject to a whole host of medically recognized conditions, whether naturally occurring or exercise-induced: heart disorders, hypertension, asthma, immune deficiencies, depression. Simply just by being an athlete, especially a competitive one, the individual can have increased risks for ill-health, particularly the incidence of impact and overuse injuries, strains and sprains is high. All that said, remedial exercise strategies can still be a key part of managing and overcoming such problems.

Exercise addiction and overtraining (which can often be accompanied by eating disorders) are very real problems, especially in these days where exercise is reputed in some quarters to be a cure for almost anything from depression or stress to obesity or physical inadequacy. Unfortunately, some people who turn to exercise to help solve their problems can become obsessed with it, to the point where excessive exercise is to the definite detriment of their health. The sports therapist should always try to be sensitive to the reasoning behind a person's involvement with exercise; after all, everyone has their own reasons, problems, interests and objectives.

TIP

Sports therapists can help people who are unaccustomed to regular exercise by: assessing their current level of fitness; planning an appropriate training programme with their approval and understanding; demonstrating, observing and coaching the correct performance of the selected exercises; monitoring their response during exercise and over a period of time.

TIP

Sports therapists can help to improve the performance of athletes by: assessing the athlete's strengths and weaknesses, goals and objectives; helping to design or improve upon a skills-related programme of training; helping to refine exercise techniques; working on sports-specific skills; working one to one; providing nutritional advice; providing supportive taping and strapping if required; providing sports massage; providing sports injury treatment; providing on-going advice and encouragement.

It is important to encourage safe participation, and this obviously means guiding people towards keeping on the right track with their training. Reinforcing the correct strategies for your client's improvements, even in the short term, should bring about the benefits that they desire, and this must include rest and recovery, or at least easy days.

If we can acknowledge the dangers of exercise alongside all the benefits, then the potential for problems will be greatly diminished.

PRINCIPLES OF EXERCISE AND FITNESS TRAINING

Objectives

Any exercise programme will be more focused, individualized and ultimately more effective if its main objectives have been well identified and defined beforehand, otherwise it will be almost aimless. Therefore, before the client begins their remedial exercise programme, they should spend time with the sports therapist discussing and agreeing upon the achievable objectives. By setting realistic, achievable and relatively short-term targets, the client is much more likely to keep to their training as recommended, and also they stand a better chance of achieving their ultimate, more long-term, objectives.

Overload

Overload, a key training principle, is a term used to describe exercise that is performed at a greater level or intensity than one is normally accustomed to. By overloading the body with particular exercises, beneficial adaptations (improving fitness) can occur. Without incorporating specific overload into training, fitness will **plateau** or simply decline.

Progression

To continually improve upon fitness, the overload placed upon specific body regions and systems must be progressively increased. Progressive overload is the way in which fitness programmes are continually but gradually, over a period of time, modified and intensified so as to accommodate the individual's improving fitness and to take them on to a higher level of performance.

Specificity

All exercise benefits are specific to the type of training performed. For example, a general whole body conditioning type of training routine encourages a very rounded functional level of fitness, whereas more regularly doing only one particular type of training, such as heavy weight-training or distance running, leads the exerciser to having more limited (but specific) fitness benefits. In the gym, exercise can be specific to the body region being worked, and it is relatively straightforward to isolate specific major muscles for strength, endurance or flexibility development. Additionally, exercise should ideally be specific to the level that the individual is at, at any one time; for example, exercise should be specifically tailored to suit the beginner, intermediate, advanced or elite participant.

Reversibility

Fitness training has to be regular, progressive and maintained for improvements to continue to occur. If training becomes less regular or less intensive, or stops altogether, the principle of reversibility becomes very apparent: newly attained adaptations to the training begin to reverse, and fitness levels revert back towards a pre-trained state. The reversible or regression principle is also worth keeping in mind when assisting an individual's return to activity following illness or injury, because they should not be expected to be able to perform at their previous levels.

Intensity

Intensity is how hard someone is working. In strength terms it can be the amount of weight that is being lifted, the amount of repetitions, or the speed or power of the movement. In cardio-vascular terms, it is usual to equate intensity with working heart rates. In order to achieve overload, the intensity (and duration) of exercise are increased.

Duration

Duration relates to amount of time is spent either on one particular exercise or on one particular exercise session. The duration of an exercise is selected relating to the actual intensity of the exercise, and according to the ability of the individual and their required objectives.

Frequency

Frequency relates to the number of training sessions performed per week. In order to maintain and build upon training effects, exercise must be carried out on a regular basis. It is commonly recommended, for health-related benefits, to train at least three to five times per week. Training on consecutive days should be performed with great care so as to not overwork particular regions or systems. Athletes typically train up to six days a week, but their routine will be planned and varied. The frequency of training must incorporate adequate rest and recovery time.

Recovery

If adequate recovery from intense training or competition is not incorporated into the training routine of an athlete, then overuse injuries, excess fatigue, lethargy, impaired performance, direct and indirect injuries and more are all possible. The same goes for those involved in health-related fitness training. It is not difficult to incorporate light training days, alternative types of training and days off into an effective programme, and the importance of doing so should be explained. Recovery time is also important during exercise sessions, as it will allow the body to remove metabolic wastes from worked muscles and replenish their fuel supplies, and also because highly elevated heart rates, related to extreme exertions, cannot be maintained for long periods.

Variance

The basic principle of variance suggests the importance of varying aspects of training so that any potentially deleterious effects resulting from a regular rigorous and vigorous exercise routine are minimized. By varying intensities and approaches, and alternating ways in which different exercises can work the same body regions, the potential for DOMS, exercise-related fatigue, impaired neuromuscular responses, minor injuries, emotive stresses or reducing motivation can be lessened.

Transfer

The transfer concept implies that one learned practical skill can underline, complement or reinforce another. In other words, a transfer of skills may be experienced when practising different manoeuvres, which can be especially useful when training programmes are developed for competitive sports. By employing working applications of transfer and variance, the fitness instructor can keep athletes fit, interested, free of boredom, skilled and co-ordinated.

Repetition

By carefully repeating a movement or action in training the quality of performance of that particular movement (skill) should improve (assuming that it is performed with correct biomechanics). Another aspect to be aware of is the fact that all exercise requires a certain amount of repetitive stress so as to facilitate adaptations and improvements, whether for strength, flexibility or endurance.

Periodization

The periodization principle demonstrates the way in which training programmes can be tailored towards achieving total preparation for optimal performance in competitions. Given that most competitive sports have a

---

TIP

The practice of cross-training (e.g. alternating such activities as cycling, running, swimming or aerobic classes to obtain, maintain and improve cardio-vascular fitness) is a classic modern example of incorporating the useful principles of variance and transfer into a training routine.

competitive season, or at least a series of competitive events spread out over a year, the majority of serious athletes will undertake a well-planned training programme that is designed to prepare them for their main events, so that they are in a peak condition, primed and ready for their best performance, just when it is needed. Periodization typically employs three phases of preparation: a conditioning phase where the emphasis is on working hard to build up a strong level of foundational fitness; a transitional phase where, alongside general conditioning, the athlete focuses on intense skill and technique development; and a competition phase where the focus is on peak performance in competition.

Each sport has different requirements. In football, for example, players undertake pre-season training which will include much general fitness work, working towards regaining match fitness, and incorporating 'friendly' matches. The season that follows is long and arduous (nine months or more, depending upon summer tournaments) and most players can expect to experience peaks and troughs in their match fitness during such a long season (especially in a sport fraught with injury), and will be continually having to work on aspects of their condition. Once the season is over, after a short break of a month or so, the cycle begins again. Other athletes such as elite runners and cyclists are perhaps the best examples of sports performers who periodize their training over one, two or more years, in the case of major championships such as the Olympics.

COMPONENTS OF FITNESS TRAINING

Warm-up

A **warm-up** is all about preparing the body for the more strenuous activities that are to follow. Typically, incorporating low-intensity aerobic activity, safe and easy-range mobility movements and short-duration preparatory stretches, a warm-up for general exercise will normally take about 10–15 minutes. Warm-up for high-level competition may be of longer duration, and involve, in addition to those components previously listed, practice of the specific skills required for the sport and short bursts of power activities, such as short sprints or jumping.

> All exercise sessions should commence with a warm-up period. In some cases this may take the form of a distinct series of preparatory exercises; in other sessions it will simply involve performing the activity at a relatively low intensity to the desired level.
>
> S.R. BIRD, A. SMITH AND K. JAMES (1998)

The warm-up is actually more than just physical preparation. Prior to competitive activity, other aspects to consider include: the weather and temperature; equipment and apparel; psychological preparation; pre-event massage; and familiarity with the location.

During warm-up, at least the following should be undertaken:

- low-intensity, short duration aerobic activities, such as simple walking, easy stepping, cycling, skipping, rebounding, rowing or jogging

- safe-range mobility work, such as shoulder circling, arm and leg flexions and extensions and gentle regional shaking
- preparatory stretching, with short duration holds, not at maximal stretch
- replication of some of the movements that will follow in competitive sports.

The warm-up, featuring a combination of activities, should aim to:

- gradually raise heart and breathing rates
- increase circulation through working muscles
- raise core body temperature
- help to improve the flow of impulses through neuromuscular pathways
- increase lubrication of synovial joints.

Maintenance (aerobic)

In the case of a general fitness training session, especially a contemporary aerobic exercise class, one of the main objectives of the session, following sufficient warm-up, will be to maintain a certain level of intensity and activity during the main (middle) section of the workout. This is a basic cardio-vascular endurance-improving strategy, where it is recommended that a moderate level of typically repetitive but alternating effort be maintained continuously, in any one period, for at least 20 minutes, on a regular basis, so as to gain the required benefits. Not only are great cardio-vascular effects observed, but this type of (aerobic) effort also encourages a more effective metabolic breakdown of body fat.

Cool-down

The **cool-down** is almost as useful as the warm-up. A typical cool-down is aimed at returning the body gradually to its pre-exercising state, and reducing the potential for post-exercise dizziness, fainting or DOMS. It can be shorter in duration than a warm-up, but involves similar types of exercises. Easy walking, jogging or cycling, for example, can be performed for just a few minutes, and this will encourage a more efficient waste product removal, and reduce the possibility of blood pooling distally. The relaxed and longer-duration stretching of main muscles after exercise helps to reduce the severity of muscle stiffness.

During cool-down from strenuous exercise, at least the following should be undertaken:

- low-intensity, short duration aerobic activities
- relaxed stretching, of longer duration.

The cool-down should aim to:

- gradually reduce heart and breathing rates
- help reduce build up of metabolic waste products
- help maintain effective venous return
- help lower elevated core body temperature.

Strength training

One definition of muscular **strength** is the capacity of a muscle or group to exert force, another is the maximal force a muscle or group can exert. Strength training mainly utilizes the anaerobic pathways of energy to provide muscles with their fuel for strenuous contractions. Therefore, because of such factors as the rapid depletion of fuel supplies, the oxygen debt, and the resulting muscle fatigue, there are inherent limitations to the performance of strength-based activities. However, strength is an area that can demonstrate big gains in relatively short periods of time.

Strength is a major component of fitness training as it is a major requirement for most sports. To achieve strength improvements, progressive overload in the form of repetition must be incorporated into the programme. Strength losses, which are often observed in association with muscle **atrophy** (wastage), can occur for several reasons: following injury or immobilization; underuse or disuse; impaired neuromuscular stimulation; restrictive pain; and reciprocal inhibition.

Strength has a direct relationship with the other key fitness components: **muscular endurance**; power; speed; stability; skill. Strength can be developed and measured in a variety of ways. There are three basic types of muscular contraction: isometric; isotonic (concentric and eccentric); isokinetic. Each type of contraction can usually be performed in a variety of ways – (by altering or adapting body positions, by using different items of equipment, or by working closely with a partner or therapist). It is normally easy enough to vary the intensities of strengthening exercise to suit the differing levels of ability and the objectives. Strength testing and assessment help the therapist plan appropriate intensities and approaches for their clients. It is their responsibility to explain and instruct the selected exercises clearly, because it is so easy to injure muscles or joints that are not conditioned to cope with the demands inflicted upon them.

Isometrics and the seven second approach

Isometric training, which should always be recommended with caution for those suffering with hypertension, is mainly used in early and intermediate stage injury rehabilitation programmes because the intensity can be controlled by the individual, and it does not involve any potentially harmful movements of injured joints. The resistance in isometric exercise is angle-specific, which means that the gains achieved are relatively localized to the angle that the working joint is at. One useful way of instructing isometric strength training is to incorporate a 'seven second' approach, which involves seven seconds of contraction, followed by seven seconds relaxation, repeated seven times (i.e. seven repetitions), in one set. The number of sets and rest periods in between, and the actual intensity of each contraction can be adapted to suit the individual's abilities. This approach offers the individual an easy working protocol to follow, in the absence of any moving (isotonic) activity (which in many ways is easier to instruct). The isometric approach can be expanded to include other muscular contractions at different positions throughout the available ranges of movement, which encourage a more comprehensive strengthening.

TIP

Remember! Most exercise activities naturally incorporate a variety of fitness components: strength; endurance; stabilization; power; co-ordination; balance; agility; skill; dynamic flexibility. Although it is important to be able to separate and explain these individual components, it is the 'putting it all together' effectively in practice that really matters.

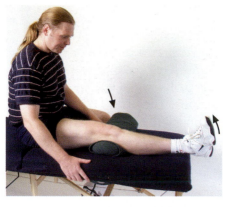

Isometric strengthening of medial quadriceps

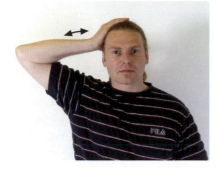

Isometric strengthening of lateral neck flexors

Performing strength exercise with the correct technique is always important, because injuries can occur, either from inappropriate overuse or from excessive overload. The concepts and aspects of demonstration, positioning, coaching and observation, amount of resistance, number of repetitions, number of sets, duration of contractions and correct rhythmic breathing must all be well considered when planning a strength programme, especially for beginners.

Isotonic work

Most strength work tends to be done in the gym, but it can be performed almost anywhere, with minimal equipment. The most common approach to strength training is through **isotonic training**, which involves the shortening and lengthening of muscles against the resistance provided by free weights, weight machines, medicine balls, resistance bands or the individual's own body weight. It is usual, when developing isotonic strength, to identify a weight that can be lifted about 10 or 12 times comfortably, with strenuous exertion but without compromising technique. Each exercise should be experimented with, starting with low weights and gradually adding more, until the suitable exercising weight is found. As fitness improves, the weights can be gradually increased. It is usual to redo the set of repetitions after a short rest period or on a second circuit of the gym. Examples of isotonic exercises include: chest press (pectoralis major); hamstring curl; abdominal curl; heel raise (gastrocnemius and soleus); leg extension (quadriceps); and bicep curl.

There are sports where the total focus is upon strength. Competitive weight-lifting and power-lifting differ from standard strength training, as emphasis is upon being able to lift heavier weights than the other competitors of a particular category. There are a variety of training strategies that are used by weight-lifters to achieve their gains. Typically, the heavier weights are lifted with lower repetitions, but through more sets, and this approach is likely to offer gains in both strength and bulk. Often, weight-lifters in training will make use of a 'spotter', someone who assists the person performing the exercise (typically the gym instructor or sports

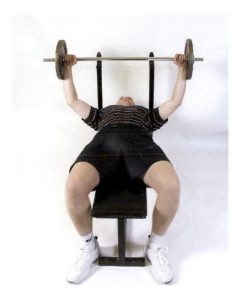

Chest press using free weights

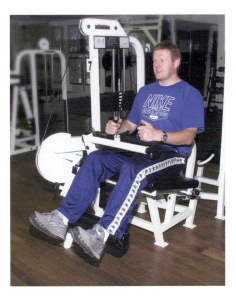

Hamstring curl using resistance machine

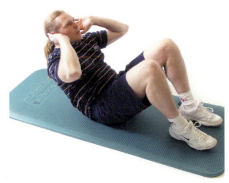

Abdominal curl, lifting own body weight

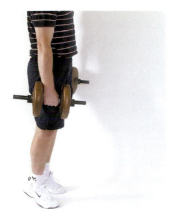

Heel raise, lifting own body weight, plus free weights

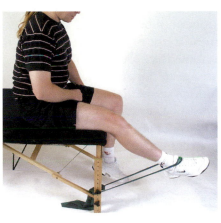

Single-leg knee extension using resistance band

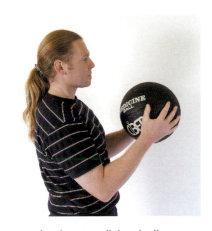

Bicep curl using medicine ball

therapist). The spotter will make sure that their own position is correct (e.g. close to their partner, balanced and prepared position, knee's off lock, back upright, hands ready to grasp and support the bar), and when requested to do so will be able to offer assistance in the lifting of the final (forced) repetitions. Weight-lifters will usually work the lower body and the upper body on different days, which allows for a more efficient recovery.

Compound training is where more than one particular exercise is performed so as to improve the strength gains in one body region (e.g. the chest press, pec dec, flat-bed and incline flyes, dips and press-ups all work the chest muscles). Pyramid training involves starting a particular exercise with relatively light weights, with high repetitions, and working up to lifting heavy weights with lower repetitions.

Some of the principles and approaches employed by weight-lifters can be used by weight-trainers, but unless the individual is particularly motivated by weight-lifting as a sport, weight-training is much the preferable approach, as the emphasis is more on functional strength development and body toning rather than pure maximal strength. There are fewer health or sports-related benefits to heavy weight-lifting, and a far greater potential for injury.

True **isokinetic training** is effectively performed only with specialized (expensive) isokinetic machines, as the resistance for such exercise needs to be constant and adapted through the speed and angle of the contractions applied. It is mainly used for intermediate and late phase rehabilitation work, and in training for sports that require fuller ranges of functional strength, or higher speed contractions such as with swimming or tennis.

Muscular endurance training

Not to be confused with cardio-vascular endurance, muscular endurance is the ability to repeat and maintain arduous muscular efforts for relatively long periods of time. Muscular endurance is obviously an important component of both functional and sporting activities, and if this area of fitness is not properly attended to then the individual can be more susceptible to exertion-related fatigue. In order to develop specific muscular endurance in the gym environment, a relatively higher number of strenuous repetitions should be performed. When weight-training (isotonically) this typically involves identifying the greatest weight that can be comfortably lifted, without strain, for between 12 and 20 repetitions. Improvements in muscular endurance also occur as a result of prolonged speed-based training, such as with run or cycle sprints. In the rehabilitation setting, muscular endurance training poses fewer risks for aggravating injuries than pure strength training, and is very much part of the recovery process. The general benefits of training for muscular endurance includes gains in strength, as well as improved muscle tone, body contours, general and functional conditioning. The risk of injuries from excessive overloading is reduced.

Power training

Muscular **power** is directly related to strength and speed. It is typically associated with performing short bursts of very strenuous activity such as: a sprint start; jumping a distance; throwing a knock-out punch; throwing a projectile (medicine ball; javelin; shot-putt; hammer; discuss; caber); serving an ace in tennis. The foundation for effective power should be built upon a well-structured and vigorous fitness routine, and certainly the athlete should have sufficient strength and flexibility to perform any one particular powerful movement. One way of improving power for particular purposes is to train the particular movement but with an additional resistance, such as a weight, medicine ball or resistance band. Plyometric exercises (plyometrics) are a particular approach to power training that involve rapid sequences of

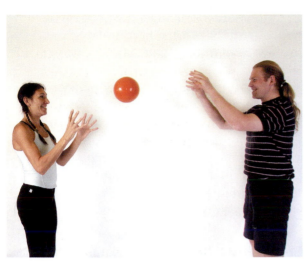

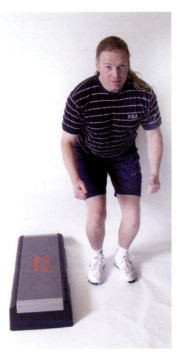

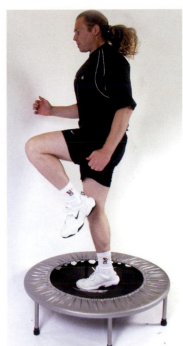

Plyometric power training of the upper body, using a medicine ball

Plyometric power training of the lower body. Lateral (side) jumps on and off or over a step

Rebound training on a mini-trampoline can be a useful method of developing power, while offering reduced impact on the body. Rebound training is also useful during rehabilitation

powerful concentric and eccentric contractions, typically variations of jumping, hopping, bounding and medicine ball tossing. This approach is considered to be explosive, and therefore a potential cause of injuries in itself, and so care should be taken to ensure that the athlete thoroughly warms-up and cools-down, and that surfaces are suitable for safe jumping and landing. Plyometric exercises, which are often worked into circuit classes for general conditioning, should be performed only when the athlete is fully fit, and not more than once or twice per week.

Speed training

Speed is a need of most competitive sports. Speed is developed by strength and power training, by having sufficient functional flexibility and biomechanical leverage, and by optimizing technique (making it more biomechanically efficient). Speed in sports may be needed at various times, such as in a game of cricket, it may be an important component of a technique, such as when throwing a discus, or it may be the prime focus, such as in a 100 m sprint. Being able to respond quickly in sport is so often crucial to the eventual outcome. Speed, therefore involves a rapidly co-ordinated sequence of: observation; processing of information; reaction; activation; and attempted performance of the desired action.

Speed is generally thought of as being anaerobically fuelled, but it should be recognized that 'speed endurance' is an all-important factor in the performance of competitive level aerobic-based activities. Speed training techniques are discussed further with regard to sports-specific training.

Mobility and flexibility training

Ideally, individual mobility and flexibility allow smooth and easy full-range movements without restriction, laxity, instability or pain. Of course, such quality of movement is compromised in the presence of injury, pathology, adaptive soft-tissue shortening (contractures) or congenital bony abnormalities. Assessment and identification of what is considered to be ideal posture, muscle balance, range of motion and gait have been discussed in detail in previous chapters, as have main methods for their improvement. Flexibility, just like any other fitness component, may be defined in both general and specific terms. Certainly, flexibility training must pay a part in all fitness routines, and it is for the sports therapist to be particularly aware of the indications for taking flexibility training beyond the basic injury prevention and recovery strategies (tightness, restriction, muscle imbalance, pain). Additionally, the therapist needs to be able to suggest variations of techniques to suit different clients and indications. It is also important to recognize the precautions and contra-indications to stretching.

It is important to be able to effectively recommend, demonstrate, provide and understand what is meant by: preparatory stretching; maintenance stretching; relaxation stretching; developmental stretching; remedial stretching; active stretching; passive stretching; assisted stretching; static stretching; ballistic stretching; MET stretching; and STR stretching.

Some sportspeople have an idea that flexibility and stretching exercises are time-consuming, boring or even a waste of time (these often tend to be the same people who do not value a warm-up). It is up to the sports therapist to point out the reasons for working on flexibility. Regular and appropriate stretching helps to: prevent injuries; increase functional performance; improve recovery from exertion; encourage relaxation; improve posture; and treat injuries.

There are some stretches which may, in some instances, be employed usefully as part of a well-structured training programme for certain sports, but if performed routinely by novices can cause injury problems. These are commonly referred to as controversial exercises, and a classic example of a controversial stretch is the 'plough' position in yoga, where the individual lies supine and then moves into a position of extreme hip, lumbar and cervical flexion, placing their feet on the floor behind their head. This may be an effective exercise for an experienced yogi or gymnast, but for many this posture places excessive stress on the vertebrae and discs of the neck and back, and should not be routinely recommended. Another possibly controversial exercise is the classic 'hurdler's hamstring stretch' which puts stress on the medial knee joint (as one leg is being stretched, the other leg is flexed outwards, at an angle). Similarly, ballistic stretching may have its place in mobility training for martial arts, and in some pre-event situations, but it should be remembered that it does little to develop flexibility.

The following pages show stretches that are basic examples, the kind that can be encouraged for the majority of clients. There are normally a selection of alternatives available for most muscle groups.

TIP

Normal sports stretching should not cause pain. For both preparatory (before sport) and relaxation (after sport) stretching, the focus should be mainly on the main muscles used in the sport. There are usually a variety of ways of stretching each region of the body.

TIP

Preparatory stretches are part of the warm-up process. They are not taken to an extreme range of motion, and are held for just a few seconds.

TIP

Developmental stretches encourage increased flexibility. They should be relaxed into, and held for 30 seconds or more.

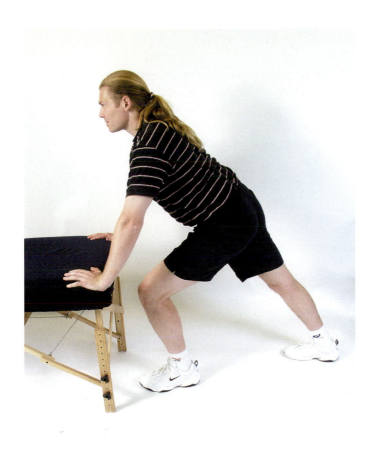

Calf stretch

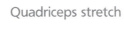

Quadriceps stretch

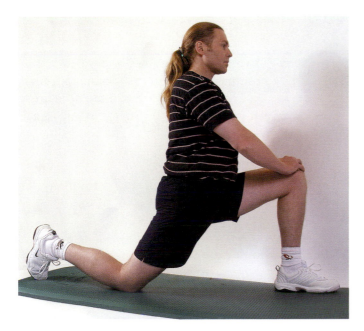

Hip flexor stretch

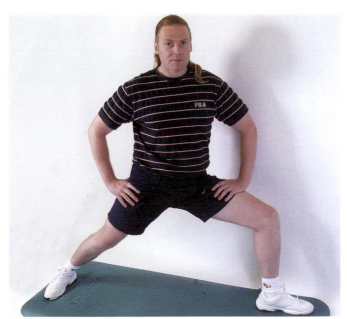

Adductor stretch

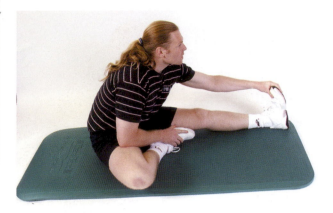

Hamstring stretch

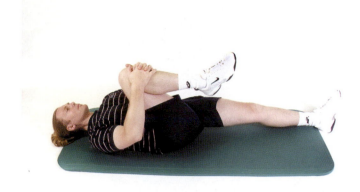

Gluteal stretch

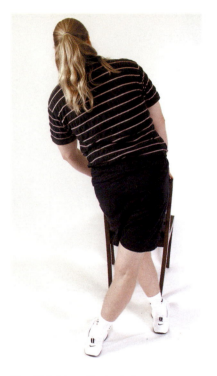

Ilio-tibial band stretch

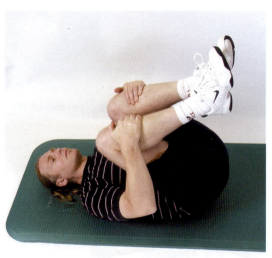

Lower back stretch

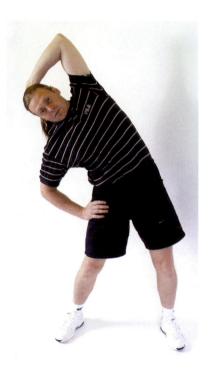

Lateral trunk and shoulder stretch

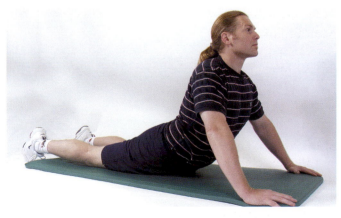

Abdominal stretch

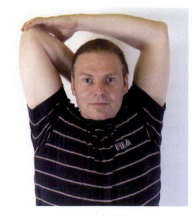

Triceps and shoulder stretch

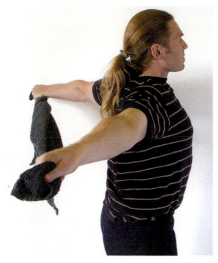
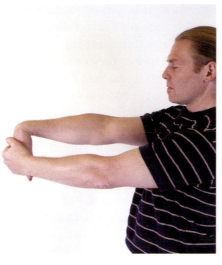
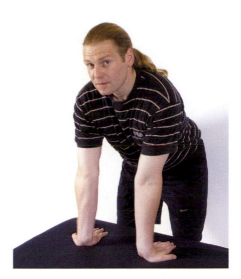

Anterior chest and shoulder stretch   Wrist extensor stretch   Wrist flexor stretch

Cardio-vascular training

Having cardio-vascular (CV) fitness, endurance or stamina is about having the capacity to effectively transport and utilize oxygen and nutrients to working muscles and to remove carbon dioxide, water and other metabolic waste products during exercise. Cardio-vascular training employs use of the aerobic pathway to supply the energy required to perform relatively longer-duration, lower-intensity activities. The development of aerobic fitness in athletes incorporates a variety of strategies, including **interval**, **continuous**, **fartlek** and cross-training (described below), all of which aim to increase the individual's capacity to perform and maintain aerobic-based exercise at a greater intensity. Even though aerobic exercise is associated with longer and slower activities, at competition standard the objective is always to be as fast as possible, and almost any high-level activity involves a combination of aerobic and anaerobic energy supply.

Typical training activities utilizing the aerobic pathway are distance walking, running, cycling, swimming, rowing and 'aerobic' exercise classes. A big part of health-related fitness development is CV endurance, and by training aerobically regularly, there are various potential benefits to be reaped: improved endurance, and increased capacity to exercise without fatigue; improved cardiac, circulatory and respiratory functioning; increased maximal oxygen uptake (aerobic capacity); increased strength of bones; increased anaerobic threshold; and improved potential to reduce elevated blood pressure and excess body fat.

The aerobic capacity of an athlete is measured as their V_{O_2}max: the maximal capability of the cardio-respiratory system to take in, distribute and utilize oxygen, in the working muscles. Various exercise tests are available to assess V_{O_2}max, and these can take the form of precise assessments under maximal exercise stress conditions (which will include specific monitoring of expired gases), or more commonly through predictive assessments, where maximal oxygen uptake is estimated from a submaximal test.

TIP ✔

To ascertain predicted maximum exercising heart rate:

$$220 - age = HR_{max} \text{ (bpm)}.$$

To ascertain target heart rate at 70 per cent of the maximum:

$$220 - age \times 70\% = THR \text{ (bpm)}.$$

For example, a person is 33 years old:

$$220 - 33 = 187 \text{ max HR (bpm)}$$

$$187 \times 70\% = 131 \text{ THR (bpm)}.$$

TIP ✔

Using the Karvonen formula to determine THR at 60 per cent of max:

$$220 - age = HR_{max} \text{ (bpm)}$$

$$HR_{max} - RHR = HRR \text{ (bpm)}$$

$$HRR \times 60\% = A$$

$$A + RHR = THR \text{ (bpm)}.$$

For example, a person is 28 years old, with an RHR of 70 bpm:

$$220 - 28 = 192 \text{ } HR_{max} \text{ (bpm)}$$

$$192 - 70 = 122 \text{ HRR (bpm)}$$

$$122 \times 60\% = 73 \text{ bpm}$$

$$73 + 70 = 143 \text{ THR (bpm)}.$$

TIP ✔

The Borg scale of perceived exertion

6   no exertion
7   very, very light
8
9   very light
10
11   fairly light
12
13   somewhat hard
14
15   hard
16
17   very hard
18
19   very, very hard
20   maximal exertion

In order to gain health-related aerobic benefits, most exercisers should be aiming to maintain a certain intensity of effort for between 20 and 60 minutes at a time (not including warm-up or cool-down), and ideally at least three to five times per week. Awareness of heart rates, especially in the response to exercise intensity, is important to the safe and effective performance of aerobic conditioning. As recommended by the American College of Sports Medicine (ACSM), for the purpose of improving aerobic fitness, an individual's (predicted) maximum heart rate (HR_{max}) is said to be 220 beats per minute (bpm) minus their age (220-age). Once the HR_{max} has been established, a target exercising heart rate can then be determined. The aerobic target heart rates (50–90 per cent of max) are sometimes also referred to as the aerobic 'training zone', which is where the benefits (improved CV endurance, calorie burning, etc.) of working at such a level are most likely to occur. The **target heart rate** (THR) is decided upon in light of all information regarding the exerciser (age; level of ability and fitness; presence or history of ill health; injuries; medical recommendations; exercise objectives). Typically, beginners, or those gradually returning to functional levels of activity, are recommended to work to around 60 per cent of their maximum heart rate. As fitness improves, target rates for general conditioning, can rise to 70 or 80 per cent of the maximum. By monitoring exercising heart rates carefully (with the aid of a heart rate monitor), the potential for danger of working unnecessarily or excessively hard is minimized, and undue stress is not placed on the heart or cardio-respiratory system. Many cardio-vascular machines in gyms now feature a built-in heart rate monitor, and exercisers should have the importance of monitoring heart rates explained to them, have their own THR worked out, and be encouraged to use heart rate monitors. When working out aerobically, the actual intensity of exercise (and therefore the exercising HR) can be increased or decreased simply by altering either or both the speed or resistance.

The '**Karvonen formula**' (heart rate reserve formula) incorporates the **resting heart rate** (RHR) into the THR equation. The heart rate reserve (HRR) is the difference between RHR and HR_{max}, and usefully incorporates an additional individual variable (RHR) to increase the appropriateness of THR. A THR determined from this formula will be higher than one determined from HR_{max} alone. It is important to note that HR_{max} formulas should not be used to determine THRs for the elderly or those suffering from cardio-vascular disorders, as the predicted rates will be too intense. In such cases, even if medical approval for exercise has been deemed unnecessary, a submaximal exercise stress test (monitoring HR, general performance, and post-exercise response) should be carefully performed so as to determine an appropriate THR.

Another way of encouraging a working awareness of how hard the individual is exercising is by use of a subjective 'scale of perceived exertion'. The well-known 'Borg scale', developed in the 1970s, is a 15 point scale running from 6 to 20, where 6 describes the feeling of no exertion, 13 describes the feeling of working somewhat hard, and 19 describes the feeling of working very, very hard. Such a scale helps reduce the possibility of overstressing the cardio-vascular system, especially if exercisers are encouraged to keep to comfortable levels of exertion.

Athletes, especially in the elite category, need to include some higher-intensity **aerobic training**, typically at 80–95 per cent HR_{max}, combined with special attention to speed and technique development, on top of their core endurance-based training.

There are a selection of standard approaches commonly incorporated into athletic training routines for the objective of developing higher-level aerobic performance.

Continuous training

Continuous training is a straightforward method of improving endurance which involves the athlete sustaining a 'steady state' of submaximal long-duration exertion. Completely aerobic, this form of training can be varied (and progressively overloaded) from session to session, for example, by increasing the performing speed over the same distance, or by incorporating increased distances.

Interval training

Interval training, which can be used to improve various fitness components, is a way of combining periods of strenuous work with periods of recovery. The work interval can be short and intense (predominantly anaerobic) or long and less intense (predominantly aerobic). The recovery period may be simply the performance of reduced intensity work, or complete rest, and the period can be from a few seconds to a few minutes. Interval training allows for replenishment of fuel supplies by aerobic mechanisms, and recovery of heart and breathing rates. Because it typically involves periods of higher-intensity training, utilizing all three energy pathways, interval training can help to develop V_{O_2} max as well as muscular strength, endurance and power, and is most suited to the types of sports requiring such a combination of performance capabilities.

Fartlek training

Fartlek training (alternating pace or 'speed-play' training) involves varying the speed of the exercise at various periods in the activity. Fartlek training is similar to interval training, but rather than there being rest intervals, there are only increases or reductions in pace. Although this approach can be used to develop all aspects of fitness and is most commonly used by runners and cyclists, it can be tailored to focus purely on aerobic development by keeping intensity to appropriate levels. Exercising in a varied undulating outdoor environment will automatically place varying demands on the athlete. A more relaxed approach to fartlek, for non-competitive athletes, is to vary the activity according to how the individual is feeling during exertion.

TIP

When working aerobically for health-related benefits, especially beginners: the intensity should allow the exerciser still to be able to talk; the exerciser should aim to gradually increase their heart and breathing rates; heart rate should be monitored, and kept near to the predetermined target rate, typically 60–70 per cent of the maximum; body temperature should gradually rise, and perspiration gradually increase; working intensity should be maintained for at least 20 minutes at a time; activity should cease or intensity reduce in the presence of adverse effects (e.g. pain; dizziness; extreme change of facial colour; loss of co-ordination); it is important to ingest adequate hydration, before and during exercise.

TIP

Because of the inherent repetitive nature of aerobic conditioning, the potential for overuse or repetitive strain injuries is increased if activities are not sufficiently varied and performed with good technique and equipment.

Pick-up speed training

Pick-up speed training is an approach used by athletes to develop both aerobic and anaerobic fitness, and in particular it improves the capacity for runners to increase speed. Beginning with a period of walking, followed by a period of jogging, the athlete then picks-up their pace to run fast and builds up to a period of sprinting. The cycle is then repeated. Technically, the duration of each phase may be timed or be performed over a pre-set distance.

Stability training

Stability training is particularly important for various reasons:

- It helps to develop proprioception and the co-ordination of movement, which means that the body's stabilizing muscles are trained to fire up and respond to the demands of any physical situation.

- It helps make body regions, and in particular joints, stronger and more able to withstand the physical stresses placed upon them, and at much less risk of injury.

- It can offer the athlete a strong base of support from which to perform strong and powerful movements.

- It helps to encourage and maintain good and fatigue-resistant posture.

- It can help improve the efficiency of powerful movements, by requiring less in the way of compensatory efforts.

- It can be employed in order to help provide dynamic support for injured, weakened, lax or unstable structures.

Stabilizing (fixator or local) muscles are those that contract in order to help prevent unwanted movements as other (mobilizing or phasic) muscles are working to produce movements. They are typically relatively deep, single-joint muscles that work within a short range of movement, often isometrically, and are predominantly made up from slow twitch fibres, favouring aerobic metabolism, which should be expected to perform sustained low-intensity contractions. Stability can and should be developed in both the core and periphery of the body, hence the terms core stability and peripheral stability. Segmental stability is another term that relates more specifically to the isolation stability training applied to the deep (core) muscles associated with segments of the spine.

The key core and peripheral stabilizing muscles of the body are: multifidus (deep lower back erector spinae muscle); transverse abdominus (TA) (deepest abdominal muscle); latissimus dorsi; diaphragm (primary respiratory muscle); internal obliques; pelvic floor muscles; trapezius; neck flexors; serratus anterior; rhomboids; rotator cuff group; quadratus lumborum; gluteals; psoas (hip flexor); piriformis (deep lateral rotator of the hip); hamstrings; and adductors.

The key principles involved in stability training are as follows:

- Awareness of correct body (biomechanical) alignment during the exercise.

- Awareness of 'neutral' alignment (i.e. good working posture, and adjusting the pelvis so that it sits comfortably between an anterior and posterior tilt).

- Keeping focused so as to activate the target muscles (i.e. in the case of transversus abdominus, which should be targeted during all core stability exercises, involves tightening the muscle, or 'sucking it in', so that it is pulled towards the spine).

- Movements are typically performed in a very controlled and slow manner, and often isometrically.

- Maintenance of smooth unstrained breathing throughout all exertions.

During stability training, as the individual gets stronger and more stable, advanced exercises can be built onto the foundational stabilizing ones: for example, as the exerciser is holding one position, they can bring in another movement or series of movements that will challenge their performance even further, this can involve a balance or isotonic strength component.

Equipment is not necessary for basic stability work, but such inexpensive items as a wobble board, fitness ball, resistance bands and free weights can greatly increase the effectiveness and variety of such training.

Training the deeper stability muscles correctly will not contribute to any undesirable situation of limited local flexibility, because they are typically 'one-joint' muscles, required to support their local region. It is the tightening or shortening of mobilizing muscles that can be the main soft-tissue cause of such restrictions.

Stability exercises should be developed to incorporate an endurance component, by way of increased duration or repetition, because endurance is a functional requirement. The sports therapist should also look for ways to provide stability exercises in a variety of positions, for example supine, prone, side-lying, sitting and kneeling (quadruped) positions.

There is evidence to suggest that core stability muscles do not function well in the presence of localized pain, particularly back pain. Additionally, deep stabilizer muscles have been shown to begin to atrophy in the absence of gravitational loading, such as that associated with prolonged bed rest. In other words, these muscles can become relatively easily inhibited, develop motor deficits and begin to waste, and therefore they require specific retraining in such situations. Stability training should be seen not only as an important general fitness component, but also as a major part of many rehabilitation programmes.

TIP
Whenever performing isometric exercises, do make sure that: the intensity is not too great to cause strain; the holding position is correct; breathing is smooth, rhythmic and unstrained; the duration of hold is no greater than 10 seconds at a time; there are no contra-indications, such as hypertension.

Co-ordination, agility, balance, reaction and sports-skills training

Being agile and able to move fluently and quickly in response to the demands of a particular situation, often in an instant, and without becoming off balance, is a main requirement of all sporting activity. It is also a most desirable requirement for general activities of daily living, and at least something to work towards. These are the refined aspects of our movements.

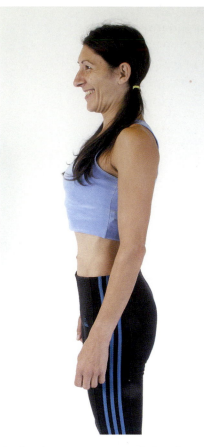

Activating transversus abdominus muscle

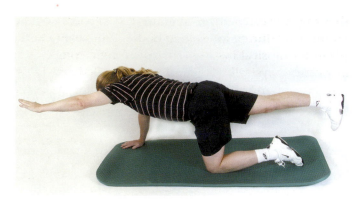

'Superman' exercise (variations for this exercise exist, depending upon the individual's ability)

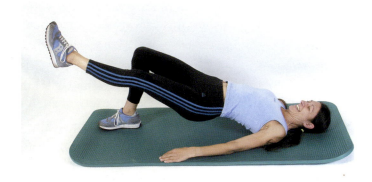

Supine 'bridge'. This exercise targets both core and lower extremity stability

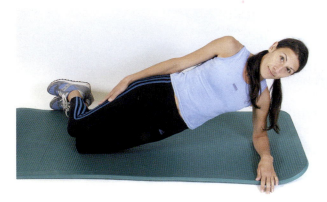

Side-lying 'bridge': repeat on the opposite side. Two points of contact with the floor. This exercise generates whole body stability, but needs to be repeated on the opposite side.

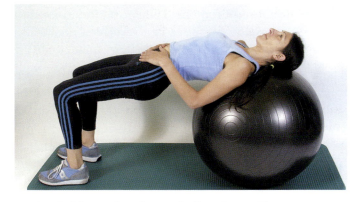

Supine bridge using fitness ball: to intensify use single-leg support

The body's nervous system controls the major aspects of all movement. In particular, the cerebrum and cerebellum are responsible for the receiving of incoming (sensory) messages, the integration and analysis of such information, and the immediate process of decision making which leads to the initiation of motor impulses that cause the required physical movements. Quite an amazing process indeed, especially when considering that this intricate course of neurological events occurs rapidly and continually during all waking hours. Whenever exercise, sport, dance, playing a musical instrument, operating a complicated piece of machinery or any other physically demanding or detailed activity is being performed, the rate and complexity of neurological functioning are almost unfathomable. The peripheral nerves supply the muscles with the information to contract and relax, and when trained the muscles are able to do this relatively well much of the time, obviously allowing for other factors such as fatigue or injury. The pattern of muscle firing and activation, the ability to make a contraction quickly, slowly, strongly or powerfully, the ability to produce the right movement at the right time, can to an extent be trained and developed.

Skill is about being able to successfully perform a precise action or combined sequence of precise actions. It is the developed combination of co-ordination, agility, balance, reaction, strength, speed, power, endurance and flexibility. Skill therefore involves the ability to perform swift and easy, responsive, harmonious, often very challenging, muscular activities, and being able to maintain a centre of gravity over a small base of support during such activities. Timing, anticipation, accuracy and economy of effort are all also components of skill.

Skill is typically goal-directed, which means that the athlete knows what they are trying to learn and why. The goals are to initially perform the skill well in practice, and eventually to be able to consistently perform the skill well. Obviously, in a competitive situation skills need to be continually adapted in response to the opposition, and this will involve being able to adjust the speed and timing of movements.

Examples of sports-related skills include: passing a ball in football; returning a backhand in tennis; and teeing-off in golf. These skills are all merely small aspects of a game, and certainly there are very many skills to each game, but to play the game competitively and successfully skills must be developed and practised, in addition to core conditioning, so as to achieve competency and ideally total efficiency.

To improve the footballer's passing of the ball, presuming there are no injuries and all other components of fitness are being trained separately, the player will, for example:

1 Practise kicking a stationary ball in a specific manner at a set target and distance, for a set number of times.
2 Practise kicking a moving ball in a specific manner at a set target and distance, for a set number of times.
3 Practise kicking a moving ball in a specific manner at a set target and distance, for a set number of times, while running.
4 Practise kicking an unpredictable moving ball in a specific manner at a moving target, for a set number of times, while running.

This basic but progressive approach can be adapted for other sports. It can easily be intensified or made more complex. The 'specific manner' in which the ball is kicked can be varied to suit the area of skill that is being honed, i.e. using instep, top of foot or outer side of foot; using left or right foot; 'trapping' the ball before it is kicked; varying the way in which the ball reaches its target. When a coach, fitness trainer or sports therapist is working with a team, players can be organized into groups and specific exercises demonstrated, practised, observed and worked so that they are improved.

All sports **skills training** should gradually progress to the forces and speeds (functional demands) that are likely to occur in the sport. In a sport where all fitness components are obviously important, methods of incorporating these into a specific training context need to be developed. For example, in rugby, football or hockey, any of the players at various points in the game will need to be able to produce a fast run instantly. The resulting sprint run is unlikely to be in a straight line, and it is likely that they will either be taking a ball with them or at least running in order to accept a pass or defend an opponent. Therefore, training to perform such specific skills, should attempt to incorporate all of the potential functional requirements. Speed, agility and co-ordination are the main fitness aspects to develop for improving the player's capacity to perform effectively at such a fast pace. Sports drills are repetitious skills-related training exercises that are employed to develop such performance.

Examples of speed and **agility training** drills:

- Short series of sprints (the 'pick-up speed' technique is useful), with short recovery periods.
- Varied distance and pace figure of eight running.
- Short series of sprints with sudden changes of direction (zig-zag pattern).
- Repetition of acceleration and deceleration patterns.
- Resisted sprints using a weighted vest, wrist or ankle weights.
- Resisted sprints, utilizing a harness held by a partner.
- Resisted sprints pulling a weighted sledge or wind chute.
- Fast paced, short distance hurdling (rapid knee lifts) over low hurdles.
- Dribbling a ball around a short circuit of organized cones.
- Running, hopping and jumping in structured patterns over a floor ladder or set of agility squares.

Skill acquisition and development occur through:

- developing a strong foundational base of fitness
- correct teaching (explanation, demonstration and observation) of skill-based techniques breaking down the various individual components of a skill, and practising each separately, before putting it all together
- regular repetition (practice) with correct technique
- the analysis and modification of the performance of a particular technique
- gradually progressing the intensity of techniques to the level expected in the sport
- developing an ability to select and execute skill-based techniques as and when required in sports
- developing an ability to remain motivated, focused and responsive throughout a game.

TIP

Skills training is best performed in the absence of fatigue. Fatigue impairs skilled performance.

REHABILITATION EXERCISE

Although exercise is the main part of getting and staying fit, it is also a major cause of injuries (sports injuries). However, even though exercise can be the cause of a problem, it is also the main component of its rehabilitation. Rehabilitation exercise incorporates all the basic principles of fitness training, but in a very specific context: that of effectively strengthening an injured body part, helping to make it functional again and restoring the player's confidence in using the affected region, while at the same time maintaining a good level of general fitness.

In order for exercise to be effective in restoring function to an injured area, it must be carefully planned and progressed. The **remedial exercise** cannot be planned effectively if a thorough physical assessment has not first been performed. The actual rate of exercise progression relates directly to the way in which the injury is responding to its treatment and rehabilitation. As discussed in previous chapters, there are three phases of healing: acute inflammatory phase; cellular proliferation phase; and remodelling and maturation phase. When prescribing rehabilitation exercise it is crucial to consider these three phases, and not to overstress the injured tissues more than they can realistically cope with. Additionally, the stages of rehabilitation are broken down, relative to the healing phases, as follows: early stage; intermediate stage; late stage; functional stage; and return to full participation.

How rehabilitation exercise is planned, modified, performed and progressed depend completely upon how the injury is responding, day to day and week to week. Most injuries will ideally receive whatever therapeutic treatment is most appropriate, whether from a doctor, therapist or surgeon (e.g. medications; cryotherapy; thermal therapy; massage therapy; electrical therapy; taping or strapping; surgery). The preferable 'conservative' approach is one that rehabilitates without the need for surgery. In some instances of severe soft-tissue injury (e.g. complete rupture of muscle or tendon), the decision whether to operate or not may be made based upon the age, fitness and normal functional requirements of the patient, and also obviously the potential for improvement. A severe strain of the Achilles tendon, for example, is often immobilized with a cast, brace or strapping, for a sufficient period of time so as to allow healing, rather than being surgically repaired. An acromio-clavicular sprain (a very common shoulder injury, often resulting from either a direct blow or fall landing on an outstretched arm) is an injury that can leave the individual with an obvious ('step') deformity on top of the shoulder (the lateral clavicle is left elevated), but will usually present little in the way of functional impairment. In such an instance, unless the affected person happens to be a high-level athlete, actor or model, it is unlikely that surgery will be offered. The conservative alternative might be to initially support the shoulder with a sling, or perhaps a spica strapping technique, and following treatment aimed at healing the injured soft-tissues, a strengthening regime focused at the muscles responsible for supporting and moving the affected region (particularly deltoids, supraspinatus, trapezius, pectorals and biceps).

> **TIP** ✔
>
> Rehabilitation exercise may also be referred to as being remedial or therapeutic exercise.

> **TIP** ✔
>
> Fitness instructors and sports therapists must be aware of the health, safety and legal implications of prescribing exercise. This is especially important when working with clients who are new to or returning to exercise, or those with known medical conditions or injuries.

Aims and aspects of rehabilitation exercise relative to each stage of recovery

1 **Early stage exercise.** It must be remembered that the key objective in this stage of healing is to minimize worsening and to encourage a fast resolution of the acute inflammatory response. If exercise is deemed to be indicated, it must be very carefully prescribed and performed so as not to aggravate the injury. Early gentle mobility work must only be performed, sub-acutely, within safe and comfortable limits, but it should include all available ranges of motion. Strength, endurance, power and flexibility should be maintained in unaffected body parts, if possible. Cardio-vascular fitness should be maintained, if possible (if the lower body is injured, then CV fitness could be maintained by use of an upper body ergometer or by swimming).

2 **Intermediate stage exercise.** Once inflammation and swelling have subsided, the intermediate stage of exercise can begin. Mobility work for the affected region must be maintained, and developmental flexibility exercises begun, but still within comfortable limits. Isometric work is usually the first stage of strengthening an injured area, normally beginning at a comfortable, mid-range position. Whether full weight-bearing (FWB) is possible depends on the location and severity of the problem. If FWB is not yet possible, partial weight-bearing (PWB) should be encouraged if safe and comfortable to do so. Stability training can be recommended if the injured person is able, and this should include proprioceptive exercise (when an injury has occurred, a weakening process naturally ensues, during the rest and recovery period, and the proprioceptive pathways become less efficient). Closed-chain balance work (see below), if pain-free, helps to improve proprioception. All other areas of fitness should be maintained as much as is possible. In some instances, such activities as cycling or hydrotherapy exercises can be included at this stage.

3 **Late stage exercise.** Mobility, flexibility, proprioception and strengthening should all be progressively increased in this stage. Unresisted, moving onto resisted, isotonic exercises can be begun. It can be very effective to separate and develop the concentric and eccentric components of the resisted isotonic exercise. Open-chain strengthening (see below) can be used to isolate muscle groups for specific strengthening. All other areas of fitness should be maintained as much as is possible. Machine and free weights, resistance bands, wobble board, medicine balls, fitness balls, treadmill, elliptical trainers, cycling, swimming and light running can all be considered for incorporation at this stage.

4 **Functional stage exercise.** This stage of exercise is looking to bring in a more vigorous regime, but still without overstressing the injured region. Supportive taping or strapping is often used, and correct biomechanical uncompensated movements must be encouraged. The emphasis is upon regaining pre-injury levels of fitness and preparing the player for a full return to sport. Strength, proprioception, stability, mobility and flexibility, speed, power, endurance, co-ordination, agility, balance and skills training should all be incorporated and developed at this stage.

5 Return to full participation. The athlete should not go back to full competitive activity until they have undertaken a specific sports-related fitness test. Their match fitness should be developed once general fitness has been regained. This will involve tentative participation in practice matches, and probably playing a role as a substitute (in team games) prior to being ready to start a full game.

Not all injuries respond quickly to even the most careful of rehabilitation programmes. If the sports therapist suspects that there might be underlying complications to the injury they should recommend a more detailed medical assessment. Also, if at any point the athlete experiences an exacerbation of symptoms, perhaps from over-enthusiastic rehabilitation exercises or from a too early return to play, then acute intervention should be applied, and a reduction in the level of activities must be encouraged.

Open-chain exercise

Open-chain exercise is that performed where the involved **kinematic** chain of muscles and joints are not in a weight-bearing position (e.g. dumb-bell bicep curls; seated leg extension). It is useful when targeting or isolating strength training to specific muscles, especially when full weight-bearing is not yet possible, but it is not very functional, as most sports or activities of daily living require the ability to support and fully weight-bear. Open-chain exercises may be concentric, eccentric or isometric.

Closed-chain exercise

Closed-chain exercise is that performed where the involved kinematic chain of muscles and joints are in a weight-bearing position (e.g. squatting; press-ups), and the body moves over its fixed distal segment. Closed-chain work is exercise close to the true functional requirements of sports and activities of daily living, and not only the muscles but joints, bones and the supportive connective tissues are all positively stressed during the exercise. Closed-chain exercises are particularly useful for developing stability and proprioception, and may be concentric, eccentric or isometric.

Eccentric work

Eccentric strengthening can be very useful in the later stages of injury rehabilitation. Eccentric (lengthening) contractions are a big part of many functional and sporting activities (e.g. decelerating from a run; running downhill; squatting; lowering a weight), and because it has been shown that there is increased potential for DOMS occurring following such activities, training for these purposes will help to improve the performance and reduce the severity of DOMS. An **eccentric contraction** typically has a greater force capacity and is

> **TIP**
>
> The sports therapist should work to continually develop their practical skill base by being able to offer a comprehensive range of progressively intensive exercises for each of the body's main regions. The main regions of the body are the: trunk; back; abdomen; neck; shoulder; upper arm; elbow; forearm; wrist; hand; hip; upper leg; knee; lower leg; ankle; and foot. This is often how the body is broken down for the purpose of describing particular protocols and strategies.

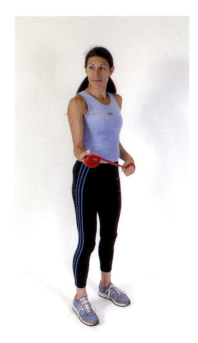

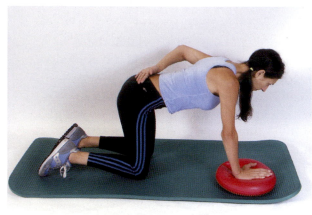

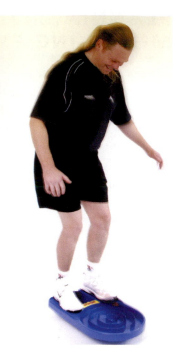

Open-chain isotonic strengthening of the lateral rotators of the shoulder, using resistance band

Closed-chain isometric strengthening/stabilizing of shoulder complex, using air-filled balance cushion

Closed chain wobble-board exercise

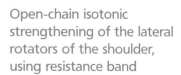

TIP

The sports therapist should be able to provide exercises aimed to develop, in a variety of ways: strength, endurance, speed, power, flexibility, stability, proprioception, co-ordination, agility, balance and sports-specific skills. Their clientele will range from complete beginners to elite athletes, and they should aim to be able to cater for all. In doing so, they will need to develop thorough understanding of exercise principles and remedial strategies.

more efficient than a **concentric contraction**, therefore in rehabilitation, when concentric contractions may not yet be sufficiently strong, eccentrics can be employed. Initial exercise might involve unresisted lowering or extending of an affected limb.

The sports therapist must try to familiarize themselves with the many and various regional rehabilitation strategies. Each of the body's regions is unique, with its own collection of assessment procedures, range of movements and exercise options. To develop essential practical knowledge and therapeutic skill, the therapist should integrate their understanding of the structural anatomy of the whole body (especially muscle positions and actions and joint movements) with their knowledge of assessment procedures (palpation; postural analysis; RoM norms; manual muscle tests; ligament stress tests; regional tests; basic neurological and circulatory tests; gait analyses; fitness tests). This should then provide the platform from which the most appropriate rehabilitation programme can be formulated and developed. Whether the injury is to the leg, trunk or arm, ankle, hip or elbow, the rehabilitation fundamentals remain the same; it is only the individual and regional adaptations that are different. However, it would be foolish to assume that rehabilitation is easy and straightforward. There are very many ways in which the rehabilitation process can be complicated, but by working with logic, caution and reservation, with explanation and feedback, and with communication or referral to other professionals when appropriate, the end result should be that the objectives have been achieved.

PLANNING, MONITORING AND MODIFYING EXERCISE PROGRAMMES

When formulating an exercise plan, remember that people come in all shapes and sizes and have different strengths and weaknesses. Individuals may also start a programme from different levels of health and training experience. In addition, individual objectives – such as losing 12lb or running the marathon 10 minutes faster – require different training methods.

PAUL STEPHEN LUBICZ (2003)

Exercise instruction can be loosely divided into three separate categories: general fitness training; sports-specific training; and rehabilitation training. The sports therapist may be involved in the provision of all of these, and each needs to be approached in different ways. General fitness training needs to be approached differently for beginners, intermediate and advanced participants, and it is quite likely that there will be particular health issues (e.g. an old injury; asthma; history of heart problems; arthritis; back pain) that need to be given full consideration when preparing the exercise programme. Sports-specific training involves a combination of core conditioning, skills work and match practice, as previously discussed. Rehabilitation exercise needs to be carefully focused on the immediate problem. Whether minor sports injury or functional stage cardiac rehabilitation, correct principles and close monitoring must be always employed. The eventual objectives of a rehabilitation programme can vary from a return to full match fitness, to being able to get back to or begin a general fitness routine, or to simply improve function and maintain performance of activities of daily living.

Nowadays, the vast majority of fitness clubs expect an obligatory **gym induction** process to be completed prior to their clients beginning their training. This will normally include a brief health-related questionnaire or consultation form, a practical induction to using the gym's various items of equipment, and an individualized exercise programme aimed at achieving identified goals. Sometimes, and ideally, a basic fitness test will also be undertaken. Fitness is measurable, and individuals will benefit from assessing their level of fitness prior to embarking on a programme so that improvements and modifications can be incorporated more effectively.

The induction allows the client to become familiar with the equipment and how to set it up for themselves, adjust the intensities, start with appropriate positionings, and perform each exercise with correct technique. This is a very important aspect to fitness instruction. New gym members, who may be new to such exercise, need to have basic principles explained to them, in simple terms, and this includes the importance of warm-up and cool-down, and awareness of keeping a good structure to their training. Exercisers are much more likely to safely achieve their objectives if they understand which exercises they need to be doing, and how hard, for how long and how often they need to be exercising. The instructor must encourage awareness of working (target) heart rates when using the aerobic equipment. When training with weights it is crucial to find a sufficiently heavy weight that can be comfortably lifted without strain for between 8 and 20 repetitions in one set, depending upon the objectives. Instructors must point out important safety aspects throughout the induction, and this should include developing awareness of signs or symptoms to stop exercising (pain, dizziness, lack of co-ordination, etc.). Although it is the job of a gym instructor to be available for advice and assistance, personal trainers will be available in some fitness clubs to closely guide, work with, encourage and monitor their clients individually through their exercises.

A typical approach to gym induction would be:

- name the particular exercise (e.g. leg press)
- explain and point to which muscles are being worked (i.e. depending upon angle of foot plate and position of feet: gluteals, quadriceps, hamstrings, adductors and calves)
- demonstrate and explain how to set up the station and adjust the weights
- demonstrate the exercise with explanation
- observe and coach the client through their execution of the exercise (with light weights)
- identify an appropriate resistance level to incorporate into their training programme.

The exercise prescription that results from the induction process will be documented on a programme card, which the client will keep with them during their exercise session. This card identifies which exercises they should be performing, and at what intensity. Periodically, the programme should be adjusted to allow for progression of their fitness.

The sports therapist who is not based at a gym will still need to be able to assess fitness, prescribe, demonstrate and coach specific exercises, monitor improvements and progress the programme. It is common for clients to pay a visit to their sports therapist and, after undergoing assessment and treatment, be given their home exercise programme. The best way to organize this is to document whichever exercises are being recommended on a programme card, and identify the particular type of exercise, intensity, repetitions, sets, duration and frequency. The drawing of simple 'stick-men' diagrams of specific exercises is not very time-consuming, and can greatly increase the client's understanding and prompt their memory very effectively. There are computer software packages that allow the therapist to personalize and print remedial exercise programmes for specific purposes. These packages, which can be a very useful investment, typically feature a clear illustration and description of how the exercise should be performed.

Although coaching sport is a specialist area of expertise, sports therapists, with their knowledge of the body and of remedial strategies and correct training principles, should be able to explain, demonstrate and coach exercise performance. Individuals need to be able to understand exercise instructions, be observed and coached into performing their techniques properly, and at the same time offered encouragement, all so that their motivation for continuing remains.

It is very important for the sports therapist to recognize the different capabilities of each individual. It must be remembered that exercise must be individually adapted to suit the beginner, the advanced, the older exerciser, the child, the teenager, the female, the disabled, the injured and those suffering all manner of health disorders. Exercise is crucial for the benefit of all, but it must be prescribed, taught and practised safely. Indeed, such

TIP

It is a responsibility of the sports therapist to encourage their clients to train with care and attention, with the right equipment and preparation, with good technique, and with appropriate intensity, duration and frequency.

prevalent conditions as chronic back pain, cardiac heart disease, hypertension, obesity, osteoarthritis, osteoporosis, stroke and post-orthopaedic surgery are very often, at least partially, managed with exercise programmes. Although a medical setting is totally appropriate for most of these conditions, especially in the early stages, there should come a point where the transition from hospital or physiotherapist arrives, and that is where the sports therapist comes in.

Ideally, medical recommendations are provided to help guide the mode of exercise. Exercise referral schemes, which are becoming more common in the UK, allow for a smoother flow of clients towards the health and fitness environment, and for exercise instructors to be suitably trained and informed of the important issues surrounding the provision of exercise for the benefit of problematic health.

EXERCISE EQUIPMENT

Some of the best, most effective and enjoyable exercise is performed with a bare minimum of equipment; indeed, for many sports all that is required is a decent pair of training shoes, T-shirt and shorts. However, as fitness has become bigger business, the industry is now served with a large product manufacturing and supply industry offering a massive array of highly technical equipment, clothing and accessories.

Most fitness centres now have a good selection of aerobic exercise stations, resistance machines, free weights and more. As exercisers themselves are generally becoming more familiar with the basic principles of training, and more focused, they are more likely to want to incorporate varied approaches to their training, and to include specific items of equipment into their workouts.

The gym environment is different from the home or outdoors, and because the sports therapist is likely to be recommending exercise in these situations (as well as the gym), they will be on the lookout for exercise equipment that is able to help clients achieve their aims and objectives both effectively and affordably.

Aerobic exercise equipment

Aerobic stations are machines that offer the facility to perform repetitive, varied intensity, endurance exercises indoors. Typically, whatever the mode, aerobic stations have in-built heart rate monitors, time and distance calculators, speed and intensity controls, and often automated programmes, all of which help to control the degree of expended effort and overall desired effect. Aerobic stations are used as part of a warm-up and cool-down, and to improve cardio-vascular fitness.

Whenever instructing the use of aerobic exercise machines, it is important to familiarize the client with the equipment, show them how to adjust their positioning, explain the control features, make sure they know how to slow

TIP
The fitness instructor working in a club will be expected to: check, clean and maintain equipment; tidy the gym and help keep it a safe environment; conduct health screening consultations with new clients; provide gym inductions for new clients; conduct fitness tests; plan and write exercise programmes; and be available for help and advice for all those exercising. Additionally, they may be required to provide personal training sessions or take exercise classes.

down and stop safely and quickly, and keep a check on them while they are exercising.

Stationary exercise bikes are very popular and easy to use. They are particularly useful for those whom repetitive or intense weight-bearing (high-impact) is not recommended, and also for those involved in rehabilitation training. Stationary bikes come in two basic categories: upright or (semi) recumbent. Some stationary cycles also feature movable arms, which offer the exerciser a simultaneous repetitive upper and lower body aerobic workout. Just as with road bikes, the stationary bike rider must be positioned correctly so as to optimize their performance and reduce the potential for injury. Particularly important is the saddle height, which should be adjusted to the height of the client. For the upright bike, this can be performed in one of two ways: ask the client to stand to the side of the bike, and make sure the saddle is about level with their hip joint; ask the client to sit on the saddle and place their foot flat on to a pedal – their leg should be slightly bent at the knee. The recumbent bikes feature a seat with back support (rather than a saddle) which some people find more comfortable and easier to use, and handlebars to the side of the seat. These bikes are easier to mount and stay on for longer periods, they improve circulation in the working leg muscles, and potentially there is less stress placed on the back. If the bike has foot straps, these should be secured properly so that feet do not slip, and because they improve the overall efficiency of pedalling, and power can be exerted in both the up and down stroke.

The treadmill is a machine with a pace-adjustable belt that is walked or run on. There are various types and features available: a wide platform is useful for larger clients or those with compensated gait patterns; some treadmills come with handrails at the front, sides or both; an incline or decline feature (which offers more functionally relevant activity and is used to alter the intensity of exercise). Easy pace walking, fast pace walking (power walking), jogging, running, fast running, plus uphill and downhill activity are all possible on good quality machines.

Using a treadmill can be difficult for some people. Try to encourage the client to begin with easy walking, striking the belt with heel first, maintaining an upright posture, looking forwards rather than downwards, staying towards the front of the machine and centre of the belt, and to try to get their arms gently swinging once they have got their balance and rhythm.

Stair climbers and step machines have many similarities: they both offer a low-impact, varied resistance aerobic workout that predominantly involves all the main muscles of the hips and legs. The main difference between the two is that the pedals on the stair climber typically have an independent action, whereas as one pedal of the step machine is pressed down, the other rises. Good stair-climbing technique requires that the exerciser takes a near full range of movement (emphasizing hip flexion on the negative phase of the stroke), which can be more comfortably performed if the resistance is set to be slightly higher rather than lower. The feet should remain flat on the pedals, and during the exercise, the client should be recommended to occasionally lift their forefoot off the pedal and flex their toes (which reduces the possibility of tingling or numbness occurring). When using step machines clients should avoid stooping forwards and also locking out their arms on the hand rails so as to off-load their legs, as this can cause excessive stress to the elbows. For both stair and step machines it is important to find the right resistance for the user: too much and it is difficult to perform full repetitions; too little and it is difficult to avoid staying low down on the pedals.

Rowing machines are popular aerobic stations employing both upper and lower body resistance to produce a whole body cardio-vascular workout. The machine replicates the action of rowing by trading oars for a central cable with handle, and the seat slides back and forth on a rail. The resistance depends on the type of machine, and commonly there are three types of machine offering either air resistance, electro-magnetic resistance, or water resistance. It is important to use the rower with good technique because regular poor technique can sometimes lead to, or exacerbate, back or knee problems. It can be difficult to master ideal rowing technique, but simply: make sure feet are strapped onto the footplates; keep shoulders in line with hips, and knees in line with feet; sit upright, holding the bar with both hands, elbows in slight flexion. The effort for the first phase of movement comes from the legs: as the handle is pulled back over the knees (by the legs), the arms take over to draw the handle to the torso as the legs are straightening, but not fully extending; as the handle and seat are returning to the start position during the final phase of the stroke, the arm extends past the knees, and then the knees begin to flex. Clients should avoid excessive wrist motion or leaning backwards from the hips.

Cross-training aerobic stations, including elliptical trainers and ski machines, are a more recent development in aerobic equipment. These provide a whole body, low-impact aerobic workout and offer a resistance that can

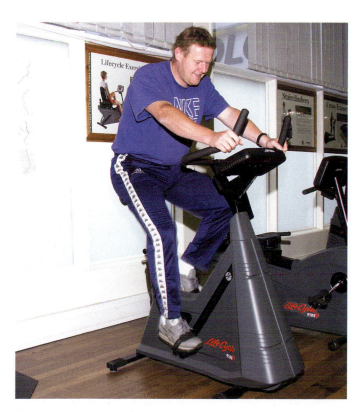

Stationary exercise bike

improve general muscle tone. They can be very useful for offering variance so as to improve performance (cross-train) in such activities as running, cycling or skiing. The ski machine simulates cross-country skiing, with its resisted sliding leg plates and arm bars. The elliptical trainer provides an elliptical-shaped stride, similar to a running stride but without the impact. The lower body works to move foot plates either forwards or backwards (a useful feature), and some of the elliptical machines also offer moving arm bars which may also be worked with the upper body.

Resistance machines

In most fitness clubs there are, alongside the aerobic stations and free weight sections, a selection of resistance or 'weight-stack' machines. The nature and style of resistance machines vary from manufacturer to manufacturer, but will involve the use of levers and pulleys, cams, hydraulics or pneumatics, and an adjustable stack of weights. This type of machinery is designed to provide a very controlled form of resistance exercise. Each station is devised so as to work a particular region of the body. There are usually adjustment settings for different sized clients, for altering the emphasis of the resistance and for altering the actual weight lifted. The movement of the machine is fixed, which takes the working regions through a set range of motion.

These machines can be considered generally safer than free weight exercises because the weight is guided throughout its movement, and there is a start and end point to the exercise, which protects the exerciser or anyone else from injury from a falling weight. However, it is still crucial to perform the exercise with correct positioning, good technique and an appropriate amount of resistance, repetitions and sets. On many machines there is opportunity to work one side of the body separately to the other, which can be particularly useful in rehabilitation settings. Additionally, isotonic concentric and eccentric and isometric work are possible, as is high-resistance, low-repetition or low-resistance, high-repetition work. The main disadvantages to resistance machines, when compared with free weights, are that they do not offer as much functional, stabilizing or proprioceptive benefit, as the weight is supported and guided on the machine through a fixed pattern and range of movement.

Common resistance machine stations include: leg press; hamstring curl; leg extension; chest press; pec dec; shoulder press; pullover; bicep curl; lat pull-down; squat; heel raise; seated row; tricep push-down; hip conditioner; seated abdominal curl; and seated back extension. Sports therapists should familiarize themselves with each of these stations and their various adjustments, recognize which muscles they target, and develop knowledge of the appropriate coaching points which need to be conveyed to the client.

Free weights

The use of free weights requires that the exerciser is in complete control of what they are lifting. Therefore, it is crucial to identify the appropriate amount of weight for each exercise. The main type of free weights come

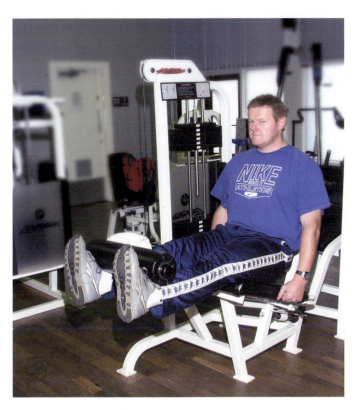

Leg extension machine

in the form of incrementally graded weighted discs or plates, which may be made variously from cast iron, steel, rubber, chrome or vinyl. These typically run in the following weights: 1.25 kg; 2.5 kg; 5 kg; 10 kg; 15 kg; 20 kg; 25 kg. Dumb-bell bars are short bars onto which an equal weight of plates are secured on each side, and these are designed for being held in one hand. Barbells are much longer (typically 1.5–1.8 m, 5 or 6 feet, long), and with these types of dumb and barbells, the weights are secured into position by use of a collar on each end (these will be either a screw or quick-release spring lock). Becoming more popular for ease of use are various types of pre-weighted dumb-bells. These are typically safely arranged on a weight rack and come in a selection of weights, typically in pairs from 2.5 kg up to 30 kg. A selection of specialized bars are also commonly found in the gym, including the bicep curl bar, the tricep extension bar, the T bar and the Olympic bar.

In addition to traditional dumb-bell and barbells, there is a variety of other types of weighted resistance equipment:

- Wrist and ankle weights: these come in a selection of weights, and they strap around the periphery of the limb (they have adjustable straps to suit different clients). They are used to increase the resistance offered when performing exercises that are using the individual's body weight and gravity as the resistance. They can also be used during aerobic-type activities such as power walking or running, thereby offering a resistance component to the workout. Wrist and ankle weights are also useful in circuit classes, the intermediate stages of rehabilitation and for the older or unconditioned exerciser.

- Weighted vests and belts: these are more likely used by conditioned athletes, adding resistance to their cardio-vascular, speed and power exercises.
- Weighted bars: these bars are available in a selection of weights, and there is no need to add weight plates as the bar itself is the weight. These can be used for performing a variety of traditional barbell type exercises, and are sometimes incorporated into conditioning exercise classes.
- Soft grip dumb-bells: these are small foam-covered, relatively light, hand-held weights, often with elasticated straps, designed mainly for use in exercise classes.
- Medicine balls: these come in a variety of weights, materials, sizes and designs and are discussed later in this chapter.

Anyone using free weights needs to be particularly careful with their technique, as there is no support from a machine; it is all down to the individual controlling their performance. The right amount of weight must be identified, and if loose weighted plates are being used, they must be secured properly. During a free weight exercise, the individual must be able to control their own body's posture in addition to the resistance of the weight and the speed and direction of the movement.

There are numerous free weight exercises. They may be performed sometimes seated on a bench, sometimes standing, sometimes single-handed, sometimes two-handed, and sometimes, when using heavy weights, with the aid of a spotter. Free weight exercises may be made more demanding by performing them in conjunction with other equipment such as a fitness ball. A sturdy, padded weight-training bench is an indispensable accessory for free weight exercises, preferably one with support rails for the barbell (for use during chest pressing), and an incline feature, which increases the range of exercises available and provides back support during some of the seated exercises (such as the incline shoulder press or incline flyes).

A very useful and versatile piece of equipment to enhance both the workout possibilities and the safety of free weight exercises is a specially designed frame (one such type is known as the 'Smith machine'), which can be used to guide and restrict the movement of a barbell through such exercises as the squat, chest (bench) press and shoulder press.

Traditional free weight exercises include: barbell and dumb-bell chest press; shoulder (military) press; shoulder press behind the neck; shoulder shrugs; barbell and dumb-bell pullovers; dumb-bell and barbell front and lateral shoulder raises; bicep barbell and dumb-bell curls; bicep hammer curls; concentration bicep curls; reverse bicep curls; squats; heel raises (double and single leg); tricep barbell and dumb-bell extensions; tricep dumb-bell kickbacks; upright rows; single-arm dumb-bell rows; barbell bent-over rows; T-bar rows; dumb-bell flyes; reverse dumb-bell flyes; dumb-bell and barbell wrist curls; reverse wrist curls; dumb-bell side bends; lunges; dead lift; power clean; snatch. Just as with resistance machine exercises, sports therapists must familiarize themselves with all major free weight exercises, and particularly the correct positioning so as to target specific muscles, and they should develop knowledge of the appropriate coaching points that need to be conveyed to the client, keeping awareness of appropriate amount of weight, repetitions and sets relative to the objectives.

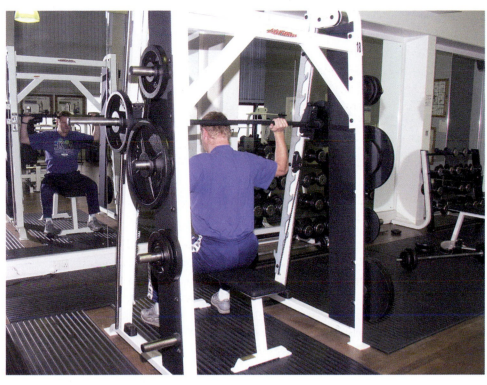

Shoulder press using the 'Smith machine'

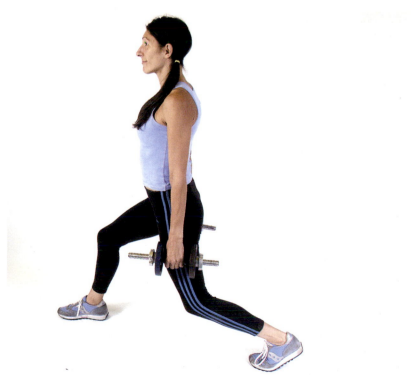

Dumb-bell lunge (gluteals, quadriceps, hamstrings and calves)

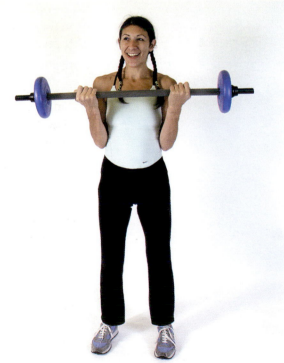

Barbell bicep curl (biceps and brachialis)

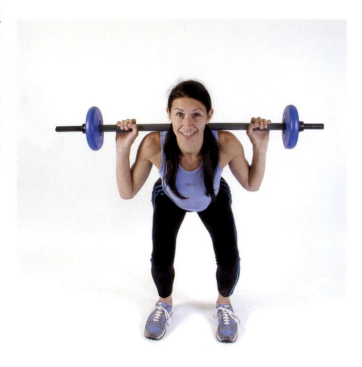

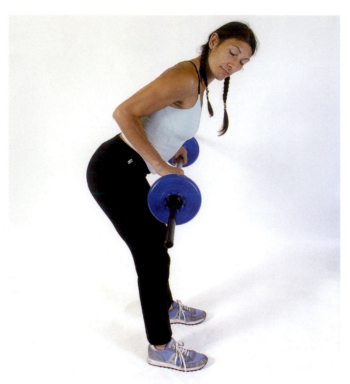

Barbell squat (works mainly gluteals, quadriceps, hamstrings, adductors and erector spinae)

Barbell bent-over rows (latissimus dorsi, teres major, posterior deltoids, trapezius, rhomboids, biceps, brachialis, brachioradialis and forearm flexors)

Other resistance stations

In the gym it is usual to find, alongside the aerobic stations, resistance machines and free weights, other stations for developing strength; these use mainly body weight and gravity as the resistance. Often simply a bench, wall-mounted or free-standing bar and frame system, some of these stations may be used in conjunction with additional resistance, others are merely a specially designed support from which to perform selected exercises. These stations include: bench or step (useful for many kinds of free weight and body weight exercises); 'Smith machine'; parallel bars (for dips or hanging bicep pull-ups/rows); chinning bars (for latissimus dorsi/bicep pull-ups and hanging leg raises); preacher curl station (for bicep curls); 'Roman chair' (for back extensions and torso side bends); incline bench (for abdominal curls and reverse curls); abdominal (cradle) trainers (providing support to the neck and encouraging good technique); and wall bars (useful for attaching resistance bands and tubing to, and for support during closed-chain rehabilitation exercises).

Resistance bands

These are specially designed, low-cost, elasticated, latex exercise bands or tubing. They come in a selection of strengths (intensities), which are usually colour-coded, they are lightweight, enabling people to take them wherever

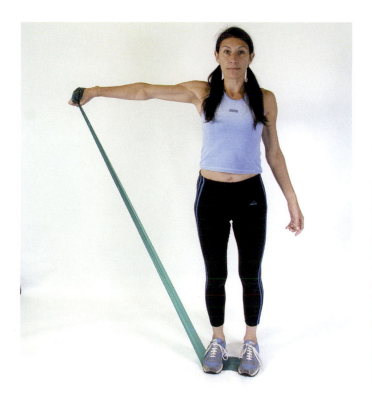

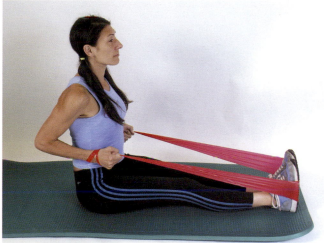

Shoulder abduction using resistance band   Seated row using resistance band

they want, and very versatile, offering an almost endless range of therapeutic exercises. Lengths can be cut by the therapist to suit the uses of their clients, and handles are available to make certain exercises a little easier. They are an ideal piece of equipment for clients to use at home. The bands tie easily onto themselves, or to a fixed stationary object, they can be wrapped around the hand, wrist or foot, and they can be used relatively unstretched and in one length for easy resistance, or slightly stretched and doubled up for greater resistance. They are especially effective for controlled rehabilitation exercises.

Medicine ball

Medicine balls are regaining their popularity. They are traditional items of gym equipment, and are great for functional strength and power development. They may be leather or plastic-cased balls, and they come in a selection of weights (typically 1–5 kg), sizes and designs. They can be used like a free weight for such exercises as chest press, shoulder press, bicep curls, tricep extensions, squats, lunges, abdominal curls or reverse abdominal curls. During this kind of exercise, medicine balls offer additional benefits in terms of the stabilizing activity that occurs as the ball is held and moved.

Perhaps the most effective use of medicine balls is in power and functional-based (plyometric) training, especially when training with a partner. Partnered medicine ball drills can allow for: simple passing of the ball to each other in a variety of ways; tossing and catching the ball; providing additional resistance against the ball during either the concentric, eccentric

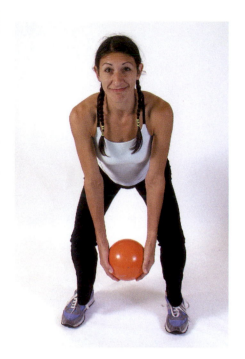

Medicine ball squat and reach 1

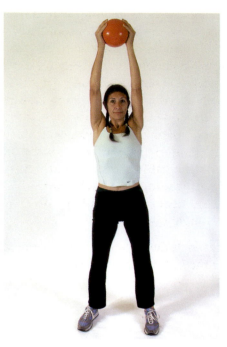

Medicine ball squat and reach 2

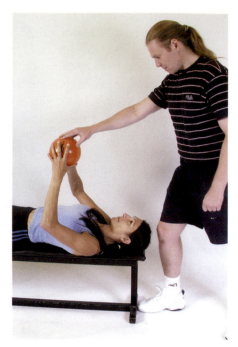

Medicine ball chest press, with additional partner resistance (which can be offered during the concentric, eccentric or both phases)

or both phases of isotonic exercises. Medicine balls can be used to provide a weighted resistance for functional exercises, such as replicating the footballer's throw-in, the rugby player's side pass or the basketball player's shot to the basket. They can help to develop skill, strength, endurance and power, but care must be taken to perform with good technique and posture.

Fitness ball

These are large, lightweight, durable, inflatable balls, also commonly known as the fit ball, Swiss ball, gym ball or stability ball. Coming in differing sizes to suit body height, fitness balls have been used for many years in the fields of physiotherapy and rehabilitation, but are now being successfully integrated into fitness programmes for all levels, from the deconditioned novice or back-pain sufferer to the elite athlete. Exercising correctly (safely) on the relatively unstable (yet supportive, comfortable and yielding) surface potentially facilitates massive improvements in balance, muscle strength and endurance, core and general stability, and flexibility. By varying the exercising posture, the centre of gravity, the amount of weight-bearing contact with the floor (one leg/arm or two), or by adding additional resistance such as free weights, resistance bands or partner resistance, the overall intensity (difficulty) of the exercises can easily be adjusted. There are a multitude of exercise possibilities, but like any other form of exercise, it is important to follow all correct principles of training, and to avoid advanced techniques until sufficiently fit. The fitness ball is by nature unstable, and as every exercise provides a balance challenge, care must be taken so as not to roll over or fall off, and to make sure that there is plenty of room to perform the exercises.

Common strength and stability fitness ball exercises include: seated balance (incorporating double and single leg support, pelvic rotations and sideways movements); supine bridge over the ball (double or single leg); abdominal crunches on the ball; rotation curls; reverse abdominal curls (lying on the floor, lifting ball with legs); side-bends; back extensions; trunk rotations; lower body rotations; hip extensions (prone over the ball); press-ups (prone over the ball, hands on floor); press-ups (prone, feet on floor, hands on ball); the 'plank' (prone, elbows resting on ball, knees or feet on floor); hip flexions (prone, hands on floor); tricep dips (from in front of the ball); supine bridge (lying on the floor, feet on the ball); hamstring curls (supine, lying on the floor, feet on the ball); squat (leaning with back against ball, against a wall, double and single leg); and heel raises (leaning with front against ball, against a wall, double and single leg).

Common flexibility fitness ball exercises include: forward bend (prone, over the ball); back extension (supine, over the ball); and side-bend (side-lying, over the ball).

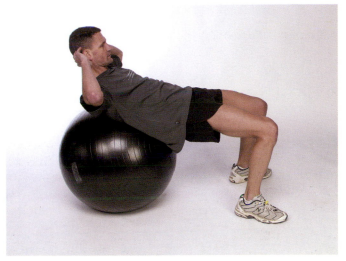

Supine abdominal crunch on fitness ball

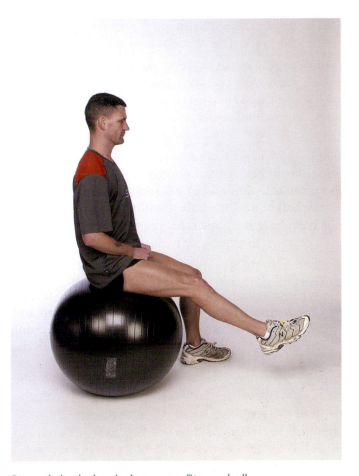

Seated single-leg balance on fitness ball

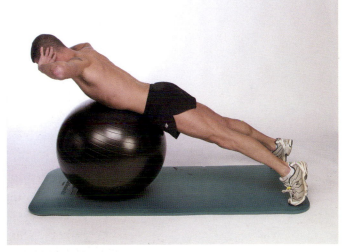

Prone back extension on fitness ball

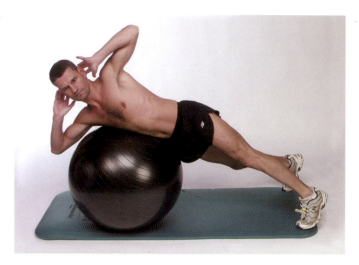

Prone trunk rotation on fitness ball

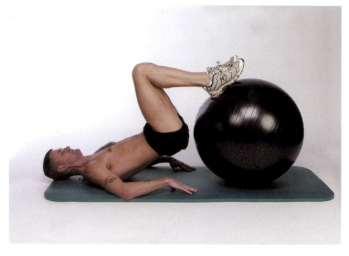

Supine hamstring curl on fitness ball

Other useful items of fitness and rehabilitation equipment

- **Exercise mat**: there are a variety of types, sizes and materials, but a professional quality exercise mat is essential for most indoor training routines.

- **Full-height mirror**: this is very useful for helping to perform exercises with correct technique. Definitely ideal, and almost essential.

- **Rebounder mini trampoline**: these can be very useful. Famously, David Beckham used one of these when rehabilitating his broken metatarsal in the build-up to the 2002 World Cup. They can be used for low-impact aerobic training, skills and **co-ordination training** and for proprioceptive training. For less able clients, a hand rail can be used.

- **Wobble board**: a well-known piece of equipment, typically used in ankle injury rehabilitation, encouraging strengthening, stabilization and proprioception. Variations include the 'rocker board' and the air-filled cushion.

- **Hand exercisers**: these are useful for all hand, wrist and forearm rehabilitation; in particular, they are used for arthritic and neurological conditions. They encourage mobility, strength, co-ordination and dexterity. There are various types of hand exercisers: squeeze balls; web disc; therapeutic putty (provides resistance through a greater range than other tools); grasp or pinch squeeze grips.

- **Skipping rope**: a traditional piece of inexpensive, portable and effective kit. Useful for developing speed, skill, agility and aerobic fitness. There are various approaches and styles. High-tech ropes are available featuring various adjustments, added weights and internal ball-bearing systems.

- **Punch bag**: often seen in gyms. Good for whole body power and endurance-based workouts. Functional in the sense that punching or kicking a bag replicates punching or kicking a (boxing or martial arts) opponent. Good stress and aggression release. Variants include the speed punch ball and the Thai boxing pad.

- **Gloves**: weight-training or cycling gloves can help protect hands from blisters and calluses. Punch bag gloves are useful for punch bag training. Hook and jab focus pads are used when training with a partner as the resistance.

- **Heart rate monitor**: it is highly recommended to keep a track on exercising heart rates, particularly for beginners and those rehabilitating from medical conditions, helping to keep them exercising at a safe level. High-level athletes benefit from being able to analyse performance more effectively. The two main types of heart rate monitor are those built into an exercise machine, and those worn around the chest with a receiver worn on the wrist.

- **Stop watch**: essential when coaching, assessing and monitoring training and fitness.

- **Pedometer**: useful for walkers, hikers, joggers and runners. Fitness can be monitored, especially time, distance, speed and endurance. They are relatively inexpensive, but care should be taken to correctly set the device up for accurate results. Some feature a heart rate monitor and calorie counter.

EXERCISE CLASSES

Exercise classes are the ideal way for some people to get their main exercise. If attending classes run by a reputable instructor, with current licensing and qualifications, the class will offer correct principles, with continual demonstration and coaching. A good contemporary instructor provides an enthusiastic, motivated and exciting workout, and the participants are encouraged both by the instructor and themselves. The workout is usually based around a musical soundtrack and is typically carefully choreographed. Exercise classes are these days getting ever more technical and conceptual, and new class systems enter the arena every year. Available at most of the larger fitness centres today will be at least some, if not all, of the following: aerobics; step aerobics; 'bums, tums and thighs'; body conditioning; body pump; body balance; body combat; body jam; spinning; yoga; Pilates; fit ball; chi ball; circuits; aqua aerobics.

Martial arts

Martial arts (from aikido to karate, kung fu, tai chi and Thai boxing) are well-disciplined, traditional cultural exercise systems. Often begun when young, or later in life out of pure interest, for self-defence or for general fitness, these classes attempt to instil in the individual a sense of respect for each and everyone, while offering many health-related benefits. Not always though are martial arts fitness principles in keeping with modern scientific fitness principles, and it is the responsibility of the leaders and instructors to remain accredited and updated on safe and unsafe training methods.

HOME EXERCISE

Most clients are offered something in the way of home exercise recommendations. If, for example, they are relatively new to exercise or recovering from injury this will involve helping to structure a weekly routine, and all the specifics need to be discussed and recorded for their easy reference. Many people are not able or do not want to attend a fitness club, and many do not have their own exercise equipment: in these instances the sports therapist has to be adaptable and resourceful. They will need to explain the appropriate way to plan an exercise session (i.e. making the area safe; basic equipment; warm-up; cool-down; etc.) and make sure that the client fully understands what to do and how to do it.

A perfectly acceptable and effective workout, for almost any level, can be performed with the minimum of equipment. An exercise mat is essential. A fitness ball, free weights or resistance bands are desirable. A recommended home warm-up can involve a short brisk walk, cycle or step-ups, combined with mobility and stretching exercises. The core of the workout, if strength, endurance and stability-based, may involve body weight exercises (e.g. press-ups, crunches, lunges, chest presses, shoulder raises). The intensity of all exercises must be adapted to suit the individual. The resistance for some of these exercises can come from standard household items, such as different sized bottles of water and cans of beans. The therapist really needs to emphasize the importance of technique, because away from the clinic, the client is left to their own devices. If aerobic-based, the emphasis has to be placed upon endurance activities. A weekly fitness routine will combine all basic conditioning components. In the clinic the therapist can demonstrate the selected exercises, and then observe and coach the client through some easy repetitions. Follow-up sessions are important so as to monitor their performance and improvements.

Rehabilitation exercise at home is possibly more complicated. Not all clients undergoing rehabilitation will be able to perform a thorough warm-up, or they may not be able to fully weight-bear. However, in the early stages, the therapist might be able to get around such factors simply by instructing very specifically progressive exercises, such as very easy localized mobility work and standard safe-range isometric repetitions. That is until such time as more activities can be safely incorporated into their programme. It is important to encourage the client to continue with their exercises so as to enhance the work done in the treatment room.

A big aspect of sports therapy is basically about helping to keep people fit enough to do the sports and activities that they love so much. Whether the exerciser is an athlete training on the track, a hiker or biker on a mountain, a jogger in the park, or a player on a pitch, outdoor exercise, for many, is what it is all about. Exercise outdoors combines the challenge and benefits of the activity, the competition, the environment and the conditions. The sports therapist is someone who can help to reinforce the importance of having good preparation, in terms of clothing, equipment and fitness. They may also be able to recommend and help plan their client's involvement in suitably supportive (general conditioning and cross-training) activities. For beginners, basic exercise activities such as walking, jogging or cycling can be easy to get into, presuming that the individual is fit enough to begin to participate, but guidance is still an issue.

RELAXATION TECHNIQUES

Rest and relaxation are vital aspects of life. If we do not get enough recovery, we can begin to experience more and longer-lasting fatigue, sustain more injuries, encounter more ailments, suffer diminishing performance and worse.

Relaxation is an aspect of rest, but it is also an exercise. Relaxation is a component of fitness. It is all very well being able to contract muscles and exercise our minds, but can we switch them off when we want to? Holding muscles in a state of tension for prolonged periods unnecessarily depletes energy supplies, restricts blood circulation, causes fatigue and hypersensitivity, exacerbates anxiety and insomnia, and can lead towards a chronically painful situation. By knowing how and being able to effectively relax, we can offer the body some respite when it needs it. Exercise is touted as being one of the best stress relievers (and it is), but strenuous energetic exercise does not allow for a calming of the mind, for contemplation and reflection, or for composing oneself in readiness for tasks ahead. Stress in the workplace and the home has now become the major problem that health analysts once predicted it would become, directly affecting our physical and mental health and well-being. As sports therapists, armed with skills and tools to help, we need to be able to guide, or at least remind, our clients of ways to help deal or cope with some of the recently found pressures of modern life.

It is a feature of many exercise classes to run through a short guided relaxation period at the end of the session, following the cool-down. This allows the body to return towards normal physiological functioning, to relax after the strenuous preceding activity, and hopefully for the client to feel refreshed, re-energized and ready to face the world again. The techniques used may include: asking the participants to lie down comfortably; playing some soothing instrumental music; encouraging smooth unforced, relaxed breathing; providing imagery and encouraging visualization; taking participants through a whole body, contract–relax sequence exercise; providing a gentle revitalizer phase at the very end, so as to awaken the body again.

Similar techniques can be used during treatment sessions, so as to enhance the relaxation component of a massage treatment. Clients, particularly those with busy, high-pressure lifestyles, and also those with stress-related health problems, can be shown simple relaxation exercises during the treatment session. Clients should be encouraged to practise one or two relaxation techniques under the sports therapist's guidance, who should make sure that they can perform them well enough so that they can practise at home.

Diaphragmatic breathing is one of the most commonly used and effective relaxation techniques.

DR EDMUND O'CONNOR (2002)

Rapid shallow breathing, where most of the respiratory effort occurs in the mid and upper chest, fails to optimize gaseous exchange and actually excites the body into an often undesirable prolonged state of arousal (increasing muscle tension, heart rate, etc.). This particular pattern of breathing might be a technique to use in immediate preparation for athletic competition, but in most other instances it is progressively detrimental to good health.

Relaxation breathing techniques

Smooth, slow and deep **diaphragmatic breathing**, where the abdomen rises (before the chest) during inspiration, helps create a relaxation (parasympathetic) response in the individual, where gaseous exchange is improved, muscle tensions decrease and blood flows improve. This is useful, not only for stress relief and general relaxation, but also it can enhance the healing rate and rehabilitation of an injury, especially when practised during treatment. Diaphragmatic breathing, which is best practised lying comfortably supine, but is also possible in a seated position, may be more effectively performed by having the client place their hands on their abdomen, where they can experience a pleasant sense of warmth, and for the rise of the abdomen during inspiration. During expiration they should aim to perform a full out-breath, reducing the chest capacity. A slightly different approach is to have the individual place their hands on either side of their lower rib cage, and feel for the smooth rise and fall of the region. By breathing in through the nose, and breathing out through pursed lips (like when whistling), the whole sequence is made more effective (pursed lip exhalation helps control the speed of the out-breath and keeps airways open for longer). It can be useful to perform breathing exercises for between 5 and 15 minutes at a time. It is important not to force or strain the breathing or to cause light-headedness.

Where a more focused remedial breathing strategy might be beneficial, it can be helpful to attempt to isolate the main respiratory muscles (diaphragm and intercostals) by having the client actively contract the accessory respiratory muscles (i.e. gently push hands together, or arms down onto the arms of a chair) while performing their deep breathing exercises. These actions can help to inhibit the muscles' respiratory function.

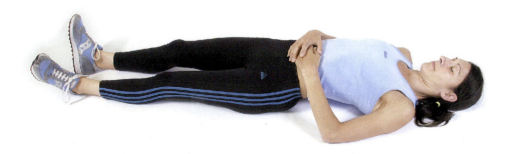

Relaxation exercises offer many benefits, and help us cope with the stresses and pressures of modern lifestyles

Progressive muscle relaxation techniques

Progressive muscular relaxation is best performed lying supine. Have the client lie down comfortably (encourage them to feel able to slightly adjust their position whenever they feel the need), perhaps with a pillow supporting the head and a blanket keeping them warm. Eyes can be shut and deep breathing performed. The client should be asked to simply lie and, for a few seconds, actively begin to identify and take muscular tensions out of their body, from the feet up to the forehead they should look for any tension to relax. Progressive muscular relaxation involves going through all of the body's main muscles, contracting them briefly (five to seven seconds, with minimal effort), and then actively relaxing them. Starting at the feet and working gradually up through the calves, thighs, hips, torso, chest, hands, arms, face and scalp is the usual approach. Once one sequence has been completed the cycle should be repeated again. By contracting a muscle group, the MET (muscle energy technique)–PIR (post-isometric relaxation) effect means that the muscles can be more efficiently relaxed.

CHAPTER SUMMARY

There is a large and growing population of physically active people at all levels of ability who are ready, willing and able to take regular exercise or to compete in sporting activities. To do this requires long-term preparation, lifestyle management, healthy living, regular varied appropriate and periodized fitness training, support, commitment, motivation, and much more.

These days the busy sports therapist will almost certainly be providing practical help and advice to all manner of sportspeople, for those who play team sports and for those who perform individual pursuits. This includes injury prevention, treatment and rehabilitation, and advice on training, technique, recovery and nutrition, and it helps if the therapist can develop their knowledge of the skills and training necessary for different sports and activities. The athletes of today now have much easier access to improved technology, training methods, facilities and sports therapy, and because of this the standards of performance continues to get better and better.

Exercise is not only for athletic types. Remedial and rehabilitation programmes help individuals recover from, or at least help to manage, a wide variety of health problems. Where health problems or injuries are an issue, the sports therapist must be very particular with what exercises and intensities are recommended. By developing a working knowledge of training principles, musculo-skeletal anatomy; assessment procedures, safety-conscious remedial strategies, exercise equipment, advice for exercising at home, and relaxation techniques, the road to improvement will be much more easily travelled.

WEBSITE @

Visit the companion website at www.thomsonlearning.co.uk/ healthandfitness/ward where you will find the answers to these questions for you to check your progress through the book.

Knowledge Review

1 What is meant by: (i) physical fitness; (ii) health-related fitness; (iii) skill-related fitness?

2 List ten beneficial effects of exercise.

3 Describe some of the key safety issues relating to the provision of exercise.

4 What is meant by: (i) overload; (ii) progression; (iii) transfer; (iv) repetition; (v) periodization?

5 Why is a thorough warm-up important?

6 Describe some ways in which power training can be performed.

7 Explain: (i) the 'Karvonen formula'; (ii) the 'Borg scale' of perceived exertion.

8 Describe some methods to develop stability and explain why it is important.

9 In what ways can sport-specific skills be developed?

10 What factors influence the planning of an injury rehabilitation programme?

chapter 13

FITNESS TESTING TECHNIQUES

Fitness assessment in the health and fitness environment can often be quite a straightforward process, which normally involves: running through selected, well-recognized physical tests; comparing the results against generally recognized norms; identifying strengths and weaknesses; and reviewing training objectives. Fitness testing can also be quite complex, where testing adaptations are implemented for a selection of specific purposes, such as assessing the injured player's return to match fitness, or analysing aspects of the elite athlete's performance. There is obviously a big difference between assessing an unconditioned individual's basic level of fitness, and performing a thorough range of functionally specific tests in an exercise laboratory. Either way, fitness testing, just like the other main methods of physical assessment, is common professional practice, and a very important area of sports therapy.

Fitness testing is very useful:

- It can help to shape a basic fitness training programme.
- Periodic testing can help to monitor fitness improvements and appropriate modifications in training routines.
- Elite athletic performance can be closely analysed, and the effectiveness of training strategies assessed.
- Post-rehabilitation and pre-match fitness testing helps to assess the functional ability of players.
- Testing fitness can be a strong competitive and motivational stimulus, and can heighten players' awareness of their responsibilities.
- Fitness tests can be used as part of team selection processes.
- Testing fitness can be a fun activity.

TIP

Tests of strength, muscular endurance, speed and aerobic fitness can be specifically organized so that they are either submaximal (not exercising with extreme effort, to exhaustion) or maximal (extreme effort). Submaximal aerobic tests are more usually performed in fitness clubs. The majority of maximal tests should only be undertaken by conditioned athletes, because of the various associated dangers.

PLANNING FOR HEALTH-RELATED FITNESS TESTING

In many fitness centres there exists, for the client under the guidance of a qualified gym instructor, personal trainer or sports therapist, the opportunity to undertake a variety of recognized fitness tests in order to help produce a fitness profile.

A sensible approach to fitness assessment, in the fitness club environment, will take the client through a logical sequence of procedures, from a relaxed, seated consultation, through taking their resting heart rate and blood pressure, height, weight, girth and postural assessments, body fat testing, to aerobic assessment (allowing for a warm-up), flexibility, strength and power tests.

A logical sequence for providing a health-related fitness test could be:

1. consultation and pre-test screening
2. resting heart rate
3. blood pressure testing
4. height
5. weight
6. BMI
7. girth assessment
8. postural assessment
9. lung function testing
10. body fat testing
11. aerobic fitness testing
12. flexibility testing
13. strength testing
14. power testing.

Ideally, a fitness test is conducted, in the main, in a quiet and relatively private atmosphere, especially for those clients who may be nervous or self-conscious (obviously, tests requiring the use of larger equipment, such as the treadmill or a resistance station, will probably need to be performed in the gym).

It is up to the sports therapist to set the scene, put the client at ease, explain the procedures and provide the opportunity for the client to ask questions. Conducting a consultation, or at least a pre-test questionnaire, allows for any relevant and important health issues (and possible contra-indications) to be detailed and identified prior to any physical activity taking place. It provides basic information regarding the client's suitability to undertake a fitness test, and allows for their initial fitness objectives to be outlined. The consultation process also offers a short period of time where the client can be encouraged to sit and relax for a while, so that more realistic resting heart rate and blood pressure readings can be taken. All tests must be performed in a manner that causes a minimum of stress or embarrassment to the client (particularly with girth assessments, and measurement of body fat).

Clearly, it is very important to make sure that all equipment required for the tests is available, functional and prepared ready for the client's appointment time. Scales and meters must be correctly and regularly calibrated, and batteries need to be checked in certain items of equipment.

The results of the fitness tests can be analysed in a variety of ways:

- against generally accepted norms
- against norms that take into consideration the age and sex of the individual
- against the same client's previous test results
- against training colleagues and team mates
- by taking into consideration the general health, lifestyle and ability of the client
- by simply looking at the positives and negatives of each of the results
- by way of a computerized analysis program.

The therapist must record all relevant information regarding the tests and results. It is usual to have a specially prepared fitness test form available, onto which the client's details and results are recorded. It is important to identify specifically which tests and protocols have been employed, so that appropriate follow-up testing can take place (this is especially important when different testers might be involved). On the fitness test form, alongside each of the particular test's results, the tester should make brief comments regarding the grading of the client's score, relative to official and validated norms. In simple terms, this can mean recording a score of excellent, very good, good, fair, poor or very poor. An overall assessment and analysis of the test results should be performed on completion. At this stage, it may be that initial fitness objectives need reviewing, and appropriate recommendations need to be made (all in the fresh light of the findings). The analysis, reviewed objectives and recommendations need to be documented on the fitness test form. There are computer programs for assessing fitness, which, although costly, can make the whole process of record keeping and analysis much easier for those who are competent with such methods.

COMMON TESTS OF FITNESS

Resting heart rate

The resting heart rate (RHR) of an individual can provide useful basic information relating to the functional health of their cardio-vascular system. Typically, as aerobic fitness is developed and improved, over a period of time RHRs can be observed to reduce. Generally, the slower the RHR (within safe limits), the less work that the heart has to do. A slower resting pulse can indicate a strong heart, and a fast resting pulse can indicate a weak heart. An average (good to fair) RHR is one between 60 and 80 beats per minute (bpm). Trained individuals and athletes commonly demonstrate RHRs of 60 bpm or less. By charting the client's RHR figures, a simple pattern of

TIP

Be aware that certain medications affect both resting and exercising heart rates, for example: beta blockers, taken for angina and hypertension, slow the heart rate (HR); nitrate (GTN) sprays, taken for angina, cause tachycardia. In such cases

- the client must be medically approved for exercise, and
- HR cannot be relied upon as a monitor of exercise intensity.

improvement (or worsening or plateauing) can be formed. The RHR figure is sometimes incorporated into certain fitness test protocols, and is also a feature of the 'Karvonen formula' for ascertaining appropriate target heart rates.

Heart and pulse rates can be measured with either a heart rate monitor, or manually, using finger tips and a stopwatch. The two most common sites to manually assess pulse rate (the wave of distension felt at superficial arterial sites) are the carotid pulse (anterior neck), and radial pulse (radial side of wrist). Light palpation of the site is sufficient, and the number of beats in 6, 10, 15, 30 or 60 seconds is counted (the first beat starts the timing). The bpm is worked out by multiplying the number of beats by the required amount (i.e. multiply the number of beats in 6 seconds by 10, 10 seconds by 6, 15 by 4 or 30 by 2).

Blood pressure testing

Blood pressure, as discussed in chapter 2, is the pressure exerted on the walls of the arteries as the heart contracts and relaxes. It is recorded as two figures (the 'upper' systolic pressure; the 'lower' diastolic pressure), which are measured in millimetres of mercury (mmHg), and a 'normal' reading is considered as being around 120/80 mmHg.

Blood pressure is affected by: hereditary factors; age (as we get older, high blood pressure can become a problem); activity (during exercise, systolic pressure tends to rise and diastolic stays pretty much the same, but over time with regular exercise, high blood pressure can, to a degree, be reduced and even controlled); inactivity; diet (e.g. excessive salt continually in the diet increases blood volume and may contribute to hypertension); obesity; smoking; alcohol; stress; arterial disease; shock; haemorrhage; heart failure; medications (various drugs, such as diuretics or beta blockers, are often prescribed to help control high blood pressure).

High blood pressure (hypertension) is a state of persistently elevated blood pressure, and where the reading is 140/90 mmHg or above. The individual is often asymptomatic, but might possibly experience headaches, nose bleeds, insomnia or tachycardia. Complications of uncontrolled hypertension can include coronary heart disease, kidney disease and stroke.

Low blood pressure (hypotension) is where the reading is 90/50 or below. It is quite a common condition, with mild symptoms including light-headedness, dizziness, occasional fainting, pallor and weakness. Postural hypotension is a transitory lowering of blood pressure caused by: the individual rising too quickly; prolonged standing in warm conditions; inadequate food; intense excitement; failure of the cardio-vascular system to adequately adjust to an altered position, which is more common in the elderly. Hypotension is also associated with excessive haemorrhage, shock and heart failure, where the danger is that insufficient blood reaches the brain.

The sports therapist needs to be aware of their clients' blood pressure so that they can gain medical approval for treatment or exercise, prepare appropriate action plans and recommendations, and monitor both their exercise and blood pressure more carefully.

Categorization of blood pressure measurements

Systolic:

- <140 mmHg normal
- 140–160 mmHg borderline isolated systolic hypertension
- >160 mmHg isolated systolic hypertension

Diastolic:

- <85 mmHg normal
- 85–89 mmHg high normal
- 90–104 mmHg mild hypertension
- 105–114 mmHg moderate hypertension
- >115 mmHg severe hypertension

Basic types of apparatus for measuring blood pressure

- The mercury sphygmomanometer, which features: a mercury pressure measurement scale; an inflatable cloth cuff (goes around the client's arm); a valve-pump (used to allow for pumping up of the cuff and controlled release of the air); two rubber tubes (one from the valve-pump to the cuff, and one from the cuff to the mercury measurement unit); stethoscope (used to listen for the return of systolic pressure, and disappearance of diastolic pressure, as the air is gradually released from the cuff).

- Aneroid (air) sphygmomanometer. These are very similar in principle to the mercury units, but make use of a calibrated dial gauge, rather than a scale.

- Digital blood pressure monitors. These are small battery-operated blood pressure units that are designed for application at either the wrist or arm. They typically feature an automatic air pump, and are able to offer a heart rate reading at the same time.

In hospital settings there may be more sophisticated equipment available for taking blood pressure, typically integrated into other units, but the portable units, although varying in cost, accuracy and ease of use, are still in general use because they tend do the job well enough. There do also exist portable ambulatory (24 hour) blood pressure monitors, which can provide a more functional evaluation, especially as blood pressure alters throughout the day according to the activities undertaken by the individual. There is a situation known commonly as 'white coat hypertension' which sometimes occurs with nervous patients, where just the thought or performance of taking a blood pressure reading, particularly in a medical setting, can cause the patient to become anxious, and their blood pressure to rise.

Unfortunately, even with resting blood pressure measurement, there is always an element of error which is related to the skill of the operator and to the equipment itself (i.e. inaccurate calibration; inappropriate cuff size; improper rate of inflation or deflation of the cuff; improper stethoscope placement or pressure; background noise).

TIP	

Because blood pressure alters throughout the day, and for various reasons, it is recommended that clients are not classified as being hyper- or hypotensive on the basis of one measurement. It is also important to not cause alarm in those clients who demonstrate high readings.

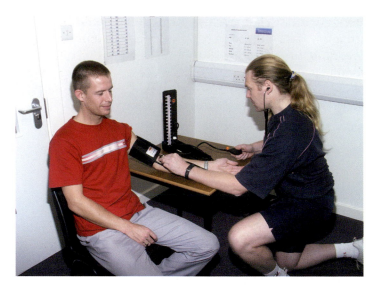

Blood pressure measurement, using a mercury sphygmomanometer

Protocol for taking blood pressure using mercury sphygmomanometer

1 The client should be seated and rested.

2 Their arm should be supported at the level of the heart on a table, with elbow slightly flexed and forearm supinated.

3 The sphygmomanometer should be released of air, and the valve closed.

4 The cuff should be applied evenly and snugly around the upper arm, about 2 cm proximal to the elbow crease (making sure it is the correct size for the arm).

5 Position the bell of the stethoscope over the brachial artery (in the medial aspect of the cubital space).

6 Inflate the cuff to between 160 and 200 mmHg (observed on the mercury scale). Do not keep the cuff inflated for any longer than is necessary.

7 Slowly deflate the cuff by slightly opening the valve.

8 Listen for the first sound of soft beating appearing (the systolic blood pressure returning after being shut off) while observing the mercury scale, and make a mental note of its reading.

9 As the cuff continues to deflate, listen for when the beating sound disappears (diastolic blood pressure), and make a mental note.

10 Inform the client of the results, and record the measurements on the test form.

11 If the measurement has not been effective (e.g. failure to obtain a reading), or if the reading appears high or incorrect, then the procedure should be repeated, but a period of about 15 minutes should be allowed between consecutive measurements. Try not to alarm the client if readings are a little high.

TIP ✔

The 'Korotkoff sounds' are the sounds heard through the stethoscope as pressure is released from the cuff. There are actually five phases as characteristic changes occur (systolic: a thud sound, a swishing sound, a soft thud; diastolic: a blowing sound, silence). To hear all the sounds clearly and to differentiate between them requires a high level of auditory acuity. The main focus for the sports therapist should be on ascertaining when the sounds first come in (systolic), and when they disappear (diastolic).

If blood pressure is observed to be relatively high, the client should be recommended to return a few days later for a follow-up assessment. If they produce another high reading, the therapist should recommend or refer the client to their GP, preferably with a clearance form for exercise participation. Remember that high blood pressure is a common problem, but it is often asymptomatic and is treatable in a variety of ways.

Lung function testing

There are two basic tools for testing lung function: the peak expiratory flow meter and the digital micro-spirometer. There are four main tests, all of which are mainly used to monitor the progression of disorders that limit airflow during expiration (e.g. asthma; bronchitis), and their response to treatment. Aside from specific respiratory disorders, other factors having a profound effect on an individual's test results will include: general state of health; heavy cold, cough or 'flu; smoking; obesity; occupation; exercise routine; environmental pollution; bad test technique.

- **Peak expiratory flow rate (PEFR)**. This extremely simple and inexpensive test measures the peak rate of air coming out of the lungs in one blow (not the volume of air). It simply requires a peak flow meter and a reference chart of normal values (norms). Typically, norms for PEFR are predicted graphically according to the individual's age, sex and height. PEFR is measured in litres per minute (l/min).

  Peak expiratory flow rate method:

  - Place a clean mouthpiece into the peak flow meter.
  - Set the gauge to zero.
  - The client is asked to stand upright.
  - They should take a deep breath in, seal lips around the mouthpiece and breathe out as powerfully as possible. It should be a short and sharp exhalation.
  - Repeat the test three times, and record the highest reading.
  - Compare the actual result with the predicted result on a graph of normal values.

- **Forced expiratory volume (FEV$_1$)**. Using a digital micro-spirometer, this test measures the proportion of vital capacity that can be forcibly expired in one second. It is measured in litres per second (l/sec).

- **Forced vital capacity (FVC)**. Also using a digital micro-spirometer, this test measures the total amount of air that can be forcibly expired after one inhalation. It is measured in litres. A high FVC score is important for exercisers, because a large amount of air is able to be utilized at any one time.

- **Forced expired ratio (FER)**. This is the ratio of air that the individual can expire in one second (FEV$_1$), to their FVC, and is expressed as a percentage. In healthy adults, the FEV$_1$ is usually at least 80 per cent of the FVC. FER can be useful for isolating problems that were detected under the FEV$_1$ or FVC tests. For example, a poor FEV$_1$ may have been scored because the FVC itself was poor. A good FER, but combined with a poor FVC, could be an indication of lung disease with chest wall rigidity.

TIP

Height, weight, BMI, girth, waist to hip ratio and postural assessments are all discussed in chapter 4. These should all be included in a health-related fitness test.

TIP

Bear in mind that peak flow rate scores from such a condition as asthma can vary significantly at different times of the day.

TIP

The peak flow meter should be cleaned regularly, according to manufacturer's instructions. Washable plastic or disposable card mouthpieces should be used.

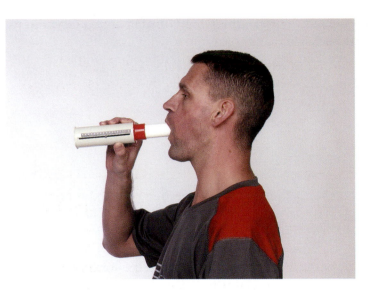

Peak expiratory flow rate test

The test results of FEV_1, FVC and FER need to be compared against recognized norms. These should be provided by the manufacturer of the equipment.

The micro-spirometer is a battery-operated unit, similar in size to the peak-flow meter. It requires a similar protocol (but needs to be switched on first). The forced exhalation should still be as strong as possible, but also for as long as possible (so that FVC can be measured). Micro-spirometry is limited in that it can measure only the rate and volume of air coming out of the lungs, not other useful respiratory information such as: total lung volume (TLV); residual volume (RV); forced inspiratory flow rate (FIFR).

As with most tests of health-related fitness, if the individual records a poor lung function test score, and they are unaware of any underlying respiratory disorder, they should be recommended to take a follow-up test a few days later. If the second test score is poor, then a referral to their GP would be appropriate, but without causing the client any undue anxiety. A good test result suggests that the individual should be able to exercise without respiratory problems.

Body fat testing

One of the key reasons for people taking up fitness training is for the improvement in body contours, body weight and body fat. If initial body fat assessment and periodic follow-up assessments are performed, improvements can be closely monitored and clients can be more likely to maintain their motivation to continue. The traditional pair of weighing scales or 'height–weight' charts cannot provide specific information regarding percentage of body fat. Muscle weighs more than fat, and if regular and appropriate exercise is undertaken, it may appear (on the scales) that body weight is not reducing (it may even be increasing), even though fat levels are reducing. Additionally, body fat testing can help to identify excessive leanness.

There are a selection of ways in which an individual's body fat percentage can be measured. The two most commonly used methods are bioelectrical impedance and skin fold measurement.

Bioelectrical impedance

> Bioelectrical impedance analysis (BIA) is based on the fact that the body contains intracellular and extracellular fluids capable of electrical conduction and cell membranes that act as electrical condensers or capacitors. Because the fat-free mass contains much of the body's water and electrolytes, it is a better conductor of electrical current than fat.
>
> VIVIEN H. HEYWARD (1991)

Bioelectrical impedance body fat monitors usually take the form of a small battery-operated unit, with a set of adhesive pads that are placed on to strategic sites on the body (typically on the right hand and foot) as the subject is lying supine. Information is analysed by the machine and readings provided digitally. It is important that the client has not performed any exercise, or eaten or drunken for several hours before the test. Also they should urinate prior to the test and not have taken any diuretic medication for a week before. The results of the test should be compared against recognized normal values, relative to the client's age, sex and body weight. There are also now available, bioelectrical impedance body fat monitors that are hand-held, or that resemble conventional scales, the reliability of these machines is improving.

TIP

Be aware that body fat percentage norms can only be used as a guide. Different people, different sports, have different ideals. However, individuals nearer the extremes of the ranges should consider remedial action.

Skin fold measurement

There are several well-used protocols for skin fold measure of body fat. The basic idea is that a selection of skin fold sites (commonly three, four or seven sites) on the body are measured using a set of fat callipers. Some protocols specify that skinfolds are only taken from one side of the body, others from both sides. The total sum of all measured sites are added together, and this gives a total skin fold measurement (in mm). This figure is then typically used to estimate, through a series of recognized equations, the client's: body fat in kg; percentage of body fat; lean (fat-free) body mass in kg; and target weight in kg. Their calculated percentage of body fat is compared against validated norms.

TIP

Lean body mass (LBM), or fat-free mass, is the estimated mass of all the non-fat body tissue. This includes muscle, bone and connective tissue. It is estimated as: total body mass (weight in kg) minus total estimated body fat (in kg).

To measure skin fold:

1 Position the client correctly according to the protocol (usually standing, relaxed).

2 Locate the specific skin fold sites.

3 Pinch the superficial tissue away at the skin fold site with finger and thumb.

4 Apply and close the callipers at the site, perpendicular to the fold.

5 Measure the skin folds accurately.

6 Record the measurement of each site.

7 Repeat each measurement three times, and record the average.

TIP

It is important to be able to perform skin fold measurement techniques skilfully and reliably each time.

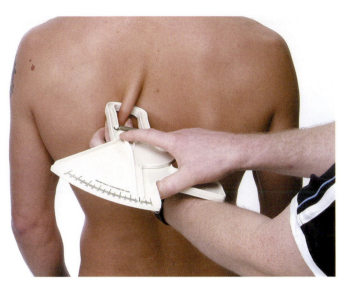

Subscapular skin fold. Skin fold callipers are used to measure superficial body fat thickness

Common skin fold sites used in protocols for estimating body fat percentages:

- Triceps: vertically, midway between the shoulder and elbow.
- Biceps: vertically, midway between the shoulder and elbow.
- Supra-iliac: diagonally, above the iliac crest.
- Subscapular: 1–2 cm diagonally, from the lower medial border of the scapula.
- Chest: diagonally, between axilla and nipple.
- Midaxillary: horizontally, at level of the xiphoid process.
- Abdominal: horizontally, 3 cm lateral and 1 cm inferior to umbilicus.
- Thigh: vertically, midway between inguinal crease and patella (weight is borne on contra-lateral limb).
- Calf: vertically, at level of maximal calf circumference on the medial aspect as the hip and knee are flexed to 90°.

Body fat percentage norms

Males:

- 6–14 per cent below average
- 15 per cent average
- 16–24 per cent above average
- >25 per cent at risk for obesity-related disorders.

Females:

- 9–22 per cent below average
- 23 per cent average
- 24–31 per cent above average
- >32 per cent at risk for obesity-related disorders.

Aerobic fitness testing

There are wide range of tests of aerobic fitness. Observing, recording and analysing exercise performance (i.e. times; exercising heart rates; pulse recovery rates; distances travelled; workloads) can usefully help to provide a functional picture of the individual's aerobic capacity. The preferred approach is to estimate (predict) V_{O_2}max by way of specific protocols and mathematical equations.

Common aerobic fitness tests are:

- cycle ergometer (e.g. Astrand Ryhming, Fox, YMCA, ACSM protocols)

- treadmill run (e.g. Bruce protocol)

- multi-stage 'bleep' test

- pulse recovery rate test

- step tests (e.g. Harvard, YMCA protocols)

- 1 mile walk (e.g. Rockport, Kline protocols)

- 12 minute run (e.g. Cooper protocol).

It is important when evaluating aerobic capacity (V_{O_2}max) that established test protocols are correctly employed. The most common gym or lab-based tests to predict V_{O_2}max involve the treadmill (e.g. Bruce protocol) or cycle ergometer (e.g. Astrand Ryhming protocol), because with such equipment it is relatively easy to control the speed and resistance. Such tests have been scientifically developed in highly controlled circumstances by experts in the field, often in university settings. Their complex, but relatively easy to use, equations have been designed to incorporate specific exertional factors (e.g. resistance, speed, timed progressive increments) and individual factors (e.g. age, sex, exertional heart rates, body weight). Single-stage tests feature no progression of intensity (a continuous workload), whereas multi-stage tests incorporate progressive increments of intensity at specific times during the test. As time goes by, tests are often re-evaluated, adjusted, refined and adapted (by either the original developers or by other experts) so as to improve their efficiency at predicting aerobic capacity.

For men aged under 19, an estimated V_{O_2}max of around 40–50 ml/kg/min can be considered good, and over 19, around 37–47 ml/kg/min. An excellent score, for men under 19 is around 55–65 ml/kg/min, and over 19, 50–60 ml/kg/min. Scores below these may be classed as poor, and scores above may be recorded by highly trained elite endurance athletes.

For women aged under 19, an estimated V_{O_2}max of around 35–45 ml/kg/min can be considered good, and over 19, around 30–40 ml/kg/min. An excellent score, for women under 19 is around 45–55 ml/kg/min, and over 19, 40–50 ml/kg/min.

The **multi-stage 'bleep' (or 'shuttle-run') test** is a maximal test, and is commonly used in group and team situations, because it is easy to organize, requires little in the way of equipment, and a number of participants can take the test at the same time. It is also a functionally relevant test for sports that involve a great deal of short distance but continual running activity. The basic protocol requires that individuals are asked to run back and forth between two lines, 20 m apart, in time to pre-recorded 'bleep' sounds from

TIP

An individual's aerobic capacity, most commonly predicted in tests as their V_{O_2}max score, is usually expressed in one of two ways: in millimetres of oxygen per kilogram of body weight per minute (ml/kg/min) or in litres per minute (l/min).

TIP

Men generally tend to have a higher aerobic capacity than women. With age, V_{O_2}max for both men and women tends to progressively reduce.

TIP

There are instances where predicted V_{O_2}max scores will be invalidated by such individual factors as: tachycardia or an erratic heart rate; cardiac medications that slow or speed-up heart rates.

FITNESS TESTING TECHNIQUES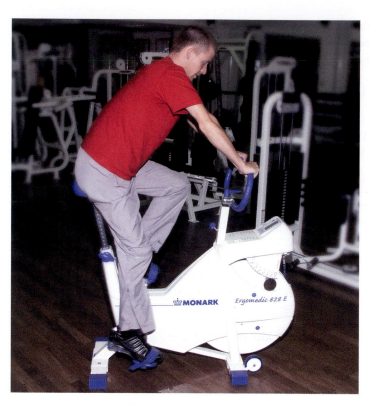

The cycle ergometer is used in tests that estimate V_{O_2}max and also for the 'Wingate test' of anaerobic endurance

TIP

The resting heart rate (RHR) and pulse recovery rate (PRR) are useful methods for monitoring general gains from regular aerobic training.

an audio tape (or preferably a CD). The time between the 'bleep' sounds decreases with each minute, with three 'bleeps' indicating a move onto the next level (the starting running speed is normally 8.5 km/h, which increases by 0.5 km/h each minute). The participants must reach the marker line before hearing the 'bleep', but if the 'bleep' has not been heard, they should wait until it is heard before continuing. Participants should continue until they can no longer keep up with the increasing speed. There are usually 23 levels (each level consisting of a series of 20 m shuttle-runs), and it is likely that only highly trained athletes will reach the upper levels. At the end of the test, a record should be made of the participants' number of shuttles and the level that they reached. The results of the test can be compared against previous tests and also norms (predicting V_{O_2}max) supplied by the manufacturer of the tape or CD.

Pulse recovery rates (PRR) are sometimes included in aerobic fitness tests, and can be an easy and useful method of self-testing for improvements. PRRs measure the decrease in pulse rate after exercise has stopped. It requires that the subject exercises sufficiently strenuously, but at relatively low intensity, so as to elevate their heart rate to a predetermined training level (typically between 70 and 90 per cent of maximum) over a period of a few minutes. A note should be made of the heart rate at the point that exercise is stopped (this is the exercise pulse). The subject should then wait for 60 seconds, and take the pulse again (this is the one minute pulse).

1 minute pulse recovery rate (bpm) = exercise pulse − 1 minute pulse

Obviously, the higher the PRR score, the better the recovery from exertion, and the higher the level of fitness. An excellent one minute PRR would be around 60 bpm or more. Good would be around 40–50 bpm, fair 20–30 and poor 10 or lower. This test can be adapted to observe and analyse the rates of recovery over a period of several minutes, but to maintain reliable comparison, the test must feature the same conditions each time (i.e. exercising to the same level of heart rate, at a similar intensity and time).

There are a selection of established submaximal step tests, the Harvard and YMCA probably being the most well known. They require minimal equipment cost and time, and can be self-administered. A step test typically involves the subject stepping up and down onto a specific height step or bench, at a specific speed dictated by a metronome, for a specific period of time, usually three or five minutes (the stepping speed for men is normally set at a slightly faster rate than for women). Recovery heart rates are taken immediately after the test, and over a period of minutes. Some step tests have been developed so as to predict V_{O_2} max, but they are most useful for assessing an individual's progress with their training programme.

One mile walk tests, the most well known being the Rockport and Kline protocols, are other easily performed fitness tests that can be used to predict V_{O_2} max. Particularly useful fitness tests for individuals of poor fitness, they simply require the individual to walk one mile as quickly as is comfortably possible, usually on an athletics track. The one mile walk must be carefully timed, the subject's immediate post-exercising heart rate taken, and these figures are then incorporated, along with other individual factors (sex, age and weight), into the protocol's equation. A predictive score can be produced, and the result is compared against the norms.

The 12 minute (Cooper) run test is a maximal test, and only recommended for individuals who are already well-trained and able to perform mid-distance running. The basic aim is to run as far as possible on a track in 12 minutes. It is a good test of endurance, with times being compared against norms, and also against the athlete's previous times.

Flexibility testing

Detailed flexibility assessment and methods of training have been discussed in previous chapters. The '**sit and reach**' test is a standard and commonly used general test of flexibility in fitness club environments. Although not specific to any one particular joint or group of muscles, the sit and reach test does allow for quick and easy assessment of back and posterior leg flexibility in one single test, and it can provide a basic impression of the subject's current level of suppleness.

There are several versions of this test. The best method involves use of a specially designed sit and reach box, which has a measured scale (in cm) printed on top. Having firstly warmed up, the subject should sit on the floor with legs fully extended and feet flat against the box. Breathing out, they should lean forward over the box, reaching with their arms (with one hand on top of the other), and the tester should note the point that the fingertips reach on the scale. Three attempts should be taken, and the best score recorded.

 TIP

When providing the sit and reach test, try to identify through observation where the subject's main tightness and suppleness lies (i.e. in the upper back, the lower back, the hamstrings or the calves).

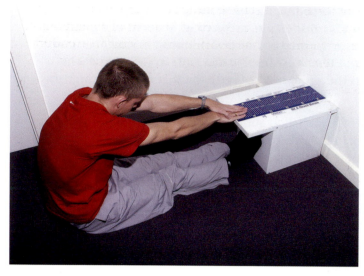

The 'sit and reach' test of back and posterior leg flexibility

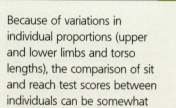

Sit and reach test norms

Males:

- >18 cm excellent
- 6–17 cm good
- 0–5 cm average
- −8–1 cm fair
- <−9 poor.

Females:

- >21 cm excellent
- 11–20 cm good
- 1–10 cm average
- −7–0 cm fair
- <−8 cm poor.

Other simple tests of flexibility include: assessment of prone lying shoulder and wrist extension (lifting a wooden pole as high as possible, with arms above head, with head and chest touching the floor); prone lying trunk and neck extension, with hands clasped behind back (measuring the maximal height of the tip of the nose); standing, place one arm behind head and the other behind the back, trying to touch finger tips to assess shoulder flexibility (if hands do not touch, measure the distance between the finger tips of each hand).

Strength testing

There are various ways of assessing muscular strength and endurance. Such tests may variously assess: maximal isotonic strength (i.e. the most amount of resistance that can be lifted in one effort); maximal isometric strength (i.e. the most amount of force that a static contraction can produce in one effort); maximal isotonic endurance (i.e. the most amount of repetitions of an exercise that can be performed in one bout); maximal isometric endurance (i.e. the most amount of time a forceful static contraction can be held).

Common muscular strength and endurance tests:

- one repetition max
- ten repetition max
- press-ups in a minute/to exhaustion
- abdominal curls in a minute/to exhaustion
- isometric grip strength
- isometric back strength
- isometric abdominal hold
- isometric press-up hold
- isometric quadriceps hold
- 30 second Wingate test.

TIP

One repetition max (1 RM) strength tests are not recommended for the majority of individuals (10 RM tests are the recommended alternative), and 1 RM tests must be avoided by those who are untrained or who have muscle or joint weakness or injuries. All isometric strength tests must be avoided by those with hypertension.

The one **repetition maximum** (1 RM) test is a test of maximum strength ability. It involves the subject lifting or pushing the most weight they can possibly manage in one single effort, typically in such exercises as the bench press, shoulder press or leg press. Because of the potential for injury associated with such an intense maximal test, the 10 RM test is the recommended alternative. This allows for maximal strength to be assessed in conjunction with a small endurance component. The maximal weight lifted will be lower than for the 1 RM test, and therefore the risk of injury is less. The subject should still be considered fit enough and sufficiently prepared (instructed) before they attempt such a test. Obviously, the position and technique must be correct. The resistance station's set-up position, resistance and test score should all be recorded. The test results can be compared against the subject's follow-up scores, thereby allowing the progression of their strength to be effectively monitored.

Upper body muscular strength and endurance are commonly evaluated by performing as many press-ups in a minute as possible. This is a functional test because body weight is being lifted. The press-up position can be adapted to suit different ability levels (i.e. box position, long box position or full press-up position), and technique must be correct. Another adaptation to this test is to perform as many press-ups as is possible (to exhaustion, with no time limit), the technique must remain correct. The subject's position and number of repetitions should be recorded. Abdominal curls in a minute (or to exhaustion) is a similar test that assesses abdominal strength and endurance. Positions for this test can also be adapted to suit different levels of ability.

A dynamometer is an isometric force measuring unit. Dynamometers are used to assess handgrip and back strength. The handgrip dynamometer typically features an adjustable grip handle (to accommodate different handgrip sizes) and either an analogue dial or digital scale which shows the maximal isometric force applied in kilograms. A reset button allows for the dial to be put back to zero following each test. The usual protocol is to: set the handle grip to suit hand size; standing, hold the dynamometer at the side of the body, with forearm in neutral; squeeze the handle as strongly as possible; record the score; repeat the procedure two more times, allowing one minute's rest between each effort; repeat same procedures on contra-lateral limb. The average score for each arm should be recorded and compared against recognized norms for age and sex.

Isometric grip strength norms

Males:

- >70 kg excellent
- 62–69 kg good
- 48–61 kg average
- 41–47 kg poor
- <41 kg very poor.

Females:

- >41 kg excellent
- 38–40 kg good
- 25–37 kg average
- 22–24 kg poor
- <22 kg very poor.

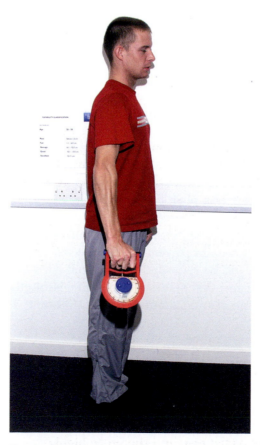

Testing isometric handgrip strength using a dynamometer

The isometric back strength dynamometer features a similar digital or analogue scale, a reset button, footstand and an adjustable length chain and handle (which is adjusted so as to allow for the correct angle of back to legs: 30°). The protocol is similar to that of the grip test, and care must be taken to create the correct testing position. Back strength should not be tested in the presence of acute or chronic back problems.

Isometric back strength norms

Males:

- >209 kg excellent
- 177–208 kg good
- 126–176 kg average
- 91–125 kg poor
- <91 kg very poor.

Females:

- >111 kg excellent
- 98–110 kg good
- 52–97 kg average
- 39–51 kg poor
- <39 kg very poor.

Other isometric strength tests include the abdominal, press-up and quadriceps hold positions. Simply, the normal exercise or test position should be correctly assumed and held for as long as possible, and the duration of the test should be accurately timed in seconds, and the result recorded.

For the abdominal test, the subject should assume the curl-up mid-position, while looking up and forward, and with bent knees. For the press-up test, the subject should assume the selected position (beginner/intermediate/ advanced press-up), and they should lower their elbows until they are at 90°. For the quadriceps test, the subject should sit against a wall and lower their body until their hips and knees are at 90°, with feet directly under the knees and arms hanging down by their sides.

Although these particular isometric tests can be useful in assessing muscular strength and endurance, and they can provide some variety to the testing routine, they are not as functionally relevant as their isotonic counterparts. Smooth rhythmic breathing must be encouraged throughout the test. It is important to remember that isometric tests should not be attempted by those suffering with hypertension.

The Wingate test is a test of anaerobic endurance. The subject cycles on a stationary cycle ergometer, pedalling as fast as they can against a pre-set resistance (relating to their body weight) for 30 seconds. Ideally, this test employs use of a computer program that can analyse the subject's performance, including their average and peak amount of power, and also the decline in power output (fatigue). Because the resistance and speed of performance is relatively high, it is a maximal test, and therefore highly strenuous and exhausting.

Power testing

The most common tests of power in the fitness environment are the standing vertical ('sargeant') jump, and the standing horizontal ('broad') jump. For the vertical jump the subject stands to the side of a high wall, and keeping their feet flat on the floor, they should reach up as high as possible and have their highest fingertip marked off on the wall. Having moved slightly away from the wall, the subject should then leap up explosively as high as possible (using both arms and legs to achieve the maximal height) and touch the wall at the highest point of the jump with their extended hand. The tester should record the height of the jump. Three attempts are usually performed, with the best score being counted. The difference between the standing height and the jump height is the test score. Test scores can be compared against those from previous or follow-up tests, and against published norms.

A similar type of test is the horizontal jump. Typically, the subject's height is measured and marked with two lines on the floor. Using the first line as the start position, the subject should attempt to leap forward, from standing, as far as is possible, landing on two feet. The best result from three attempts should be recorded and compared. It is important when conducting jump tests to make sure that the testing area is safe and free from clutter or slippy surfaces. Also, such tests should not be attempted by those individuals suffering from problematic weight-bearing joints.

Other power-based fitness tests include the medicine ball throw and the short sprint. For the medicine ball throw, the subject should lie down supine on the floor, with arms extended above their head. They should attempt to throw an appropriate weight medicine ball forward from this position as far as possible, without bringing their back off the floor. Obviously, this test requires a large open space. The tester should record the distance that the ball lands at, and the best of three attempts is the test result.

Short, set distance, timed sprints (typically 20, 30, 40 or 50 m) can be performed in a sports hall or on the running track. Functionally relevant for most sporting activities, these tests can help assess speed and power developments. Times can be compared against previous and follow-up tests, and also against team mates or training colleagues.

TESTING THE ELITE ATHLETE

Testing the fitness of elite athletes can certainly involve many of the tests previously discussed. In particular, the maximal V_{O_2}max tests, the sprint tests and the various tests of strength and power are all completely relevant tests that can be used to monitor the fitness and training routines of elite athletes. Elite athletic performance is obviously founded upon a high level of core fitness, and skill development specific to the sport in question. Therefore, testing particular aspects of the athlete's fitness and skill is very relevant. Lab-based fitness testing, by exercise physiologists and sports scientists, using exercise equipment (e.g. treadmill, bike, rowing machine), heart rate monitors, spirometers and even electrocardiograms (ECGs), all linked to specially designed computer software, are the usual methods by which cardio-vascular ability and function are now analysed. Detailed reports are formulated, and training programmes are appropriately adapted in light of the results.

PRE-MATCH FITNESS TESTING

The pre-match fitness test is quite different from the general fitness test. A pre-match fitness test simply aims to assess the ability of the athlete to perform at their normal competitive level, after having recovered sufficiently from injury. Obviously, the recovery from injury involves careful assessment and progressive rehabilitation, and the final stage of such a process involves a period of functional sport-specific training. Once both the player and coach or sports therapist is confident that a return to full competition is possible, then pre-match testing can take place. It is common for the sports therapist to be asked the question 'Can I play on Saturday?' The answer to the question must consider all the relevant factors: the healing of the injury; the amount, type and level of conditioning that the athlete has been able to undertake; the general fitness of the athlete; the sport-specific skills of the athlete; the psychological state of the athlete.

The pre-match test, which may take place a day or two before a competition, or on the morning of the event, basically aims to identify any possible weaknesses in the athlete's functioning, particularly relating to the injury that they have apparently recovered from. It must include performance of intensive moves and techniques that are a feature of their sport. In the case of football, for example, this can include, following warm-up: short bursts of fast-paced running; skipping, hopping, running backwards, zig-zags; stop and start running; explosive jumping and landing; kicking the ball in various ways (e.g. passing and volleying); heading the ball; and blocking tackles. This type of testing can take up to 30 minutes, and if no adverse reactions are reported or observed, then the player may be considered fit for consideration.

> **TIP**
>
> The athlete must be made aware that too soon a return to competition level activity can easily lead to aggravation of the existing injury, or even suffering a new one.

CHAPTER SUMMARY

This chapter has looked at the various ways in which individual fitness can be assessed and analysed. Fitness testing is important for various reasons, and is a particularly useful way of helping the sports therapist plan a programme of training. Follow-up testing helps to monitor the programme, and then build in progressions and adaptations. It is sensible to provide a fitness test with a logical order, beginning, for example, with resting heart rates and blood pressure, and finishing with tests of strength and power. Test results should always be compared against recognized norms (where available) and also against follow-up results. Great care must be taken by the sports therapist to perform the tests correctly and in the same way each time, so as to allow for accurate results and comparison. On completion, the results of the fitness test need to be explained clearly to the client, and their weaknesses and strengths highlighted. It is often that the initial objectives for fitness development are reviewed and altered in light of a set of test results. Elite athletes also commonly undertake many of the standard fitness tests available in health clubs, but they will also periodically undergo more specialized testing in a sports performance laboratory. The pre-match fitness test is a different type of test that aims simply to assess the athlete's fitness to return, following injury, to full competition.

WEBSITE @

Visit the companion website at www.thomsonlearning.co.uk/ healthandfitness/ward where you will find the answers to these questions for you to check your progress through the book.

Knowledge Review

1 Why is fitness testing useful?

2 What would be a logical sequence to a health-related fitness test?

3 In what ways can fitness test results be analysed?

4 Describe the procedure for taking blood pressure.

5 What is: (i) PEFR, (ii) FEV_1, (iii) FVC, (iv) FER?

6 Describe the procedure for measuring body fat using skin fold callipers.

7 List five different tests of aerobic fitness.

8 Describe the 'multi-stage of bleep' test.

9 Describe three different tests of muscular strength and endurance.

appendix 1
case studies

CASE STUDY NUMBER ONE

Mr Owen, the semi-professional footballer: a sports therapy scenario

Mr Owen plays centre forward for a semi-professional football club. He is aged 31, married, and works full-time as a delivery driver. He has played a good level of football since leaving school, his career highlight being a good run with his previous club in the FA Cup, where he scored the winning goal against a well-known first division side, a game that was featured on 'Match of the Day'. Obviously, Mr Owen has suffered a variety of injuries over the years, but fortunately nothing too serious, the worst case being the torn cartilage he suffered about six years ago, which required surgery and a lengthy period of rehabilitation. Mr Owen takes his training very seriously, and has used the services of a masseur regularly over the years. Because his sports therapist has moved away from the area, he is looking for someone else to help him with his training, recovery and minor injuries. He has come to see you two weeks before pre-season training begins.

Task

1 During the initial consultation, in addition to the standard questions, what else do you think it would be important to ask Mr Owen?

2 How might you approach the first treatment session?

3 What after-care advice might you choose to discuss with Mr Owen?

CASE STUDY NUMBER TWO

Mrs Noakes, the long-distance runner: a post-event sports massage treatment scenario

You are part of a small team, at a large marathon event, in a marquee providing post-event sports massage for the competitors. The majority of competitors have received sports massage previously and know what to expect, and the service is proving popular. Mrs Noakes, aged 47, although apparently a keen and experienced runner, informs you that she has never experienced such treatment before. She is clearly a little apprehensive, but has been recommended to try it by one of her running colleagues. She is also obviously very tired and achy following her exertions, having finished the race half an hour ago (in 4 hours 20 minutes).

Task

1 How would you go about putting Mrs Noakes at ease?

2 What information would you require from Mrs Noakes prior to providing any form of treatment?

3 What treatment do you think would be most appropriate on this particular occasion?

CASE STUDY NUMBER THREE

Mr Johnson, the squash player: a minor injury assessment, treatment and after-care advice scenario

Mr Johnson is aged 46, married, with two young children, and runs his own shop-fitting business, which involves a lot of organizational skills as well as manual work. Playing squash twice a week is his main form of exercise and stress relief. Mr Johnson recently undertook a health-related fitness test at the fitness club where he plays, which revealed that he has a BMI of 25 and a WHR of 0.94, suggesting that he is a little overweight (and possibly in the 'at risk' category for CHD). His flexibility was shown to be 'poor', his aerobic fitness to be 'fair', but his strength tests showed 'good' results. Two weeks ago, while playing squash, Mr Johnson felt a sharp pain and 'snapping' sensation in his calf. The leg did not feel right, so he abandoned the game and has not played since. He applied ice to the leg intermittently for a couple of days, which appeared to help with the pain. He did not think that there had been any swelling or bruising, and, during the past fortnight, the pain has reduced considerably, only hurting when he stands on tip-toes or tries to run. Mr Johnson freely admits that he does not undertake any fitness training as such, and that his idea of a warm-up is the 'knock-up' prior to the game.

Task

1 Explain what further information you might require before beginning assessment or treatment for Mr Johnson.

2 Discuss the physical assessment techniques which might be appropriate for him.

3 Explain your treatment strategy.

4 Explain how you would prepare a remedial exercise programme for Mr Johnson.

5 What after care advice would be most appropriate for Mr Johnson?

CASE STUDY NUMBER FOUR

Miss Bell, the amateur footballer: a functional fitness test, treatment and action plan scenario

Miss Bell is aged 23, she has always had a keen interest in watching football, and after seeing an advert for players for the new season for a local women's football team, she decided to give it a try. Her exercise background is limited to sporadic periods of gym training and the occasional aerobics class. She has never played competitive football before. Her general health is good, and the only significant injury that she has sustained was a moderate ankle sprain four years ago, which does give her a little bit of trouble from time to time. She does not smoke, and only drinks alcohol socially. Her job as a social worker is full time and demanding. She is not married and has no children. Seeing the notice board at the gym, she noticed the services of a sports therapist, and thought it might be a good idea to get some advice regarding her training for football. The team trains on Wednesday evenings and plays its games on Sunday afternoons.

Task

1 Explain what further information you might require before beginning any further assessment or treatment for Miss Bell.

2 Discuss the physical assessment techniques which might be appropriate for her.

3 Explain how you would assess her fitness.

4 Explain how you would prepare a programme of regular sports therapy treatment for Miss Bell.

5 Prepare a functionally relevant training programme for Miss Bell.

CASE STUDY NUMBER FIVE

Mr James, the motor mechanic: a post-medical rehabilitation scenario

Mr James, a 38-year-old motor mechanic, was recommended by his GP to visit a physiotherapist following a five day history of left-sided lower back pain and paraesthesia radiating down the left leg (especially on the lateral aspect of the leg and ankle and into the sole of the foot). The pain developed several hours after lifting an engine. The problem was aggravated by sitting, coughing, sneezing and straining at the toilet. It was relieved by resting and lying down. Mr James has had a long history of non-specific backache, but had 'learnt to live with it'. The latest episode had been the worst yet. His GP had prescribed analgesic and anti-inflammatory medication and referred him to a state-registered physiotherapist in private practice.

Initial physiotherapy consultation

Observation: Scoliosis and relative loss of lumbar lordosis.

Palpation: Tender over L5 spinous process. Paravertebral muscle spasm. Trigger points in lumbar erector spinae (referring into left buttock).

RoM: Restricted and painful active flexion, extension and bilateral lateral flexion (more so on left side).

Special tests: Positive straight leg raise – 30° on left. Left foot eversion weakness. Difficulty walking on toes on left side. Sluggish left ankle reflex. Posterior pelvic tilt. X-ray of lumbar and sacral region normal.

Initial diagnosis

L5–S1 intervertebral disc prolapse causing S1 nerve root compression. A high irritability problem.

1st physiotherapy treatment

- Interferential therapy.
- Positional release techniques.
- Manipulation absolutely contra-indicated.
- Continue with GP-prescribed medication.
- Recommended rest from all aggravating physical activities, and adopting positions of maximal comfort.

2nd physiotherapy treatment

- Improvement on initial discomfort.
- RoM still restricted.
- Musculature still very sensitive.
- Manual spinal traction.
- Positional release techniques.
- Gentle massage techniques.
- Acupuncture to lumbar and sacral regions and points on left hip and leg.
- Rest still advised, and supported prone lumbar extension.

3rd physiotherapy treatment

- Spasm and sensitivity reduced.
- Massage (including neuromuscular technique) to lumbar, sacral and hip regions.
- Muscle energy techniques to erector spinae, quadratus lumborum, piriformis and hip flexors.
- Acupuncture techniques.

- Remedial exercises recommended (prone lumbar extension, rotation and flexion, and easy supine, core stability exercise).
- Recommended applications of warmth/heat.

4th physiotherapy treatment

- Symptoms dramatically improved.
- Massage (including neuromuscular technique) to lumbar, sacral and hip regions.
- Muscle energy techniques to erector spinae, quadratus lumborum, piriformis and hip flexors.
- Manual spinal (lumbar) manipulation.
- Recommended visit to sports therapist for exercise guidance, lifestyle and dietary advice and remedial massage therapy.

Initial sports therapy consultation

Mr James revealed that he never takes any form of structured exercise other than his physical occupation. His diet 'is not as balanced or nutritious as it could be'. His height is 1.65 m and weight 95 kg. He smokes about ten cigarettes per day and regularly drinks about two to four pints of beer per day. He rarely drinks water – preferring tea, coffee and fizzy drinks. His resting pulse rate is around 75 bpm. His blood pressure is around 130/90. He is married with two young children. He used to enjoy swimming and cycling as a teenager. He lives two miles from his work. Mr James is pleased with the results of his three week course of physiotherapy. He now is keen to reduce the potential for further episodes. He is excited about the prospect of embarking on a healthier lifestyle with professional sports therapy guidance. He has the full support of his family.

Task

1 Work out Mr James's BMI and compare against accepted norms.
2 Discuss how you would assess your client's physical condition.
3 Outline your proposed therapeutic objectives.
4 Draw up a treatment and action plan. Explain how you would instigate a programme of remedial actions. Your plan and advice should relate to: flexibility, mobility, strengthening and endurance exercise; injury prevention; massage techniques; protective clothing/equipment; diet; thermal therapy. The action plan should be in agreement with your client and tailored to suit his preferences and working commitments.

appendix 2
major muscles: origin (O), insertion (I), action (A) tables

MUSCLES OF THE HEAD, FACE AND NECK

FRONTALIS
O: Cranial aponeurosis
I: Facial muscles of forehead
A: Draws scalp anteriorly, raises eyebrows
Notes: Causes horizontal 'wrinkling' of the forehead, and is also known as the 'occipito-frontalis' muscle.

OCCIPITALIS
O: Occipital bone and mastoid process
I: Cranial aponeurosis
A: Draws scalp posteriorly
Notes: Also known as the 'occipito-frontalis' muscle.

CORRUGATOR
O: Frontal bone (superior and medial to the orbit)
I: Deep skin of medial eyebrow
A: Draws eyebrow medially and inferiorly
Notes: Causes the expression of frowning.

BUCCINATOR

O: Maxilla and mandible, at side of mouth

I: Orbicularis oris

A: Compresses cheek

Notes: Enables the blowing of air out of the mouth, and sucking in.

RISORIUS

O: Fascia overlying the masseter muscle

I: Skin at the angle of the mouth

A: Retracts angle of mouth

Notes: Contributes to the actions of smiling and grinning.

MASSETER

O: Maxilla and zygomatic arch

I: Mandible

A: Elevation, protraction and lateral movements of the mandible

Notes: A main mastication muscle, strongly closing lower jaw and clenching teeth.

ORBICULARIS OCULI

O: Frontal bone and maxilla (orbit)

I: As above

A: Closing of the eye

ZYGOMATIC MAJOR

O: Zygomatic bone

I: Skin at angle of mouth and orbicularis oris

A: Draws superiorly, and retracts angle of mouth

Notes: Contributes to the actions of smiling and laughing.

MENTALIS

O: Mandible

I: Skin of chin

A: Elevates and protrudes lower lip

Notes: Causes wrinkling of the skin of the chin.

ORBICULARIS ORIS

O: Maxilla, nasal septum, mandible and other muscles of mouth

I: As above

A: Closes, compresses and protrudes lips

Notes: Contributes to speech and mastication.

TEMPORALIS

O: Temporal, frontal and parietal bones

I: Mandible

A: Elevation, retraction and lateral movements of the mandible

Notes: A main mastication muscle, closing the lower jaw and clenching the teeth.

STERNOCLEIDOMASTOID

O: Superior sternum and medial clavicle

I: Mastoid process

A: Cervical flexion, protraction and rotation

Notes: When one side contracts, it causes rotation; when both sides contract, they cause flexion and protraction. Also an accessory muscle of respiration.

PLATYSMA

O: Fascia overlying deltoid and pectoral muscles

I: Mandible and fascia overlying the muscles of the chin and jaw

A: Depresses mandible, draws lateral lip posteriorly and inferiorly, and draws superiorly the skin of upper chest

SPLENIUS

O: Ligament nuchae, C7–T6

I: Mastoid process, occiput, C1–C3

A: Cervical extension and rotation

Notes: There are two muscles (splenius capitus and cervicus), which overlie the posterior neck.

SCALENES

O: C2–C7

I: Ribs 1 and 2

A: Elevation of ribs during inspiration, cervical flexion, lateral flexion and rotation

Notes: There are three muscles (scalene anterior, medius and posterior), which are situated at the side of the neck, they are also accessory muscles of respiration.

MUSCLES OF THE BACK AND SHOULDER

TRAPEZIUS

O: Occiput, C7 and all T vertebrae

I: Lateral clavicle, acromion process, spine of scapula

A: Shoulder elevation, cervical extension, scapula retraction, depression and rotation

Notes: Upper, middle and lower segments, forming a trapezoid shape. As the scapula rotates, it contributes to the final component of shoulder abduction.

LEVATOR SCAPULAE

O: C1–C4

I: Upper, medial scapula

A: Elevation and rotation of the scapula, cervical lateral flexion

DELTOIDS

O: Lateral clavicle, acromion process, spine of scapula

I: Deltoid tuberosity, along lateral humerus

A: Shoulder abduction, flexion, extension, medial and lateral rotation.

Notes: Three components (anterior, medial and posterior).

RHOMBOID MINOR

O: C7–T1

I: Upper medial border of scapula

A: Scapula retraction, rotation and fixation

Notes: Situated above rhomboid major.

RHOMBOID MAJOR

O: T2–T5

I: Middle and lower medial border of scapula

A: Scapula retraction, rotation and fixation

Notes: Situated below rhomboid minor.

TERES MINOR

O: Upper lateral border of scapula

I: Greater tubercle of humerus, at the inferior facet

A: Lateral rotation and stabilization of shoulder

Notes: One of the four rotator cuff muscles, situated above teres major. Works closely with infraspinatus.

TERES MAJOR

O: Lower lateral border of scapula

I: Anterior medial humerus at bicipital groove, below the head

A: Medial rotation, adduction and stabilization of the shoulder

Notes: Situated below teres minor, but not considered part of the rotator cuff group.

SERRATUS ANTERIOR

O: Lateral borders of ribs 1–9

I: Anterior surface of medial scapula

A: Protraction, rotation and fixation of scapula

SUPRASPINATUS

O: Supraspinous fossa of scapula

I: Greater tubercle of humerus

A: Initial abduction and stabilization of the shoulder

Notes: One of the four rotator cuff muscles. Runs underneath the acromion process.

INFRASPINATUS

O: Infraspinous fossa of scapula

I: Greater tubercle of humerus

A: Lateral rotation and stabilization of shoulder

Notes: One of the four rotator cuff muscles. Works closely with teres minor.

SUBSCAPULARIS

O: Subscapular fossa (anterior scapula)

I: Lesser tubercle of humerus

A: Medial rotation, adduction and stabilization of shoulder

Notes: One of the four rotator cuff muscles.

LATISSIMUS DORSI

O: T6–L5, iliac crest, inferior angle of scapula, and inferior ribs

I: Bicipital groove of humerus

A: Adduction, medial rotation, extension and depression of shoulder

Notes: Broad origin, narrow insertion, making the latissimus a relatively powerful muscle.

ERECTOR SPINAE

O: Variously: sacrum, iliac crest, spinous and transverse processes of vertebrae and ribs

I: Variously: Spinous and transverse processes, ribs, occiput and mastoid process

A: Extension, rotation and stabilization of the vertebral column

Notes: A large and complex group of muscles, also known as the sacrospinalis, the erector spinae includes: the iliocostalis, longissimus, spinalis and semispinalis (including multifidus) muscle groups.

MUSCLES OF THE UPPER ARM

BICEPS BRACHII

O: (Long head) supra-glenoid tubercle of scapula, (short head) coracoid process

I: Radial tuberosity and bicipital aponeurosis of ulna and forearm flexors

A: Elbow flexion, and supination of forearm

Notes: Two heads (long and short), crosses two joints (shoulder and elbow) and contributes to the synergy of shoulder flexion.

BRACHIALIS

O: Distal half of anterior humerus

I: Coronoid process and ulnar tuberosity

A: Elbow flexion

Notes: Situated underneath the biceps.

CORACOBRACHIALIS

O: Coracoid process of scapula

I: Middle 3rd of medial humerus

A: Shoulder flexion and adduction

Notes: 'Coraco' relates the coracoid process, 'brachial' relates to the upper arm.

TRICEPS BRACHII

O: (Long head) infra-glenoid tubercle, (lateral head) upper, posterior humerus and (medial head) lower, posterior humerus

I: Proximal olecranon process

A: Elbow extension

Notes: Three heads (long, lateral and medial), also contributes to shoulder adduction and stabilization.

BRACHIORADIALIS

O: Lateral humerus

I: Styloid process of radius

A: Elbow flexion

MUSCLES OF THE LOWER ARM AND HAND

SUPINATOR

O: Lateral epicondyle of humerus, lateral collateral ligaments of elbow and proximal ulna

I: Upper lateral radius

A: Supination of forearm

Notes: Contributes to the synergy of elbow flexion.

PRONATOR TERES

O: Medial epicondyle of humerus and coronoid process of ulna

I: Lateral middle radius

A: Pronation of forearm

Notes: Contributes to the synergy of elbow flexion, helps to stabilize the superior radio-ulnar joint and works closely with pronator quadratus.

PRONATOR QUADRATUS

O: Distal anterior surface of ulna

I: Distal anterior surface of radius

A: Pronation of forearm

Notes: Helps to stabilize the inferior radio-ulnar joint and works closely with pronator teres.

COMMON FLEXORS

O: Medial epicondyle of humerus, upper and middle radius and ulna

I: Metacarpals and phalanges

A: Flexion of the wrist and fingers

Notes: This complex group includes: flexor carpi radialis, flexor carpi ulnaris, palmaris longus, flexor digitorum superficialis and flexor digitorum profundus.

COMMON EXTENSORS

O: Lateral epicondyle of humerus and upper, middle and lower radius and ulna and interosseous membrane

I: Metacarpals and phalanges

A: Extension of the wrist and fingers

Notes: This complex group includes: extensor carpi radialis longus, extensor carpi radialis brevis, extensor digitorum communis, extensor digiti minimi, extensor carpi ulnaris and extensor indicis.

POLLICIS GROUP

O: Middle and lower radius and ulna, carpals and 2nd and 3rd phalanges

I: Proximal and distal thumb

A: Extension, abduction, adduction and opposition of thumb (pollex)

Notes: This complex group includes: extensor pollicis brevis, extensor pollicis longus, adductor pollicis, abductor pollicis longus, abductor pollicis brevis, flexor pollicis brevis and opponens pollicis.

MUSCLES OF ANTERIOR TORSO AND ABDOMEN

PECTORALIS MAJOR

O: Clavicle, sternum, six superior costal cartilages and abdominal aponeurosis

I: Greater tubercle and lateral bicipital groove of humerus

A: Adduction, medial rotation and flexion of the shoulder, also assists in flexion

Notes: Broad origin, narrow insertion making the pec major a relatively powerful muscle.

PECTORALIS MINOR

O: Ribs 3–5

I: Coracoid process

A: Protraction, depression and stabilization of scapula

Notes: An accessory muscle of respiration, with three origins (at the ribs).

RECTUS ABDOMINUS

O: Xiphoid process and costal cartilages 5–7

I: Pubic symphasis and pubic crest

A: Flexion of the trunk and compression of the abdominal viscera

Notes: Two heads, either side of the linea alba, sectioned by tendinous aponeurosis (the '6 pack').

TRANSVERSUS ABDOMINUS

O: Ribs 7–12, lumbar fascia, iliac crest and lateral inguinal ligament

I: Linea alba and pubic crest

A: Compression and support of the abdominal viscera, and forced expiration

Notes: The deepest abdominal muscle, fibres run across (transversely), greatly contributes to core stability, is important for back support and strength, and also is an accessory muscle of respiration.

EXTERNAL OBLIQUES

O: Ribs 5–12 (external surfaces)

I: Linea alba, pubis, anterior iliac crest and abdominal aponeurosis

A: Rotation, lateral flexion and flexion of the trunk, and support of the abdominal viscera

Notes: The fibres of the 'outer obliques' run down, diagonally from the ribs to the midline, they are also accessory muscles of respiration.

INTERNAL OBLIQUES

O: Thoracic and lumbar fascia, anterior iliac crest and lateral inguinal ligament

I: Ribs 10–12, linea alba and abdominal aponeurosis

A: Rotation, lateral flexion and flexion of the trunk, and support of the abdominal viscera

Notes: The fibres of the 'inner obliques' generally run up from the inguinal and iliac region to the midline and ribs. They are also accessory muscles of respiration.

QUADRATUS LUMBORUM

O: Ilio-lumbar ligament and fascia, and iliac crest

I: Rib 12 and L1–4

A: Elevation of pelvis, lateral flexion of trunk, and assists in forced expiration

Notes: The fibres run up from iliac crest to bottom rib and lumbar vertebrae.

MUSCLES OF THE HIP AND UPPER LEG

PSOAS

O: T12–L5

I: Lesser trochanter of the femur

A: Hip flexion

Notes: Psoas and iliacus (also referred to as iliopsoas) join together at the same insertion.

ILIACUS

O: Iliac fossa, anterior sacral ligament and anterior hip capsule

I: Lesser trochanter of the femur

A: Hip flexion

Notes: Iliacus and psoas (also referred to as iliopsoas) join together at the same insertion.

GAMMELI

O: Ischium

I: Trochanteric fossa (medial aspect of greater trochanter)

A: Lateral rotation of the hip

Notes: Two muscles (superior and inferior), part of the six lateral hip rotator group of muscles.

PIRIFORMIS

O: Anterior sacrum

I: Superior aspect of greater trochanter of femur

A: Lateral rotation of the hip

Notes: Sciatic nerve runs over or through piriformis, one of the six lateral hip rotator group of muscles.

QUADRATUS FEMORIS

O: Lateral ischium
I: Greater trochanter of femur
A: Lateral rotation of the hip
Notes: One of the six lateral hip rotator group of muscles.

OBTURATORS

O: Obturator foramen of the ischium
I: Trochanteric fossa (medial aspect of the greater trochanter)
A: Lateral rotation of the hip
Notes: Two muscles (internus and externus), part of the six lateral hip rotator group of muscles.

GLUTEUS MAXIMUS

O: Medial iliac crest, posterior superior iliac spine, sacrum and coccyx
I: Gluteal tuberosity, ilio-tibial band and posterior femur
A: Hip abduction, extension, assists lateral rotation
Notes: Broad origin and insertion, making gluteus maximus a relatively powerful muscle.

GLUTEUS MEDIUS

O: Lateral ilium (just inferior to crest)
I: Greater trochanter of femur
A: Hip abduction, assists in lateral and medial rotation
Notes: Situated underneath maximus and over minimus.

GLUTEUS MINIMUS

O: Inferior lateral ilium (over and around acetabulum)
I: Greater trochanter of femur
A: Hip abduction, assists medial rotation
Notes: Deepest and smallest glute.

TENSOR FASCIA LATA

O: Anterior ilium and anterior superior iliac spine
I: Iliotibial band (at middle, upper third)
A: Abduction, medial rotation and flexion of the hip
Notes: TFL contributes to knee extension and stability, via ITB.

ILIOTIBIAL BAND

O: Tensor fascia lata and gluteus maximus

I: Lateral tibial condyle

A: Knee stabilization

Notes: Strong long tendon running down the lateral aspect of the thigh.

GRACILIS

O: Medial inferior pubis

I: Upper medial tibia

A: Hip adduction, assists in knee flexion

Notes: A long thin muscle that inserts into the pes anserine tendon (along with sartorius and semitendinosus). One of the five hip adductor muscles.

PECTINEUS

O: Pubis

I: Medial femur (just below lesser trochanter)

A: Hip adduction, assists in hip flexion and lateral rotation

Notes: The most superior of the five hip adductor muscles.

ADDUCTOR BREVIS

O: Pubis

I: Upper medial aspect of femur

A: Hip adduction, assists in flexion and lateral rotation

Notes: 'Brevis' means small. One of the five hip adductor muscles.

ADDUCTOR LONGUS

O: Pubis

I: Medial aspect of middle femur

A: Hip adduction

Notes: One of the five hip adductor muscles.

ADDUCTOR MAGNUS

O: Pubis and ischial tuberosity

I: Middle third of medial femur and medial condyle

A: Hip adduction and assists flexion and medial rotation

Notes: 'Magnus' means large. One of the five hip adductor muscles.

SARTORIUS

O: Anterior superior iliac spine

I: Upper medial tibia

A: Assists in hip flexion and medial rotation, and knee extension

Notes: Overlies the quadriceps, and runs from hip to medial knee. Shares insertion at the pes anserine tendon with gracilis and semitendinosus.

RECTUS FEMORIS

O: Anterior inferior iliac spine

I: The tibial tuberosity, via the patella tendon

A: Knee extension, and assists hip flexion

Notes: Covers two joints (the hip and knee), and is the most superficial of the four quadriceps muscles.

VASTUS LATERALIS

O: Greater trochanter, gluteal tuberosity and lateral border of femur

I: The tibial tuberosity, via the patella tendon

A: Knee extension

Notes: The most lateral of the four quadriceps muscles.

VASTUS INTERMEDIUS

O: Anterior and lateral shaft of the femur

I: The tibial tuberosity, via the patella tendon

A: Knee extension

Notes: The deepest of the four quadriceps muscles.

VASTUS MEDIALIS

O: Intertrochanteric line (between the greater and lesser trochanters), and along the medial aspect of femur

I: The tibial tuberosity, via the patella tendon

A: Knee extension

Notes: The most medial of the four quadriceps muscles.

BICEPS FEMORIS

O: (Long head) ischial tuberosity, and (short head) lower aspect of the posterior femur

I: Lateral tibial condyle and head of fibula

A: Knee flexion, and assists in hip extension

Notes: The most lateral of the three hamstring muscles, has two heads (long and short), and covers two joints (hip and knee).

SEMIMEMBRANOSUS

O: Ischial tuberosity

I: Posterior aspect of medial tibial condyle

A: Knee flexion, and assists hip extension

Notes: A medial hamstring muscle.

SEMITENDINOSUS

O: Ischial tuberosity

I: Medial tibia, just inferior to the condyle

A: Knee flexion, and assists hip extension

Notes: A medial hamstring.

MUSCLES OF THE LOWER LEG AND FOOT

GASTROCNEMIUS

O: Lateral condyle of femur, and popliteal surface, superior to medial condyle

I: Calcaneum, via Achilles tendon

A: Plantarflexion, and assists knee flexion

Notes: The largest and most superficial calf muscle, it has two heads, covers two joints (knee and ankle), and joins the soleus and plantaris at the Achilles tendon.

SOLEUS

O: Posterior head of fibula, upper fibula and medial border of tibia

I: Calcaneum, via the Achilles tendon

A: Plantarflexion

Notes: Lies underneath the gastrocnemius on the lateral side of the lower leg. It shares its insertion into the Achilles tendon with the gastrocnemius and plantaris.

PLANTARIS

O: Superior to the lateral condyle of the femur

I: Calcaneum, via the Achilles tendon

A: Assists plantarflexion and knee flexion

Notes: A small, short calf muscle, sharing its insertion into the Achilles tendon with the gastrocnemius and soleus.

POPLITEUS

O: Lateral epicondyle of femur and lateral meniscus of the knee

I: Upper aspect of the posterior tibia

A: Assists in knee flexion

Notes: Its fibres run down from the lateral to medial aspect of the knee joint. It helps to 'unlock' the lateral meniscal cartilage of the knee, drawing it back as the knee is flexed.

TIBIALIS POSTERIOR

O: Interosseous membrane, the posterior tibia and fibula

I: Plantar aspect of the tarsals and metatarsals

A: Assists plantarflexion and inversion

Notes: Its fibres run centrally between the tibia and fibula, and medially under the medial malleolus to the tarsals.

TIBIALIS ANTERIOR

O: Anterior, lateral tibia

I: Medial tarsal (cuneiform) bone, and base of 1st metatarsal

A: Dorsiflexion and assists inversion

Notes: Lies anteriorly on lateral shin, crossing over to the medial foot at distal tibia.

COMMON FLEXORS

O: Posterior tibia and fibula, tarsals and metatarsals

I: Metatarsals and phalanges

A: Plantarflexion and metatarsal and phalangeal flexion, assisting variously in inversion, eversion, abduction and adduction

Notes: This complex group, which also provides support to the longitudinal arches, includes: flexor digitorum longus, flexor hallucis longus and the intrinsic foot muscles.

COMMON EXTENSORS

O: Lateral tibia, anterior fibula and interosseous membrane

I: Phalanges

A: Dorsiflexion and phalangeal extension

Notes: This complex group includes: extensor digitorum longus, extensor hallucis longus and the intrinsic foot muscles.

PERONEUS TERTIUS

O: Inferior third of the anterior fibula and interosseous membrane

I: Base of 5th metatarsal (on the dorsal aspect)

A: Dorsiflexion, and assists in eversion

Notes: The most anterior peroneal muscle, its fibres run down just in front of the lateral malleolus.

PERONEUS LONGUS

O: Head of the fibula, and superior 2/3 of the lateral aspect of the fibula

I: Base of 1st metatarsal and medial cuneiform (on the plantar aspect)

A: Eversion, and assists in plantarflexion

Notes: The longest peroneal muscle, it runs laterally under the lateral malleolus to the underside of the foot.

PERONEUS BREVIS

O: Inferior 2/3 of the lateral aspect of the fibula

I: Base of 5th metatarsal (on the dorsal aspect)

A: Eversion and weak assister of plantarflexion

Notes: The shortest, most lateral peroneal muscle, its fibres run down behind the lateral malleolus to the outside of the foot.

MAIN MUSCLES OF RESPIRATION

DIAPHRAGM

O: Xiphoid process, costal cartilages of inferior six ribs and L1–3

I: Central tendon

A: Draws the central tendon down inferiorly during inspiration

Notes: When relaxed the diaphragm is dome shaped, as it contracts, it flattens, increasing the volume of the thoracic cavity.

EXTERNAL INTERCOSTALS

O: Inferior border of (superior) rib

I: Superior border of (inferior) rib

A: Elevation of ribs during inspiration

Notes: When they contract, the eternal intercostals increase the lateral and anteroposterior volume of the thoracic cavity.

INTERNAL INTERCOSTALS

O: Superior border of (inferior) rib

I: Inferior border of (superior) rib

A: Draw ribs together during forced expiration

Notes: The internal intercostals are considered accessory respiratory muscles, helping to decrease the volume of the thoracic cavity during forced expiration.

appendix 3
measurement
conversions

Although conversions from metric to imperial can be useful, it is best to think and work with metric. These days, it is rarely necessary to convert a metric value to imperial for technical purposes. However, older clients may still think in imperial terms and some fitness tests still use an imperial base (the one mile walk test, for example). The BMI equation requires metric weight and height measurements, therefore a conversion chart can be useful. Being more aware of lengths, distances and weights (in real terms), both imperial and metric, better prepares the therapist for interpretation and analysis of test results, exercise recommendations and basic communication skills during consultations. A calculator is also an important piece of basic equipment!

METRIC/IMPERIAL COMPARISONS

- 1 METRE IS GREATER THAN 1 YARD (1 m > 1 yd)
- 1 KILOGRAM IS GREATER THAN 1 POUND (1 kg > 1 lb)
- 1 CENTIMETRE IS LESS THAN 1 INCH (1 cm < 1 in)
- 1 KILOMETRE IS LESS THAN 1 MILE (1 km < 1 mile)

LENGTH/DISTANCE CONVERSIONS

- 1 km = 1000 m = 0.62137 mile
- 1 m = 1000 mm = 100 cm = 0.001 km
- 1 m = 39.37 in = 3.281 ft = 1.0936 yd
- 1 cm = 10 mm
- 1 cm = 0.3937 in
- 1 mile = 1.609 km
- 1 mile = 1760 yd
- 1 ft = 0.3048 m

- 1 yd = 0.914 m = 91.44 cm
- 1 yd = 3 ft
- 1 ft = 12 in
- 1 in = 2.54 cm = 25.4 mm

WEIGHT CONVERSIONS

- 1 kg = 1000 g
- 1 kg = 2.2046 lb
- 1 g = 0.035 oz
- 1 st = 14 lb
- 1 lb = 0.454 kg
- 1 oz = 28.35 gm

DIVISION FACTORS: IMPERIAL TO METRIC

(Divide the imperial number by the given value)
- inches to centimetres: 0.3937
- feet to metres: 3.281
- yards to metres: 1.0936
- pounds to kilograms: 2.2046

HEIGHT AND WEIGHT METRIC/IMPERIAL CONVERSIONS

| Height | | Weight | |
Ft'in"	cm	lb	kg
4'10"	147.3	100	45.4
4'11"	149.9	110	49.9
5'0"	152.4	120	54.5
5'1"	154.9	130	59
5'2"	157.5	140	63.6
5'3"	160	150	68.1
5'4"	162.6	160	72.6
5'5"	165.1	170	77.2
5'6"	167.6	180	81.7
5'7"	170.2	190	86.3
5'8"	172.7	200	90.8
5'9"	175.3	210	95.3
5'10"	177.8	220	99.9
5'11"	180.3	230	104.4
6'0"	182.9	240	109
6'1"	185.4	250	113.5
6'2"	188		
6'3"	190.5		
6'4"	193		

appendix 4
sample forms

FORM 1. SPORTS THERAPY CONSULTATION FORM

The sample consultation form allows the therapist to document all the client's relevant personal details, including: name; date of birth; age; address; contact phone numbers; medical history; medications; recent treatments and consultations; doctor's name and surgery details; height and weight; occupation; exercise routine; specific problems and injuries; general lifestyle notes; informed consent to treatment. It is recommended that, where relevant, particular details can be circled and appropriate notes written in the adjacent space. Take care to identify, for example, which body part (i.e. left or right) is affected. Both client and practitioner should date and sign at the foot of the document.

FORM 2. SPORTS THERAPY RECORD CARD

Therapists are required by law to keep up to date, legible and accurate records. The client's record card must be safely and confidentially stored (along with the consultation form and any other forms filled in with regard to their personal details, including: physical assessments, fitness tests, exercise programmes and action plans). By keeping up-to-date client records, a more effective evaluation of progress is enabled and, also, the appropriateness of the strategies being employed can be better assessed. Client records must be written up (in permanent ink, and using no correction fluid – any corrections should be initialled) after every treatment, and within 24 hours. All entries should be dated and signed by the therapist.

FORM 3. PHYSICAL ASSESSMENT FORM (THREE SEPARATE PAGES)

In the sports therapy clinic, it can be helpful to use physical assessment forms that have all main tests and assessments already listed. All that then remains for the therapist is to: correctly provide the assessments; record the results (ticking where appropriate, stating any measurements and making comments); compare the results against previous results and against recognized norms; explain the results to the client; make particular recommendations in light of the results. Both client and therapist should date and sign at the foot of the document.

FORM 4. FITNESS TEST FORM

The sample fitness test form provided allows for the results of three fitness tests to be documented (for ease of comparison). Whichever particular test protocol being utilized must be specifically documented, and any comments relating to the client's results must be made (e.g. poor, fair; good; excellent; better than last time). The positives and negatives of each test should be identified, objectives reviewed (in light of the test results), and recommendations made. If a particular test is not being taken, write 'n/a' (not applicable). Both client and practitioner should date and sign at the foot of the document.

FORM 5. SPORTS THERAPY ACTION PLAN

The sample sports therapy action plan should help the therapist and client to identify and agree on the main objectives, decide the best methods to achieve these objectives, and plan for the provision of appropriate activities. The client can be given a copy of the (detailed) action plan to take home. Both client and therapist should date and sign at the foot of the document.

SPORTS THERAPY CONSULTATION FORM

Date:

Client name: | DoB: | Age:

Address: | Height (m):

| Weight (kg):

Home Tel No: | Work Tel No: | Mobile Tel No:

Doctor name: | Surgery: | Tel No:

Occupation:

Exercise routine:

Have you recently visited: doctor/consult/physio/osteo/sporther/chiro/acup/pod/msg/other:
Details:

Are you currently taking any medications?
Details:

Main reason for attending:

Any current problem or known history of the following:
Musculo-skeletal problems:

Arthritis; Osteoporosis; Fractures; Joint replacement; Pins and plates:
Heart/Circulatory/Arterial/Blood pressure:

Thrombosis/Embolism/Varicose veins:

Diabetes/Epilepsy/Asthma/Allergy:

Skin conditions:

Cuts/Bruises/Burns/Rashes/Scars/Warts/Moles:

Pregnancies:

Major/Recent illnesses:

Major/Recent operations:

Digestive/Urinary/Endocrine/Respiratory/Neurological problems:

Specific aches, pains, problems and injuries: Head/Neck/Thoracic/Lumbar/
Sacral/Coccygeal/Abdominal/Shoulder girdle/Upper arm/Elbow/Lower arm/
Wrist/Hand/Fingers/Pelvic girdle/Hip/Upper leg/Knee/Lower leg/Ankle/Foot/Toes

General notes: accidents; sports injuries; headaches; migraines; vision; audition; olfaction; sinuses; fatigue; depression; sleep; stress; energy; well being; diet; fluid intake; smoking; alcohol.

I confirm that the above information is correct to the best of my knowledge. If there is any change in my condition I will notify the therapist at the earliest opportunity. I understand that this therapy service may involve a combination of techniques, including: physical assessment; sports massage; remedial massage; heat and cold applications; electro-therapy; remedial exercise. I understand that all treatment methods will be explained to me, and I give my consent to the treatment provided.

Client signature: | Date:
Therapist signature: | Date:

SPORTS THERAPY RECORD CARD

Client name: DoB: Age:

Date/Review/Therapy provided today/After Care/Therapist comments/Therapist signature

PHYSICAL ASSESSMENT FORM (PAGE 1)

Date: Client name: Contra-indications: Y/N Details:

Current objectives:

Height (m) _____ Weight (kg) _____ BMI _____ Body fat (mm) _____ Body fat (%) _____
Comments:

Body circumferences (cm): Chest ___ Waist ___ Hips ___ Upper Arm L ___ R ___ Upper Leg L ___ R ___ Lower Leg L ___ R ___
WHR: _____
Comments:

Body type: Ectomorph ___ Mesomorph ___ Endomorph ___ **Comments:**

POSTURAL ASSESSMENT/BODY ALIGNMENTS

HEAD/NECK: Tilted left ___ Tilted right ___ Rotated left ___ Rotated right ___ Forward ___ Flat Lordotic curve ___
Excessive Lordotic curve ___ Other:
EYES: Level ___ Other:
EARS: Level ___ Other:
MUSCULATURE:
Comments:

SHOULDERS: Level ___ Right high ___ Left high ___ Rounded ___ Other:
SCAPULAE: Even ___ Adducted ___ Abducted ___ Winged ___ Rotated ___ Other:
CLAVICLES: Level ___ Other:
MUSCULATURE:
Comments:

UPPER EXTREMITIES: Hang evenly ___ Rotated ___ Other:
ELBOWS: Even ___ Cubitus Varus ___ Cubitus Valgus ___ Cubitus Recurvatus ___ Other:
WRISTS: Even ___ Other:
FINGERS: Even ___ Other:
MUSCULATURE:
Comments:

SPINE: Normal ___ Kyphosis ___ Lordosis ___ Flat back ___ Scoliosis ___ Other:
MUSCULATURE: Even ___ Other:
Comments:

HIPS: Even ___ Pelvic tilt ___ Coxa Vara ___ Coxa Valga ___ Other:
MUSCULATURE: Even ___ Other:
Comments:

KNEES: Even ___ Genu Valgus ___ Genu Varus ___ Genu recurvatum ___ Patella squint ___ Excess Q Angle ___
Reduced Q Angle ___ Other:
MUSCULATURE: Even ___ Other:
Comments:

ANKLE/FOOT/TOES: Even ___ Tibial torsion ___ Varus heels ___ Valgus heels ___ Pes Planus ___ Pes Cavus ___
Hyper Pronation ___ Hallux Valgus ___ Plantar-flexed first ray ___ Splay foot ___ Hammer-toes ___ Other:
MUSCULATURE: Even ___ Other:
Comments:

LEG LENGTH: Even ___ Discrepancy ___ True ___ Apparent ___
Comments:

Client signature: Date:
Therapist signature: Date:

PHYSICAL ASSESSMENT FORM (PAGE 2)

RANGE OF MOVEMENT ASSESSMENTS (DEGREES OR CM)

CERVICAL: Flexion _____ Hyperextension _____ Left Rotation _____ Right Rotation _____
Left Lateral Flexion _____ Right Lateral Flexion _____
Comments:

THORACIC/LUMBAR: Flexion _____ Hyperextension _____ Left Rotation _____
Right Rotation _____ Left Lateral Flexion _____ Right Lateral Flexion _____
Comments:

SHOULDER: Left Flexion _____ Right Flexion _____ Left Hyperextension _____
Right Hyperextension _____ Left Abduction _____ Right Abduction _____
Left Medial Rotation _____ Right Medial Rotation _____ Left Lateral Rotation _____
Right Lateral Rotation _____ Left Horizontal Abduction _____ Right Horizontal Abduction _____
Left Horizontal Adduction _____ Right Horizontal Adduction _____
Comments:

ELBOW/FOREARM: Left Flexion _____ Right Flexion _____ Left Extension _____
Right Extension _____ Left Pronation _____ Right Pronation _____ Left Supination _____
Right Supination _____
Comments:

HIP: Left Flexion _____ Right Flexion _____ Left Hyperextension _____
Right Hyperextension _____ Left Abduction _____ Right Abduction _____ Left Adduction _____
Right Adduction _____ Left Medial Rotation _____ Right Medial Rotation _____
Left Lateral Rotation _____ Right Lateral Rotation _____
Comments:

KNEE: Left Flexion _____ Right Flexion _____ Left Hyperextension _____
Right Hyperextension _____
Comments:

ANKLE: Left Dorsiflexion _____ Right Dorsiflexion _____ Left Plantarflexion _____
Right Plantarflexion _____ Left Inversion _____ Right Inversion _____ Left Eversion _____
Right Eversion _____
Comments:

Client signature: Date:
Therapist signature: Date:

PHYSICAL ASSESSMENT FORM (PAGE 3)

GAIT ASSESSMENT

HEAD: Upright ___ Forward flexed ___ Deviated laterally ___ Other:
Comments:

TRUNK: Upright ___ Forward flexed ___ Deviated laterally ___ Other:
Comments:

SHOULDERS: Free and even movement during stance and swing ___ Other:
Comments:

ARMS: Reciprocal swing ___ Even motion ___ Other:
Comments:

HIPS: Free and even movement during stance and swing ___ Other:
Comments:

LEGS: Free and even movement during stance and swing ___ Other:
Comments:

KNEES: Free and even movement during stance and swing ___ Other:
Comments:

ANKLES/FEET: Heel strike ___ Propulsion ___ Excess pronation ___ Excess supination ___ Foot slap ___
Excess dorsiflexion ___ Other:
Comments:

GENERAL GAIT PATTERN: Step length even ____ Normal Stride width ____ Normal Foot Angle ____ Pain-free gait ____
Steady gait ____ Normal cadence ____ Other:
Comments:

ANALYSIS OF MOVEMENT PARAMETERS

REVIEWED OBJECTIVES

RECOMMENDATIONS

Client signature: Date:
Therapist signature: Date:

FITNESS TEST FORM

Client name: DoB: Age: Date 1.   2.   3.

Pre-test screening: Y/N Contra-indications: Y/N
Details:

Current objectives:

Height (m): _____ Weight (kg): 1. _____ 2. _____ 3. _____
BMI: _____ Comments:

Body fat (mm): 1. _____ 2. _____ 3. _____
Body fat (%): 1. _____ 2. _____ 3. _____
Comments:

Blood pressure: 1. _____ 2. _____ 3. _____
Comments:

Lung function test: 1. _____ 2. _____ 3. _____
Comments:

Flexibility test: 1. _____ 2. _____ 3. _____
Comments:

Strength test A: 1. _____ 2. _____ 3. _____
Comments:

Strength test B: 1. _____ 2. _____ 3. _____
Comments:

Strength test C: 1. _____ 2. _____ 3. _____
Comments:

Power test: 1. _____ 2. _____ 3. _____
Comments:

Aerobic test A: 1. _____ 2. _____ 3. _____
Comments:

Aerobic test B: 1. _____ 2. _____ 3. _____
Comments:

Positives:

Negatives:

Reviewed objectives:

Recommendations:

Client signature: Date:
Therapist signature: Date:

SPORTS THERAPY ACTION PLAN

Client name: Date: DoB: Age:

OBJECTIVES: Increase postural awareness ___ Amend body contours ___ Improve body position ___ Improve muscle tone ___ Decrease skeletal stress ___ Increase range of movement ___ Injury prevention ___ Restore function ___ Strengthen muscles ___ Improve endurance ___ Improve flexibility ___ Improve speed ___ Improve power ___ Improve balance ___ Improve coordination ___ Improve proprioception ___ Improve agility ___ Improve full functional ability ___ Improve general fitness ___ Improve sports performance ___ Increase energy levels ___ Improve well-being ___ Reduce stress ___ Other:
Comments:

METHODS TO ACHIEVE OBJECTIVES: Modification of current physical activities ___ Training alterations ___ Protective equipment ___ Exercise equipment ___ Sports equipment ___ Taping/Strapping ___ Supports/Bracing ___ Orthotics ___ Cryotherapy ___ Heat/Electrical treatments ___ Remedial massage ___ Remedial exercise ___ Nutritional strategies ___ Self-massage ___ Relaxation techniques ___ Other:
Comments:

EXERCISE TYPE: Early phase ___ Intermediate phase ___ Late phase ___ Functional phase ___ Sport specific ___ Aerobic ___ Isometric ___ Isotonic ___ Isokinetic ___ Concentric ___ Eccentric ___ Core stability ___ Open chain ___ Closed chain ___ Flexibility ___ Static stretching ___ MET stretching ___ Gym based ___ Class based ___ Hydrotherapy based ___ Home based ___ Outdoor ___ Other:
Comments:

EQUIPMENT: Free weights ___ Machine weights ___ Resistance band ___ Wrist/Ankle weights ___ Medicine ball ___ Fitness ball ___ Step ___ Rebounder ___ Treadmill ___ Stationary bike ___ Rower ___ Cross trainer ___ Elliptical trainer ___ Stepper ___ Upper body ergometer ___ Wobble board ___ Other:
Comments:

DETAILED ACTION PLAN: This should include specifically documented exercises and other recommendations, relating to the client's *current* condition, and to the information stated above.

Continue on another sheet if necessary

Client signature: Date:
Therapist signature: Date:

appendix 5
useful contacts

PROFESSIONAL ASSOCIATIONS, AGENCIES AND TRAINING PROVIDERS

Data Protection Agency
Information Commissioner Wycliffe House
Water Lane
Wilmslow
SK9 5AF
Tel: 0162 554 5740
www.dataprotection.gov.uk

Federation of Holistic Therapists (FHT)
3rd Floor
Eastleigh House
Upper Market Street
Eastleigh
SO50 9FD
Tel: 023 8048 8900
www.fht.org.uk

Fitness Professionals Ltd (Fit Pro)
Kalbarri House
107–113 London Road
London
E13 0DA
Tel: 08705 133 434
www.fitpro.com

Focus Training Ltd
5 Cannons Court
Institute Street
Bolton
BL1 1PZ
Tel: 01204 388 330
www.focus-training.com

ILAM (Institute of Leisure and Amenity Management)
ILAM House
Lower Basildon
Reading
RG8 9NE

Tel: 01491 874800
www.ilam.co.uk

Institute for Optimum Nutrition
Blades Court
Deodar Road
London
SW15 2NU
www.ion.ac.uk

International Therapy Education Council (ITEC)
4 Heathfield Terrace
Chiswick
London
W4 4JE
Tel: 020 8994 4141
www.itecworld.co.uk

London School of Sports Massage
28 Station Parade
Willesden Green
London
NW2 4NX
Tel: 020 8452 8855
www.lssm.com

Northern Institute of Massage
14–16 St Mary's Place
Bury
BL0 0DZ
Tel: 0161 797 1800
www.nim56.co.uk

Premier Training and Development Ltd
Parade House
70 Fore Street
Trowbridge
BA14 8HQ
Tel: 01225 353574
www.premierglobal.co.uk

Sports Massage Association
40 Nottingham Place
London
W1U 5NX
Tel: 020 7908 3639
www.sportsmassageassociation.org

Sports Rehab and Education Services Ltd
16 Royal Terrace
Glasgow
G3 7NY
Tel: 0870 240 7417

SPRITO (Sport and Recreation Industry Training Organization)
24–32 Stephenson Way
London
NW1 2HD
Tel: 020 7388 7755
www.sprito.org.uk

The Register of Exercise Professionals (REPS)
Charter House
29a London Road
Croydon
CR0 2RE
Tel: 020 8686 6464
www.reps-uk.org

The Society of Sports Therapists
16 Royal Terrace
Glasgow
G3 7NY
Tel: 0845 600 2613
www.society-of-sports-therapists.org

The Wright Foundation (Exercise Referral Training)
PO Box 159
Dundee
DD1 9HF
Tel: 01382 451188
www.wrightfoundation.com

Vocational Training Charitable Trust (VTCT)
Unit 11
Brickfield Trading Estate
Chandlers Ford
SO53 4DR
www.vtct.org.uk

YMCA Fitness Industry Training
111 Great Russell Street
London
WC1B 3NP
Tel: 020 7343 1850
www.ymcafit.org.uk

TRADE JOURNALS AND MAGAZINES

International Therapist
Dept. I T
3rd Floor Eastleigh House
Upper Market Street
Eastleigh
SO50 9FD
Tel: 023 8048 8900
www.fht.org.uk

Massage World
5–6 Newman Passage
London
W1T 1EH
Tel: 020 7323 5821

Peak Performance
67–71 Goswell Road
London
EC1V 7EN
www.pponline.co.uk

SportEx
Centor Publishing Ltd
86 Nelson Rd
Wimbledon
London
SW19 1HX
Tel: 020 9287 3312
www.sportex.net

TRADE SUPPLIERS

Allsport Medical
15–17 The Garrick Centre
Irving Way
London
NW9 6AQ
Tel: 020 8203 1441
www.allsportmedical.co.uk

Bodycare Products
Northfield Road
Southam
CV47 0RD
Tel: 01926 816 155
www.bodycare.co.uk

JPM Products Ltd
Units 11–12
Crane Mead Business Park
Crane Mead
Ware
SG12 9PZ
Tel: 01920 468 380
www.jpmproducts.co.uk

Physio-Med Services Ltd
7–12 Glossop Brook Business Park
Glossop
SK13 7AJ
Tel: 01457 860444
www.physio-med.com

Physique Management Company Ltd
Jackson Close
Grove Road
Drayton
Portsmouth
PO6 1UP
Tel: 0870 60 70 381
www.physique.co.uk

ProActive Health Ltd
Quarry Court
Bell Lane
Cassington
OX29 4DS
Tel: 01865 886 300
www.proactive-health.co.uk

glossary

acupuncture A therapeutic technique involving the insertion of needles. Used by some physiotherapists and doctors (and acupuncturists). Practitioners claim beneficial effects for such problems as: pain management; impaired circulation; hypertonicity; trigger points; low energy.

acute injury The immediate and early stage of an injury, typically described as being the initial 24–72 hours following trauma, and marked by the presence of an inflammatory response.

adenosine triphosphate ATP is a chemical compound containing adenine, ribose and three phosphate groups. ATP provides the energy for muscular contractions. The muscle myofilaments (actin and myosin) use this energy to cause their process of cross-bridging during the contraction of muscle fibres. This compound is involved in all three pathways of energy supply: the two anaerobic pathways (creatine phosphate and lactate systems) and the aerobic system.

adhesions Fibrous infiltration of soft-tissue as a result of trauma or pathology. Involves a binding together of normally separate tissues, resulting in restricted mobility.

aerobic training Relatively long-duration, low-intensity exercise. Fuelled by the aerobic pathway of energy.

agility training A key component of fitness. Developing balance, co-ordination, speed, reaction and generally fluid movement.

agonist Prime mover or protagonist. A muscle whose action is the main mover of a joint.

anabolism The metabolic process of building up simple substances into more complex compounds.

anaerobic training Exercise activity performed without utilizing the oxygen (aerobic) energy pathway. Fundamentally, relatively short-term strength, speed and power-based activities.

antagonist Muscle whose action opposes that of its agonist. Major muscles tend to work in antagonistic pairs across joints (e.g. biceps and triceps).

ante- Prefix meaning before or forward (e.g. antenatal; anterior; anteversion).

anti- Prefix meaning against (e.g. anti-inflammatory; antibiotic; antigen).

arthroscopy 'Key-hole' examination of a joint through a tiny camera, with visuals on a screen. The procedure may incorporate a trimming and cleansing operation of the joint.

articulation (a) Where two or more bones meet to form a joint (e.g. the knee joint; the scapulo-thoracic articulation). (b) The movement of a joint, whether active or passive.

atrophy Wasting of muscle due to disuse, disease, injury or malnutrition.

audiosonic (AS) A hand-held percussor massage machine. Produces a gentle agitation of tissues at a depth under the skin.

balance (physical) The ability to maintain the body's centre of gravity over its base of support.

balance training Exercise techniques designed to encourage physical balance, such as standing on one leg, on a wobble board, or maintaining positions using a fitness ball.

ballistic stretching 'Bouncing' type mobility exercise. Not usually recommended for developing flexibility, but possibly useful as part of the warm-up for certain sports.

basal metabolic rate (BMR) The lowest rate of metabolism (energy use) that can sustain life. Measured after overnight sleep and fast.

beats per minute (bpm) A common and simple method for evaluating the intensity of training, and for basic fitness assessment.

blood pressure (BP) The pressure exerted on the walls of the main arteries as the heart is contracting (systolic) and relaxing (diastolic).

body fat percentage The estimated proportion of body fat in the body. Typically assessed by use of skin fold measurements or bioelectrical impedance, and the associated mathematical formulae.

body mass index (BMI) Body mass index is a rather limited, but commonly used estimate of an individual's fatness. A simple formula takes the individual's weight (in kg) and divides this by their height (in m) squared. BMI = weight (kg)/height (m^2), and the resulting figure is compared against a small scale of generalized norms.

bone Hard, dense, connective tissue. Two basic types: compact and cancellous. Five classifications of bone: short; long; irregular; flat; sesamoid.

bone marrow Contained within the inner cavity of many bones. Red bone marrow produces new blood cells. Yellow bone marrow stores fat cells.

bursa A fluid-filled, sac located around joints, and whose purpose is to help reduce the friction between moving tissues.

bursitis Inflammation of a bursa, due to mechanical irritation (e.g. constant rubbing of tendons; excessive compression), or infection.

calorie A unit of energy measurement used to measure heat-producing, or energy producing value in food.

cardio-vascular (CV) The combined functional aspects of the circulatory (in particular the heart) and respiratory (in particular the lungs) systems.

cartilage Resilient connective tissue. Provides additional protection and support for the skeletal system. Three types: articular; fibro; elastic.

catabolism The metabolic breakdown of complex compounds into simpler substances.

cavity An anatomical space. Commonly described cavities are the: cranial; spinal; thoracic; abdominal; pelvic. Cavities are defined by the skeletal and soft-tissue structures that surround them, and also contain areolar and adipose connective tissue. Four particular anatomical spaces, commonly described due to their vulnerability and the important structures that they house, are: the femoral triangle (below the groin); the popliteal space (behind the knee); the cubital space (in the elbow crease); the axillary space (the armpit).

cell The basic unit of life.

chiropody/podiatry Allied medical professions, involving treatment of the feet by a chiropodist or podiatrist, for such a variety of foot-related problems as corns, calluses, pes planus, hallux valgus, structural malalignments and impaired gait.

chiropractic One of the mainstream complementary therapies. Principally involves the application of joint manipulative techniques aimed at improving structural alignment.

chronic injury A long-standing injury problem.

closed-chain exercise Exercise in a weight-bearing position that produces predictable movement through the associated kinematic chain.

code of ethics An official set of rules as agreed and instigated by a professional organization. Guided by legal regulations, and designed to promote high standards of practice, it will state clearly the obligations of its members.

cold pack An easy method of applying cryotherapy to an injured region. Typically made from frozen gel or silicone.

collagen A connective tissue, and there are several types. Gives strength and resilience to structures, and is predominant in ligaments, tendons, cartilage and scar tissue.

complementary Therapy or 'medicine' that may either be recommended in conjunction with conventional allopathic medicine, or sought privately by the individual. The mainstream complementary therapies (e.g. osteopathy; chiropractic; acupuncture; sports therapy; aromatherapy; reflexology) have in recent years gained much greater respect and utilization.

concentric contraction An isotonic muscle contraction, with shortening of the primary muscle(s).

condyle A rounded protuberance that occurs on some bones, either for muscle attachment or stability (e.g. medial and lateral femoral condyles).

connective tissue The most abundant basic tissue. Binds together, supports, strengthens and protects. The main classes of connective tissue are: areolar; adipose; white fibrous; elastic fibres; reticular fibres; cartilage; blood; bone.

continuous training A key component of aerobic fitness training that involves the athlete sustaining a 'steady state' of submaximal long duration exertion.

cool-down A key component of fitness training. Designed to help return the body to its pre-exercising state and to reduce the potential for poor recovery or delayed onset muscle soreness.

co-ordination training A key component of fitness development. Involves skills practice (repetition).

creatine phosphate (CP) A substance found in skeletal muscle used for very short-term maximal energy.

cryotherapy The use of cold or ice for therapeutic purposes, typically to help calm inflammation, swelling and pain.

cyto- Prefix relating to the study of cells (e.g. cytology; cytoplasm; cytotoxic).

dehydration Loss of body fluids.

delayed onset muscle soreness (DOMS) Characteristic muscle aching, tenderness, oedema and weakness following excessive or inappropriate exercise activity.

derm- Prefix relating to the skin (e.g. dermis; epidermis; dermatome).

dermatome An area of skin supplied by one sensory spinal nerve. Typically, a strip of skin, about an inch or two (2–5 cm) wide, either running around the torso or down the limbs. Each relates to a particular spinal segment.

developmental stretching Relatively long duration, relaxed and progressive stretching. Helps to improve flexibility.

diagnosis Educated assessment of the nature of an injury or illness, made by a medical expert.

diaphragmatic breathing A relaxation and breathing training exercise. Conscious full breathing, involving controlled activation of the diaphragm during inspiration.

diffusion Process whereby small molecules pass through the semi-permeable cell membrane, from an area of high concentration to an area of lower concentration. Diffusable substances include water, oxygen, carbon dioxide, glucose, amino acids, fatty acids, glycerol, vitamins and minerals.

direct injury An extrinsic injury, typically involving an impact trauma.

diuretic A substance that promotes water excretion.

duration A key aspect of sports therapy. Duration means 'period of time'. In any particular treatment or exercise, the duration may be a few seconds, minutes, or more.

dynamometer A strength testing machine. Most common are for hand grip strength or back strength. The grip strength dynamometer usually incorporates an adjustable grip handle and a dial, which shows the amount of force produced during a single (isometric) exertion.

dys- Prefix meaning abnormal, problematic (e.g. dysfunctional; dyspepsia; dyslexia).

ease-bind A palpatory soft-tissue assessment technique, used to ascertain the relative amount of easy movement and eventual restriction in connective tissues and muscles.

eccentric contraction An isotonic muscle contraction, with lengthening of the involved muscle.

electrical muscle stimulation (EMS) Muscles may be electrically stimulated, by way of a low-frequency interrupted direct current, to encourage increased tone, and to gently massage an area. Can be useful in early and intermediate stage rehabilitation.

electro-massage Massage techniques applied by a machine. There are a variety of units, each offering different effects and applications.

end-feel The quality of feel at the end-range of a joint's movement, as assessed and palpated by the therapist.

endo- Prefix meaning within, inner, containing (e.g. endomycium; endocrine; endogenous).

endocrine gland Hormone-secreting ductless gland. Hormones are chemical messengers and are released directly into the bloodstream. The endocrine system works with the autonomic nervous system to regulate most bodily functions.

endorphin A variety of opioid peptide hormones secreted in the CNS. Their most well-known action is in the mediation of pain.

enzyme A biological catalyst. Enzymes are protein compounds that speed up the rate of physiological reactions, but do not themselves alter in the process.

The main two factors involved in enzyme activity are the body's working temperature and the pH (measure of acidity) of the involved solution.

epi- Prefix meaning upon, following (e.g. epimycium; epicondyle; epithelium).

epicondyle A protuberance above a condyle on a bone (e.g. medial and lateral humeral epicondyles).

epithelium Tissue that covers the inner surfaces of the body. Several types, with various functions. It lines vessels and organs, forms membranes, and glands are made up of epithelial tissue.

ergogenic Able to improve work or performance.

erythema A reddening of the skin, due to increased superficial circulation and vasodilation.

essential When used to describe a nutrient: necessary for growth and well-being, but cannot be produced in the body so must be provided by food.

extra- Prefix meaning outside, beyond or in addition to (e.g. extracellular; extracapsular; extraction).

extrinsic injury An injury related to external factors, such as the nature of the training, equipment, environment or competition.

facilitated region An abnormal situation, where neurologically related soft-tissues become hypersensitive or hyperirritable due to constant dysfunctioning.

fartlek training Fartlek training, or 'speed-play' training, involves varying the speed of the exercise at various periods in the activity.

fascia Fibrous connective tissue. Covers, supports and separates muscles.

fibrosis Process of scar tissue formation.

first aid The initial help and assistance offered to an injured or affected person.

fitness test (health-related) A series of basic tests and controlled exercises, designed to gain assessment of the subject's physical and functional capabilities.

fixator Stabilizing muscles, whose main action is to provide support to assist in holding the body in position during posture and while movement takes place. Core stabilizing muscles can be trained to support the back and torso during movements of the body. Stabilizing muscles are predominantly slow twitch (Type 1) muscle fibres, and are deep and close to joints.

flat back A postural malalignment demonstrating a reduced lumbar curvature, often associated with posterior pelvic tilt.

flexibility The relative suppleness or ability to stretch all major muscle groups towards a near normal range. May be measured by use of a tape measure or goniometer.

foramen A hole in a bone or group of bones (e.g. ischial and vertebral foramen).

fracture A break in a bone. Various types, e.g. compound; comminuted; greenstick; avulsion; stress.

frequency A key aspect to sports therapy. Frequency is typically taken to mean 'how often' (e.g. three sets of ten repetitions of one particular exercise in one workout, and three exercise sessions or treatments per week). In treatment situations, electrical frequencies need to be carefully selected and adjusted when using electrical muscle stimulation, transcutaneous electronic nerve stimulation or ultrasound.

gait The quality and style of walking (or running). Two basic components: stance phase and swing phase.

glycaemic index (GI) A measurement of the degree to which carbohydrates in different foods raise blood sugar levels, compared with pure glucose.

glycogen The form of carbohydrate stored in the body, mostly in the muscles and liver.

glycogenesis The conversion of protein or fat to glucose.

glycogenolysis The conversion of glycogen to glucose.

goniometry The measurement of specific angles and ranges of movement, using a goniometer (a type of protractor).

gym induction The process of guiding a new gym member through all the essential safety issues, and instructing the use of equipment (stations, machinery and free weights).

G5 machine A free-standing massage machine, with a selection of applicator heads for different effects.

haemo- Prefix relating to blood (e.g. haemoglobin; haemophilia; haemostasis).

holistic An approach to health improvement which considers the 'whole' of the person: their mental (mind), physical (body) and spiritual (spirit) well-being.

homeostasis State of internal physiological balance or equilibrium, despite variations in the external environment.

hormone Chemical messenger produced by endocrine glands. Typically released directly into the bloodstream.

hot pack Any type of small heated pack that might be heated in boiling water, in the microwave, or electrically. May be applied onto the body, post-acutely, to provide superficial warmth, increased circulation, relaxation, pain relief or preparation (pre-heat) for further treatment.

hydrotherapy The use of water to provide therapeutic benefit. May involve: jacuzzi/whirlpool; steam bath; water jet massage; exercise in water.

hyper- Prefix meaning above normal or excessive (e.g. hypertonic; hypertension; hyperextension).

hyperaemia Increase in blood circulation through a region.

hypertrophy Increase in size of muscle fibres due to specific resistance training.

hypo- Prefix meaning below normal or deficient (e.g. hypoglycaemia; hypothermia; hypoxia).

impact injury An injury resulting from an impacting force, for example having a heavy fall, head clash with an opponent, or being struck by a ball.

indirect injury An intrinsic injury, typically resulting from excessive forces generated within.

inflammation The body's typical acute response to a musculo-skeletal injury. The five classic signs and symptoms are: pain; swelling; redness, warmth; and impaired function.

infra-red lamp A useful form of thermal therapy. Provides increased circulation, relaxation and possibly pain relief. Many safety issues apply.

insertion Point(s) on a bone that a muscle runs to. On concentric contractions the insertion moves towards the origin.

insulin A hormone produced by the pancreas that assists glucose entry into cells.

intensity A key aspect of sports therapy. Intensity means 'how hard'. In training, the intensity should always be appropriate to the individual's ability. In treatment, the intensity might relate to the strength of electrical stimulation, or to the amount of pressure applied through a massage technique, for example. Intensity should always be increased with caution.

inter- Prefix meaning between (e.g. intermuscular; interstitial; interosseous).

interval training A form of aerobic training that combines periods of strenuous work with periods of recovery.

intra- Prefix meaning within (e.g. intramuscular; intracellular; intra-articular).

intrinsic injury An injury resulting from, individual, anatomical or pathological factors.

isokinetic training Muscle training that maintains tension on a muscle across its available range of movement at a controlled speed with an accommodating resistance.

isometric training Isometric means same length. Muscle contractions without shortening or lengthening, a static contraction. Particularly useful in early stage rehabilitation strengthening.

isotonic training Isotonic means same tension. Muscle contraction with shortening and lengthening. Most gym machine and free weight strength exercises involve isotonic contractions.

joint An articulation. The contact point between two or more bones and/or cartilage. Joints are either synovial (freely movable), cartilaginous (slightly movable) or fibrous (immovable).

karvonen formula The 'heart rate reserve (HRR) formula' incorporates the resting heart rate into the training heart rate (THR) (220 − age = HR_{max}) equation. The Karvonen formula: HR_{max} − RHR = HRR (bpm). HRR × (percentage exercise intensity) = A. A + RHR = THR (bpm). (RHR = resting heart rate.)

kinematic The dynamics of movements. The 'kinematic chain' is the complete series of muscles, bones and joints involved in any particular movement.

kinesthesia Usually taken to mean conscious awareness of body position and movement rates.

kyphosis Postural malalignment demonstrating exaggerated or pronounced thoracic curvature.

legislations Official and legally binding laws, rules and regulations.

ligament Tough, relatively inelastic band of connective tissue. Ligaments are predominantly composed of collagen fibres, and attach, link and hold bone to bone at joints. They also form part of the synovial capsule. Like tendons, they have a relatively poor blood supply.

ligament stress test (LST) A basic structural integrity test of a suspected ligamentous injury. Involves the therapist passively stressing the affected ligament along its length. Excess laxity or pain can be indicative of injury.

lordosis Postural malalignment demonstrating exaggerated or pronounced cervical or lumbar curvature.

manual muscle tests (MMT) Tests aimed at assessing the contractile ability of muscles. MMTs help to differentiate between a muscle injury, neurological impairment and damage to related tissues.

manual therapy Any treatment predominantly performed by the therapist without much in the way of equipment, such as massage or mobilization.

martial arts Oriental disciplines of fitness, self-defence and personal development.

massage Manipulation of the soft-tissues of the body for a selection of effects and benefits.

massage medium Lubricant used to help perform certain massage techniques, including: oils; creams; lotions; balms; talcs.

membrane A thin layer of tissue. Surrounds a cell, tissue or organ, or lines a cavity. A mucous membrane, such as in the respiratory or digestive tract, secretes mucus for protection and lubrication. Serous membranes line the larger cavities of the body, such as the abdomen (peritoneum) or chest (pleura). These comprise two layers, lubricated by a thin plasma-like (serous) fluid, which encourages a freer movement of the organs within.

metabolism The chemical and physical changes that take place within the body to facilitate continued growth and functioning.

mobility The measurable amount of movement available at a joint, or range of joints. Mobility may also be seen as the individual's functional ability to move, either specific joints or generally.

multi-stage bleep test A classic test which allows for evaluation of an individual's aerobic capacity. Involves timed runs between two points, and as the test progresses, the time increases. The subject attempts to run and keep up with the sound of pre-recorded 'bleeps'.

muscle Contractile tissue, for motion, posture, heat production and movement of substances within the body. Three types: striated (skeletal or voluntary); smooth (involuntary); cardiac (heart).

muscle tone/tonus Normal state of partial contraction in a resting muscle.

muscular endurance A key aspect of fitness development. The ability to perform and maintain relatively strenuous muscular activity.

myo- Prefix relating to muscular system (e.g. myofibril; myoglobin; myositis).

myotome A group of muscles innervated by a single nerve root.

nerve A bundle of fibres responsible for transmitting impulses of sensation to the CNS, or motor impulses from the CNS to muscles and organs.

neuro- Prefix relating to nervous system (e.g. neurology; neuromuscular; neurotransmitter).

neurotransmitter Chemical released at nerve endings to transmit impulses across synapses to other nerves or to the muscles, organs or glands that they supply.

observation Visual inspection or analysis.

oedema Swelling as a result of abnormal accumulation of fluids within tissues. Can be local or general, acute or chronic. May be lymph or synovial based. Can result from problematic lymphatic drainage, trauma to tissues or secondary to underlying pathology such as coronary heart disease. Chronic oedema may be accompanied by thin, fragile or thickened sclerosed skin.

open-chain exercise Exercise where the working limb (or kinematic chain) is not in a weight-bearing position (e.g. seated leg extension). It is often employed during intermediate stages of rehabilitation.

organ Body part of two or more tissues forming a specific function. The organs of the body are known as viscera.

origin Point(s) of attachment for a muscle, via its tendon(s), to its bone(s).

orthopaedics The area of medicine involved in the detail assessment, surgical intervention, and recommendation for treatment and management of musculo-skeletal problems.

orthotics The science involved in the making and fitting of orthopaedic supports, braces and shoe inserts and modifications.

osteopathy One of the mainstream complementary therapies. Involves detailed physical assessment, followed by such techniques as massage, muscle energy, positional release and joint manipulation.

overload A key training principle. In order to gain improvements (adaptations) in fitness, training levels should be (progressively) overloaded (at appropriate intervals).

overtraining A condition typified by such symptoms as excessive fatigue, higher incidence of injuries, poor sleep, persistently elevated heart rate, amenorrhoea, weakened immune system, etc.

overuse injury An injury resulting from excessive, repetitive or inappropriate training.

palpation Physical assessment of tissus through educated touch and feel.

para- Prefix meaning near, beside, resembling or abnormal (e.g. parathyroid; parasympathetic; paraesthesia).

paraffin wax (PW) Thermal (heat) therapy using molten paraffin wax, applied to the affected region either by brush or by repeated immersion into a specialized wax bath.

pathology The study of disease processes.

peak expiratory flow rate (PEFR) A simple test of lung function. The subject blows forcefully into a tube, and their score is recorded. Provides basic information regarding the peak rate of air coming out of the lungs in one blow.

perceived exertion (scale of) The Borg scale of perceived exertion allows the exerciser to report, subjectively, on how hard they feel they are exercising. A scale of 6 (no exertion) to 20 (maximal exertion) is typically used.

percussor machine Electrical massager, which produces rapid tapotement-like movements. Helps to increase circulation and relax muscle tension.

peri- Prefix meaning around (e.g. pericardium; perimycium; periosteum).

periodization A key training principle, involving the tailoring of fitness programmes towards achieving total preparation for optimal performance in competitions. Periodization typically employs three phases of preparation: a conditioning phase; a transitional phase; and a competition phase.

periosteum A vascular, fibrous membrane – the outer protective covering for bone. Gives attachment for muscles and ligaments and contains many osteogenic and osteoblast cells (the bone-forming cells that deposit new bone tissue). Also contains nerves, lymph vessels and capillaries which serve the marrow and cancellous bone.

periostitis Inflammation of the periosteum, typically resulting from excessive physical stress from exercise (e.g. 'shin splints').

permeability The ability of membranes to allow soluble substances to pass through them.

phasic muscles More responsible for explosive movements through gravity. Tend to be uniarticular (crossing just one joint), but not always. Have greater proportion of fast twitch (Type II) fibres and, therefore, contract quickly but are more prone to fatigue. They are also more prone to such activity injuries as musculo-tendinous junction problems and tendonitis.

physical activity readiness questionnaire (PARQ) Used for basic pre-exercise screening of clients.

physical assessment A selection of manual tests designed to form a basic assessment of the client's physical state, which then guides the sports therapist towards being able to provide the correct treatment and advice. Involves observation and palpation, and can include assessment of: height; weight; body circumferences; posture; range of motion; gait; and muscle, joint, nerve and circulatory integrity.

physical fitness Defined variously as being: the ability to comfortably perform particular physical tasks; the ability to carry out daily tasks without undue fatigue; the ability to function well under exercise conditions; the capability of the cardio-respiratory and muscular systems to function at optimum efficiency.

physiotherapy A major allied medical profession involving assessment, treatment and prescriptive exercises for a wide variety of health problems. Main methods include rehabilitation exercise, manual therapy and electro-therapy. There are many specialist areas within the field of physiotherapy.

pick-up speed training An approach used by athletes to develop both aerobic and anaerobic fitness, and, in particular, speed. Beginning with a period of walking, followed by a period of jogging, the athlete then picks-up their pace to run fast and builds up to a period of sprinting.

planes Three main ways in which sections of the body can be viewed or body movements described. The frontal plane, with a straight vertical line, divides the body into anterior and posterior portions. The sagittal plane divides the body into left and right sides. If the particular plane in question is central, on a midline between each section, it is known as either the midsagittal or midfrontal plane. The transverse plane, with a horizontal line, divides the body into superior and inferior portions. The planes of the body enable specific description of a view of the body. Cross-section anatomical diagrams, photographs and scans are described in terms of planes. Frontal plane movements include lateral flexion and extension and abduction and adduction. Sagittal movements include flexion and extension. Transverse movements are rotational.

plateau A key training principle. If fitness training is not gradually and progressively overloaded, it will reach a plateau (levelling off).

plumb-line assessment Method of assessing postural alignment. Client stands beside a full-height, weighted string.

poly- Prefix meaning many or excessive (e.g. polyarthritis; polymyalgia; polyuria).

post- Prefix meaning after, behind or beyond (e.g. post-natal; post-isometric; post-operative).

postural muscles More responsible for posture and support of the body in gravity. Tend to be biarticular (crossing two joints) and have greater proportion of slow twitch (Type I) fibres. They are slower to contract but less prone to fatigue. Tend to shorten and increase their tension when under strain and are more prone to cramp and trigger point development.

posture The physical attitude of the structural body during standing, sitting and movement. Good body alignment and posture should be encouraged and developed.

power A key training component, associated with performing short bursts of very strenuous activity. Combines strength and speed. Power-based exercises usually involve plyometric activities.

preparatory stretching Basic short duration major muscle group stretches, prior to fitness training or competition. Forms part of the warm-up.

prognosis Probable long-term outcome, regarding an injury or other medical condition.

progression A key training principle. Training must be progressively (gradually, but sufficiently) overloaded so as to achieve adaptations safely and effectively.

proprioception The body's ability to maintain awareness of its positioning, through its specialized sensory receptors (proprioceptors), enabling rapid neuromuscular responses to the ever-changing environment.

pulse The alternating wave of expansion and recoil within an artery that relates to the contraction (systole) of the left ventricle of the heart.

pulse recovery rate (PRR) A simple test of cardio-vascular fitness. Typically, the one minute PRR is taken from the exercising heart rate to ascertain the individual's efficiency of recovery from exertion.

range of movement (RoM) The degree of movement at a particular joint or region. There are recognized norms which should be compared against when assessing an individual's RoM.

recovery A key training principle. All well-considered training programmes should incorporate sufficient recovery periods, days and techniques.

referral The professional process of recommending additional, alternative or specialist attention, assessment, treatment or exercise. Involves documented discussion, explanation and agreement with all those concerned.

reflex tests Simple neurological tests that involve gently striking certain tendons on the body with a reflex hammer in order to assess their response, and therefore their nerve supply. Most commonly tested reflexes are: patella tendon; biceps; triceps; and Achilles.

rehabilitation The recovery programme that is carefully prepared and planned for, by a physiotherapist, sports therapist or other professional, for an injured client. Each stage (early stage to the full functional stages) requires a carefully planned approach.

relaxation The act of effectively resting, or being able to relax. Relaxation exercises, such as diaphragmatic breathing or progressive relaxation, are recommended so as to allow the body its necessary recovery time from exertions, to offset stresses and fatigue, and to replenish energy levels.

remedial exercise Specially selected exercises designed to help achieve agreed achievable objectives, such as increasing specific flexibility, reducing body fat or improving aerobic endurance.

remedial massage Advanced application of massage and mobilization techniques to achieve specific objectives such as: freer, fuller RoM; muscle relaxation; pain reduction; formation of optimal scar tissue.

repetition A key training principle. By repeating particular exercises, athletes improve skills and functional endurance.

repetition maximum (RM) The most amount of weight that can be lifted in one lift (1 RM), or for ten lifts (10 RM).

research Systematic, scientific and ethically sound investigation into a particular area of practice. Research is often designed to support or negate a particular hypothesis, and therefore further the knowledge (and evidence) base of a subject.

resisted movement Specific movement made against the measured resistance of the therapist or exercise equipment such as free weight. It may be isometric or isotonic.

resting heart rate (RHR) Typically between 50 and 80 beats per minute. A lower HR tends to suggest that the individual is aerobically trained, and that their heart is working less hard at rest.

retinaculum Fibrous connective tissue holding tissues into position.

reversibility A key training principle. As the amount of training reduces or is stopped, fitness levels reduce.

RICES Rest, Ice, Compression, Elevation, Support.

sauna A dry heat treatment. Clients sit in a timber construction, and the air is heated to between 70 and 110 °C. Encourages relaxation, perspiration (skin cleansing and elimination of waste products) and increased blood circulation.

scar tissue New tissue laid down as a repair following trauma. The restoration of an injured tissue depends upon the severity of the trauma and upon which type of cell – stromal or parenchymal – is active in the repair. Stromal repair is performed with the cells from the supporting connective tissue and is predominantly collagen and non-functional. Parenchymal repair is with the injured tissue's functional cells.

scoliosis A postural malalignment, demonstrating an 'S-shaped' curvature of the spine, often featuring pelvic girdle or leg length imbalance, and associated malalignments.

sign An objective finding relating to an assessment of an individual (e.g. pallor; swelling; bleeding; malalignment).

'sit and reach' test A simple test of back and leg flexibility. The subject sits with feet against a sit and reach box. They lean forward as far as is possible, and their best score from three attempts (measured on the scale on top of the box) is recorded.

skill A trained, well-performed action.

skills training The act of developing good ability to perform particular tasks and actions. Sports-specific training involves varied repetitions of actions relevant to the sport.

somatype Basic body type categorization. Three basic somatypes: ectomorph; mesomorph; endomorph.

specialized tissues These include all special and vital organs (e.g. eyes; nose; heart; lungs; genitalia).

specificity A key principle of training, which suggests that all exercise benefits are specific to the type of training performed. Exercise should also be specific to the level that the individual is currently at.

speed A need of most competitive sports, speed is developed by strength and power training, by having sufficient functional flexibility and biomechanical leverage, and by optimizing technique (making it more biomechanically efficient).

sphygmomanometer Equipment used to measure blood pressure. Features a mercury scale, two rubber tubes, a small air pump and a cuff.

sports massage The application of specific massage techniques, designed to help improve sports performance or recovery from training and competition. Sports massage can be adapted to be used in pre-event, during-event or post-event situations, and for general maintenance.

sprain An injury to a ligament. Three grades of sprain: first degree (mild); second degree (moderate); and third degree (severe).

stability training A key component of fitness and functional ability. Stability training helps to keep the body strong enough to withstand the rigours of training and competition. Stability exercise involves targeting the body's (core and peripheral) stabilizing muscles.

static stretching Basic stretching that involves simply stretching and then holding the position, whether actively or passively performed.

steam bath A wet heat treatment that involves the recipient's body being seated in an enclosed fibreglass bath, with their head situated outside of the unit (which many find more preferable, being able to breathe comfortably). Water is heated inside the cabinet by an electrical element, and the resultant steam circulates around the unit at a temperature of around 45–50 °C. A thorough heat treatment that encourages relaxation and increased circulation.

steam room A wet heat treatment, similar to a steam bath, but where the client's head is also exposed to the steam.

strain An injury to a muscle or tendon. Three grades of strain: first degree (mild); second degree (moderate); and third degree (severe).

strength The capacity of a muscle or group to exert force.

symptom Subjective information revealed by the individual regarding their condition (e.g. pain; nausea; numbness; cold).

synergists Muscles that work with the prime mover to perform specific movements. Also called neutralizers because they may help to neutralize unwanted motion from the prime mover, in order to refine a particular movement.

synovitis Inflammation of the synovium of a synovial joint. May be due to impact or repetitive trauma, or infection.

system Group of organs functioning together for the same general purpose.

taping The use of adhesive rolls of tape, whether elasticated, non-elasticated, permeable to air, water resistant, hypoallergenic or tearable, for the purpose of supporting injured, weak or vulnerable joints or muscles.

target heart rate (THR) An individual's (aerobic) THR is calculated by firstly working out their maximal HR (220 − age), and then working out an appropriate percentage of this figure, according to their fitness level. Beginners typically exercise at between 50 and 70 per cent of their max, and more advanced may work at between 70 and 90 per cent.

tendinosis Chronic degeneration of tendon fibres.

tendon Strong cord of connective tissue that attaches muscle to bone. Like ligaments, they have a poor blood supply and are relatively inelastic (only around 10 per cent movement). They effectively transmit muscular force to the bones, and therefore very little muscle force is lost stretching the tendon.

tendonitis Inflammation of a tendon.

thermal therapy The application of heat as a method of increasing relaxation or improving the healing rate of injuries. Common methods include: infra-red lamp; paraffin wax bath; sauna; steam bath; steam room; and moist hot packs.

tissue Group of similar cells that perform a specific function.

tissue fluid Extracellular or interstitial fluid. Similar in composition to blood and lymph. Surrounds and nourishes living cells.

transcutaneous electronic nerve stimulation (TENS) An electrical method for helping to relieve pain. A low-intensity, high-frequency current is applied through pads placed strategically on the skin. TENS can be used by clients unsupervised, once guided.

transfer A key training principle that suggests that the benefits gained from one particular exercise regime may cross-over to another.

trigger point (TP) A very localized area of hypersensitivity, typically housed within postural muscle. When 'active' they characteristically refer aching in a particular pattern away from the point.

triglycerides The body's most concentrated energy source and the form in which most fats are stored in the body.

trochanter A large protuberance. Provides for prominent muscle attachment and additional structural stability (e.g. greater and lesser trochanters of the femur).

tuberosity A large protuberance on a bone. Mainly for prominent muscle attachment (e.g. tibial, ischial, gluteal and radial tuberosities).

Type I fibres Slow-twitch (ST) or slow-oxidative (SO) muscle fibres. Associated with endurance activities (aerobic exercise and postural control).

Type II fibres Fast-twitch (FT) muscle fibres. Two types: fast-oxidative-glycolytic (FOG) Type IIA; fast-glycolytic (FG) Type IIB. These two types of fibres are associated with short-term, forceful, anaerobic activities, but are prone to fatigue.

ultrasound (US) Electrical therapy equipment, commonly used in the treatment of strains, sprains and tendonitis. Employs inaudible, high-frequency sound waves that occur as an alternating electrical current is imposed onto a piezo-electric crystal within a transducer (applicator) head. By varying the frequency, intensity, transducer head and duration, the effects can be altered to suit the nature of the presenting condition.

variance A key training principle that involves varying aspects of training so that any potentially deleterious effects resulting from any regular rigorous and vigorous training routines are minimized.

vaso- Prefix relating to blood vessels (e.g. vasodilation; vasoconstriction; vasomotor).

vasoconstriction A decrease in the diameter of blood vessels, reducing blood flow through a region.

vasodilation An increase in the diameter of blood vessels and, therefore, blood flow.

V_{O_2}max Maximal oxygen uptake. The maximal amount of oxygen that can be taken in and utilized by the working muscles during exercise. There are a variety of tests available, most of which attempt to predict/estimate the individual's V_{O_2}max or aerobic capacity.

waist to hip ratio (WHR) The WHR helps to identify patterns of fat distribution in the upper and lower body.

warm-up A key component for all fitness activities. May involve gradually raising heart rate, performing mobilizing and stretching exercises, and movements that replicate those of the activities that are to follow.

yoga Means 'union'. An ancient Indian discipline offering a variety of styles and approaches to health improvement. Most common in the West is Hatha yoga, which has an emphasis on generating strength and suppleness in combination with calmness and body awareness.

bibliography and recommended reading

Anderson, M.K. and Hall, S.J. *Fundamentals of Sports Injury Management* Williams and Wilkins (1997) Maryland, USA

Apley, A.G. and Solomon, L. *Physical Examination in Orthopaedics* Butterworth Heinemann (1997) Oxford, UK

Austin, K.A., Gwynn-Brett, K.A. and Marshall, S.C. *Illustrated Guide to Taping Techniques* Wolfe (1994) London, UK

Bird, S.R. and Smith, A. and James, K. *Exercise Benefits and Prescription* Stanley Thornes (1998) Cheltenham, UK

Briggs, J. *Sports Therapy: Theoretical and Practical Thoughts and Considerations* Corpus Publishing (2001) Chichester, UK

Bruckner, P. and Khan, K. *Clinical Sports Medicine* 2nd edition McGraw-Hill (2001) Sydney, Australia

Cameron, M.H. *Physical Agents in Rehabilitation: From Research to Practice* WB Saunders (1999) Philadelphia, USA

Cash, M. *Sports and Remedial Massage Therapy* Ebury Press (1996) London, UK

Cassar, M.P. *Handbook of Massage Therapy* Butterworth Heinemann (1999) Oxford, UK

Chaitow, L. *Muscle Energy Techniques* Churchill Livingstone (1996) Edinburgh, UK

Chaitow, L. *Neuromuscular Techniques* Churchill Livingstone (1997) Edinburgh, UK

Chaitow, L. *Positional Release Techniques* 2nd edition Churchill Livingstone (2002) Edinburgh, UK

Davis, R.J., Bull, C.R., Roscoe, J.V. and Roscoe, D.A. *Physical Education and the Study of Sport* Wolfe (1991) London, UK

Dick, F.W. *Sports Training Principles* 4th edition A and C Black (2002) London, UK

Fox, S. and Pritchard, D. *Anatomy, Physiology and Pathology for the Massage Therapist* Corpus Publishing (2001) Chichester, UK

Fritz, S. *Mosby's Fundamentals of Massage Therapy* 2nd edition Mosby (2000) Missouri, USA

Greenman, P.E. *Principles of Manual Medicine* 2nd edition Williams and Wilkins (1996) Maryland, USA

Hall, C.M. and Brody, L.T. *Therapeutic Exercise: Moving Toward Function* Lippincott, Williams and Wilkins (1999) Philadelphia, USA

Heyward, V.H. *Advanced Fitness Assessment and Exercise Prescription* 2nd edition Human Kinetics (1991) Champaign, IL, USA

Hudson, M. *Sports Therapy: A Practical Approach* Stanley Thornes (1998) Cheltenham, UK

King, R.K. *Performance Massage* Human Kinetics (1993) Champaign, IL, USA

Kisner, C. and Colby, L.A. *Therapeutic Exercise: Foundations and Techniques* FA Davis (1996) Philadelphia, USA

Le Quesne, S. *Nutrition* Thomson Learning (2003) London, UK

Lubicz, P.S. *The Sunday Times* 3 August (2003)

McArdle, W.D., Katch, F.I. and Katch, V.L. *Exercise Physiology: Energy Nutrition and Human Performance* 5th edition Lippincott, Williams and Wilkins (2001) Philadelphia, USA

McGuinness, H. *Holistic Therapies* Hodder and Stoughton (2000) London, UK

McLatchie, G., Harries, M., King, J. and Williams, C. *ABC of Sports Medicine* BMJ Publishing Group (1995) London, UK

Mellion, M.B. *Sports Medicine Secrets* Hanley and Belfus (1994) Philadelphia, USA

Micheli, L.J. and Jenkins, M. *The Sports Medicine Bible* HarperCollins (1995) New York, USA

Moffat, D.B. and Mottram, R.F. *Anatomy and Physiology for Physiotherapists* Blackwell Scientific Publications (1987) Oxford, UK

Nordmann, L., Appleyard, L. and Linforth, P. *Professional Beauty Therapy* Thomson Learning (2001) London, UK

O'Connor, E. *SportEx Magazine* January (2002)

Olson, T.R. *ADAM Student Atlas of Anatomy* Lippincott, Williams and Wilkins (1996) Philadelphia, USA

Palmer, M.L. and Epler, M. *Fundamentals of Musculoskeletal Assessment Techniques* 2nd edition Lippincott-Raven (1998) Philadelphia, USA

Parsons, T. *An Holistic Guide to Anatomy and Physiology* Thomson Learning (2002) London, UK

Peterson, L. and Renstrom, P. *Sports Injuries* Martin Dunitz (1986) London, UK

Prentice, W.E. *Rehabilitation Techniques in Sports Medicine* 3rd edition McGraw-Hill (1999) Pubuque, IA, USA

Rosser, M. *Sports Therapy: An Introduction to Theory and Practice* Hodder and Stoughton (1997) London, UK

Sherry, E. and Wilson, S.F. *The Oxford Handbook of Sports Medicine* Oxford University Press (1998) Oxford, UK

Shultz, S.J., Houglum, P.A. and Perrin, D.H. *Assessment of Athletic Injuries* Human Kinetics (2000) Champaign, IL, USA

Stafford-Brown, J., Rea, S. and Chance, J. *BTEC National in Sport and Exercise Science* Hodder and Stoughton (2003) London, UK

Stone, R. and Stone, J. *Atlas of Skeletal Muscles* 2nd edition McGraw-Hill (1997) New York, USA

Tortora, G.J. and Grabowski, S.R. *Principles of Anatomy and Physiology* 8th edition HarperCollins (1996) New York, USA

Werner, R. *A Massage Therapist's Guide to Pathology* Lippincott, Williams and Wilkins (1998) Maryland, USA

index